COUNSELING ABOUT CANCER

COUNSELING ABOUT CANCER
STRATEGIES FOR GENETIC COUNSELING

THIRD EDITION

KATHERINE A. SCHNEIDER, MPH

Center for Cancer Genetics and Prevention
Dana-Farber Cancer Institute

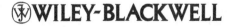

A JOHN WILEY & SONS, INC., PUBLICATION

Published by John Wiley & Sons, Inc., Hoboken, New Jersey

Published simultaneously in Canada

For general information on our other products and services or for technical support, please contact our Customer Care Department within the United States at (800) 762-2974, outside the United States at (317) 572-3993 or fax (317) 572-4002.

Wiley also publishes its books in a variety of electronic formats. Some content that appears in print may not be available in electronic formats. For more information about Wiley products, visit our web site at www.wiley.com.

Library of Congress Cataloging-in-Publication Data:
Schneider, Katherine A.
    Counseling about cancer : strategies for genetic counseling / Katherine A. Schneider.
— 3rd ed.
        p. ; cm.
    Includes bibliographical references and index.
    ISBN 978-0-470-08150-1 (paper)
    1. Cancer—Genetic aspects. 2. Cancer—Patients—Counseling of. 3. Genetic counseling.
I. Title.
    [DNLM: 1. Neoplasms—genetics. 2. Neoplasms—psychology. 3. Genetic Counseling.
4. Neoplasms—nursing. QZ 200]
    RC268.4.S355 2012
    616.99'4042—dc22

                                                                                    2011010973

oBook ISBN 9781118119921
ePDF ISBN 9781118119891
ePub ISBN 9781118119914
eMobi ISBN 9781118119907

Printed in the United States of America

*This book is dedicated to
my father, Donald G. Daviau
and
my three sons
Nicholas, Christopher, and Jordan*

Contents

FOREWORD, XI
PREFACE, XIII
ACKNOWLEDGMENTS, XV

CHAPTER 1: CANCER EPIDEMIOLOGY, 1

1.1. CANCER STATISTICS, 1

1.2. CANCER ETIOLOGY, 10

1.3. CASE EXAMPLES, 18

1.4. FURTHER READING, 21

CHAPTER 2: CANCER DETECTION AND TREATMENT, 23

2.1. THE DIAGNOSIS OF CANCER, 23

2.2. TUMOR CLASSIFICATION, 31

2.3. CANCER TREATMENT, 37

2.4. FURTHER READING, 45

CHAPTER 3: CANCER BIOLOGY, 47

3.1. THE MALIGNANT CELL, 47

3.2. CARCINOGENESIS 52

3.3. ONCOGENES, 59

3.4. TUMOR SUPPRESSOR GENES, 64

3.5. EPIGENETIC MECHANISMS, 70

3.6. FURTHER READING, 73

CHAPTER 4: HEREDITARY CANCER SYNDROMES, 75

4.1. ATAXIA TELANGIECTASIA, 75

4.2. AUTOIMMUNE LYMPHOPROLIFERATIVE SYNDROME (ALSO CANALE–SMITH SYNDROME), 77

4.3. BECKWITH–WIEDEMANN SYNDROME (ALSO EXOMPHALOS MACROGLOSSIA GIGANTISM [EMG] SYNDROME), 78

4.4. BIRT–HOGG–DUBÉ SYNDROME, 80

4.5. BLOOM SYNDROME, 82

4.6. BLUE RUBBER BLEB NEVUS SYNDROME (ALSO TERMED BEAN SYNDROME), 83

4.7. BREAST–OVARIAN CANCER SYNDROME, HEREDITARY, 84

4.8. CARNEY COMPLEX, TYPES I AND II (INCLUDES NAME SYNDROME AND LAMB SYNDROME), 87

4.9. DIAMOND–BLACKFAN ANEMIA, 89

4.10. FAMILIAL ADENOMATOUS POLYPOSIS (ALSO ATTENUATED FAP, GARDNER'S SYNDROME, TURCOT SYNDROME, AND HEREDITARY DESMOID DISEASE), 90

4.11. FANCONI ANEMIA, 93

4.12. GASTRIC CANCER, HEREDITARY DIFFUSE, 95

4.13. GASTROINTESTINAL STROMAL TUMOR, FAMILIAL (ALSO MULTIPLE GI AUTONOMIC NERVE TUMORS), 97

4.14. JUVENILE POLYPOSIS (INCLUDES HEREDITARY MIXED POLYPOSIS), 98

4.15. LEIOMYOMATOSIS RENAL CELL CANCER, HEREDITARY, 100

4.16. LI–FRAUMENI SYNDROME, 101

4.17. LYNCH SYNDROME (ALSO TERMED HNPCC), 105

4.18. MELANOMA, CUTANEOUS MALIGNANT (INCLUDES FAMILIAL ATYPICAL MOLE-MALIGNANT MELANOMA SYNDROME, DYSPLASTIC NEVUS SYNDROME, AND MELANOMA–ASTROCYTOMA SYNDROME), 109

4.19. MULTIPLE ENDOCRINE NEOPLASIA, TYPE 1 (ALSO WERMER SYNDROME), 111

4.20. MULTIPLE ENDOCRINE NEOPLASIA, TYPE 2 (ALSO SIPPLE SYNDROME, FAMILIAL MEDULLARY THYROID CARCINOMA SYNDROME), 113

4.21. MYH-ASSOCIATED POLYPOSIS, 115

4.22. NEUROBLASTOMA, FAMILIAL, 116

4.23. NEUROFIBROMATOSIS, TYPE 1 (ALSO VON RECKLINGHAUSEN DISEASE), 118

4.24. NEUROFIBROMATOSIS, TYPE 2, 119

4.25. Nevoid Basal Cell Carcinoma Syndrome (Also Gorlin Syndrome, Basal Cell Nevus Syndrome), 121

4.26. Paraganglioma–Pheochromocytoma Syndrome, Hereditary (Including Carney–Stratakis Syndrome), 123

4.27. Peutz-Jeghers Syndrome, 125

4.28. PTEN Hamartoma Syndrome (PHS) (Also Cowden Syndrome; Includes Bannayan–Riley–Ruvalcaba Syndrome and Proteus Syndrome), 127

4.29. Renal Cell Carcinoma, Hereditary Papillary, 130

4.30. Retinoblastoma, Hereditary, 131

4.31. Rothmund–Thomson Syndrome, 133

4.32. Tuberous Sclerosis Complex (TSC), 134

4.33. Von Hippel Lindau Syndrome, 137

4.34. Werner Syndrome (Also Termed Progeria of the Adult), 139

4.35. Wilms Tumor, Familial (Includes Denys-Drash Syndrome, Frasier Syndrome, WAGR Syndrome), 141

4.36. Xeroderma Pigmentosum (Includes XP/CS Complex, XP Variant), 143

4.37. Further Reading, 145

CHAPTER 5: ALL ABOUT BREAST CANCER, 151

5.1. Overview of Breast Cancer, 151

5.2. Breast Cancer Management: Screening, Diagnosis, and Treatment, 162

5.3. Breast Cancer Syndromes, 171

5.4. Further Reading, 184

CHAPTER 6: ALL ABOUT COLORECTAL CANCER, 187

6.1. Overview of Colorectal Cancer, 187

6.2. CRC Management: Screening, Diagnosis, and Treatment, 199

6.3. CRC Syndromes, 207

6.4. Further Reading, 218

CHAPTER 7: COLLECTING AND INTERPRETING CANCER HISTORIES, 221

7.1. Collecting a Cancer History, 221

7.2. Challenges to Collecting an Accurate History, 242

7.3. Interpreting a Cancer History, 246

7.4.   CASE EXAMPLES, 255

7.5.   FURTHER READING, 266

CHAPTER 8: CANCER RISK COMMUNICATION, 267

8.1.   GENETIC COUNSELING AND RISK PERCEPTION, 267

8.2.   THE COMMUNICATION OF RISK, 278

8.3.   COUNSELING CLIENTS AT VARIOUS RISKS, 289

8.4.   CASE EXAMPLES, 298

8.5.   FURTHER READING, 306

CHAPTER 9: GENETIC TESTING AND COUNSELING, 309

9.1.   THE LOGISTICS OF ARRANGING TESTS, 309

9.2.   PRETEST COUNSELING, 325

9.3.   RESULTS DISCLOSURE AND FOLLOW-UP, 337

9.4.   CASE EXAMPLES, 346

9.5.   FURTHER READING, 356

CHAPTER 10: PSYCHOSOCIAL ASPECTS OF CANCER COUNSELING, 357

10.1.   THE PSYCHOSOCIAL FEATURES OF CLIENTS, 357

10.2.   MAKING A PSYCHOSOCIAL ASSESSMENT, 379

10.3.   PROVIDING ADDITIONAL EMOTIONAL SUPPORT, 394

10.4.   CASE EXAMPLES, 400

10.5.   FURTHER READING, 407

CHAPTER 11: ETHICAL ISSUES IN CANCER GENETIC COUNSELING, 409

11.1.   BIOETHICAL PRINCIPLES AND GUIDELINES, 409

11.2.   STRATEGIES FOR RESOLVING ETHICAL DILEMMAS, 423

11.3.   TYPES OF ETHICAL DILEMMAS IN CANCER GENETIC COUNSELING, 431

11.4.   ISSUES OF JUSTICE, 442

11.5.   FURTHER READING, 443

APPENDIX A: SPECIFIC TUMOR TYPES AND ASSOCIATED SYNDROMES, 445

APPENDIX B: REVIEW OF BASIC PEDIGREE SYMBOLS, 457

INDEX, 459

Foreword

When Katherine Schneider wrote the first edition of *Counseling About Cancer*, cancer genetics was an emerging area of research and patient care. Today, it is an established subspecialty within genetics and oncology, with important interactions with many other medical specialties. In cancer centers and other academic centers, genetic counselors provide comprehensive information across a range of conditions. They assess individuals and families for the hereditary component of cancer risk, arrange molecular evaluations, facilitate enrollment to a complex menu of research studies, and provide counseling to patients and families as to the implications of their genetic test results, whether positive, negative, or inconclusive. They see patients with an ever-expanding range of conditions for which susceptibility genes have been identified, from rare pediatric bone marrow disorders to common adult cancer syndromes. In the more common adult hereditary cancer syndromes, genetic counselors assist medical oncologists and surgeons to help patients consider whether genetic information will influence options for managing their cancers. At the same time, health-care providers without formal genetics training have been doing very focused genetic testing, encouraged and supported by the genetics diagnostics industry. The contrast serves to highlight the breadth and depth of the knowledge base that genetic counselors must master, in addition to their expertise in counseling and their required organizational talents.

In this expanded volume, Kathy has once again provided a comprehensive and accessible resource. She has expanded all of the previous chapters, from epidemiology and molecular biology to the 36 conditions detailed in the most encyclopedic chapter. She has added two chapters focusing in detail on breast and colorectal cancers. These chapters reflect her understanding of the need for genetic counselors to become familiar with the data on the efficacy and limitations of options for screening, surgical treatment, and prophylactic surgeries, not to take the place of surgeons, gastroenterologists, or oncologists, but to help make clear the places where a germline mutation can affect medical options and decisions.

Genetics continues to be an exploding area, perhaps even faster than before. The fourth edition of this book will almost certainly include information about the implications of SNPs identified in genome-wide association studies, the issues associated with the use and results of full sequencing, and the challenges of making sure that the power of genetics is accessible to all. Genetic information from analyses of tumors and germline will increasingly be used to guide cancer therapies. Pharmacogenetic data will likely be considered in the personalization of cancer care. However, all of these frontiers are not yet ready for prime time, and do not yet reach the level of practical importance to merit inclusion in the third edition. Genetic counselors will surely remain on the front lines of the ongoing genetics revolution, helping to translate this explosive scientific progress to patients and to educate their providers as well. Fortunately, they have a new version of the Kathy Schneider resource to guide them.

JUDY E. GARBER, MD, MPH
Director, Center for Cancer Genetics and Prevention
Dana-Farber Cancer Institute
February 2011

Preface

Clinical cancer genetics has grown by leaps and bounds since the last edition of this textbook was published almost 10 years ago. There are more hereditary cancer syndromes, clinical genetic tests, cancer monitoring options, and a great many more cancer genetic providers. Advances in molecular and clinical cancer genetics continue to occur at a dizzying pace, providing hope that the future will indeed hold better ways to detect, treat, and prevent inherited forms of cancer.

As noted in a *Spider-Man* comic, "With great power comes great responsibility." Despite all the clinical and scientific changes in cancer genetics, the primary aim of cancer genetic counseling, which is to help clients and their families, has stayed the same. In fact, clients continue to ask the same types of questions: Will I develop cancer? Will my child develop cancer? What can I do to protect myself and my child from getting cancer?

Our responsibility as cancer genetic counselors is to find the best way to educate clients and families about their cancer risks and their options for genetic testing and cancer monitoring. To provide quality cancer genetic counseling, one must:

- provide clients with information that is both useful and accurate
- identify clients and families who are at increased risk for hereditary cancers
- assist clients through the genetic testing process
- help clients, their relatives, and their health-care providers to understand the implications of genetic test results
- provide support to clients during emotionally laden discussions
- facilitate the referral of clients to the appropriate medical providers

The earlier versions of *Counseling About Cancer* were borne out of a need to create a useful resource for a new genetic counseling specialty. At this point in time, cancer genetic counseling has established itself as a critically important medical specialty and serves as a model of excellence for other adult-onset genetic disorders.

Counseling About Cancer, Third Edition reflects the growing sophistication of our profession and offers an expanded discourse on all facets of the cancer genetic counseling process.

Chapters 1–3 provide detailed background information regarding cancer statistics, risk factors, cancer biology, cancer terminology, and detection and treatment strategies. Each chapter has been substantially revised. Chapter 4 describes 36 hereditary cancer syndromes, including cancer risks, diagnostic criteria, genetic testing options, and links to resources for families.

Since most cancer genetic counselors provide counseling about breast cancer and/or colorectal cancer, this edition has added two new chapters. Chapter 5 focuses on hereditary breast cancer and Chapter 6 focuses on hereditary colorectal cancer. These chapters provide detailed information about these two forms of cancer, including normal anatomy, common types of tumors, possible hereditary cancer syndromes, and suggestions for monitoring high-risk individuals.

Chapters 7–9 provide greatly revamped discussions regarding the collection of family history information, cancer risk communication, and pre- and posttest genetic counseling. Each chapter includes definitions, discussions about potential challenges, as well as the strategies with which to meet these challenges.

Chapters 10 and 11 offer detailed looks at the complex psychological and ethical issues that cancer genetic counselors may encounter. These two chapters have been largely rewritten and provide a much more in-depth look at these important arenas.

Counseling About Cancer, Third Edition also includes an increased number of tables and figures to supplement the text as well as an appendix that contains tables of possible cancer syndromes by organ type. This edition also offers 14 new case stories that illustrate the strategies listed in each chapter and demonstrate the complexities of this type of genetic counseling.

I hope that this textbook serves as a useful resource for practicing genetic counselors, other clinicians who work in cancer genetics or other specialty areas, as well as genetic counseling students.

KATHERINE A. SCHNEIDER, MPH
Center for Cancer Genetics and Prevention
Dana-Farber Cancer Institute
August 2011

Acknowledgments

I am grateful for the many wonderful people in my life who helped me with the completion of this book. First, thank you to my editor, Thomas H. Moore, and to my four reviewers—Robert Resta, Janice Berliner, Anu Chittenden, and Vickie Venne—who faithfully read the chapters and provided such invaluable feedback.

I owe a huge debt to the wonderful group of genetic counselors with whom I work—Emily Brown, Anu Chittenden, Monica Dandapani, Carly Grant, Claire Healy, Elaine Hiller, Shelley McCormick, and Irene Rainville. Thanks also to Sapna Syngal, Elena Stoffel, Frederick Li, Lisa Diller, Andrea Patenaude, Perrin Schilling, and Jennifer Wiernicki for your assistance. And a special thank you to Judy E. Garber who granted me with protected time to write—I would not have been able to complete this edition without your understanding and support.

I am also grateful for the other colleagues who helped me along the way, including Robin Bennett, Saundra Buys, Charis Eng, Meredith Keenan, and June Peters. And I am grateful for the many special clients and families with whom I have worked over the years. Thanks also to the Ethics Advisory Board at the Dana-Farber Cancer Institute and for the Ethics Fellowship Award allowing me to further my study of ethics.

Thank you to my friends who encouraged and supported me along the way: Elisabeth Daniels, Daniel Hulub, Bradford Kinne, Donna McCurdy, and Sabrina Popp; my siblings, Robert, Thomas, and Julia; and especially my loving mother, Patricia E. Daviau.

Lastly I remain indebted to the Jane Engelberg Memorial Fellowship for awarding me the grant to allow the development of the first edition of this book. It was the opportunity of a lifetime.

K.A.S.

CANCER EPIDEMIOLOGY

The problem may be briefly stated: What does: "median mortality of eight months" signify in our vernacular? I suspect that most people, without training in statistics, would read such a statement as "I will probably be dead in eight months"—the very conclusion that must be avoided, since it isn't so and since attitude matters so much. . . . When I learned about the eight-month median, my first intellectual reaction was: fine, half the people will live longer, now what are my chances of being in that half.

(Gould, 2004, pp. 139–140)

Cancer epidemiologists seek to answer the question, "Why did these people develop these particular cancers at this time?" Cancer epidemiology is the study of cancer incidence and mortality within a population. This chapter provides current cancer statistics and a description of the many known or suspected causes of cancer.

1.1. CANCER STATISTICS

This section describes the incidence and mortality rates of specific cancers, and the differences in cancer rates by ethnic group and geographic location. First, here is a brief review of the terminology commonly used in cancer statistics.

- *Incidence*—This refers to the number of new events (i.e., cancer diagnoses or deaths) that have occurred in a defined population during a specified period of time. This is the term most frequently used in reports of cancer statistics. For example, in the fictitious city of Madison, there were 14,000 new cases of lung cancer in 2008. Therefore, the 2008 incidence of lung cancer in Madison is 14,000.

- *Prevalence*—This is the number of disease cases (i.e., cancer cases) in a defined population at a designated time. Prevalence includes both individuals newly diagnosed with cancer (incidence) and those who are survivors of the disease. Thus, cancers with high survival rates will have higher prevalence within a population than malignancies that cause rapid mortality. For example, in Madison, there were 14,000 new cases of lung cancer in 2008 and 5000 lung cancer survivors. Thus, the 2008 prevalence of lung cancer in Madison is 19,000.

- *Rate*—This is a way of measuring disease frequency that allows comparisons between populations or subsets of populations. Frequently used examples include the incidence rate, prevalence rate, and cancer survival rate. To obtain the incidence rate, divide the number of new cases over a fixed time interval by the number of people in the population during that time. It is also conventional to use a denominator of fixed size in order to compare the rate to other disorders or populations. For example, 14,000 new cases of lung cancer were diagnosed in Madison, which has a total population of 2 million. This means that the incidence rate of lung cancer in Madison is 0.7 or 700 cases per 100,000 people (14,000 [incidence] divided by 2 million [population]).

- *Relative risk*—This is a ratio of risk between two populations or groups. A value of 1.0 means that there is no difference in the risks of cancer in two groups, while a value above 1.0 means that there is a higher risk in one group. For example, in the neighboring city of Jefferson, the incidence rate of lung cancer is only 300 per 100,000 people. Therefore, the people in Madison (with a lung cancer incidence rate of 700 per 100,000) have a relative risk of lung cancer that is 2.3 times higher than those living in Jefferson.

1.1.1. CANCER INCIDENCE IN THE UNITED STATES

Almost everyone has a relative or friend who has developed cancer. A glance at the 2011 cancer rates in Table 1.1 explains why: cancer is a very common disease. In the United States, lifetime cancer risks are 1 in 3 for women and 1 in 2 for men. Nearly 1.6 million new cases were diagnosed in 2011, and this number seems to increase each year.

Cancer types and rates differ for men and women. In the United States, the leading sites of cancer in 2011 were prostate cancer for men (see Table 1.2) and breast cancer for women (see Table 1.3). For both sexes, lung cancer ranks second and colorectal cancer ranks third.

TABLE 1.1. PROBABILITY THAT MEN AND WOMEN IN THE UNITED STATES WILL DEVELOP CANCER OVER THEIR LIFETIME

	Birth to 39	40–59	60–69	70–79	Ever
Men	1 in 70	1 in 12	1 in 6	1 in 3	1 in 2
Women	1 in 50	1 in 11	1 in 9	1 in 4	1 in 3

Source: American Cancer Society (2011, p. 14).

Excludes nonmelanoma skin cancer.

TABLE 1.2. MOST COMMON FORMS OF CANCER FOR MEN IN THE UNITED STATES: 2011 ESTIMATES

Cancer	Number of New Cases	Percentage of Cases
Prostate	240,890	29%
Lung and bronchus	115,060	14%
Colon and rectum	71,850	9%
Urinary bladder	52,020	6%
Melanoma of the skin	40,010	5%
Kidney and renal pelvis	37,120	5%
Non-Hodgkin lymphoma	36,060	4%
Oral cavity and pharynx	22,710	3%
Leukemia	25,320	3%
Pancreas	22,050	3%

Source: American Cancer Society (2011, p. 10).

TABLE 1.3. MOST COMMON FORMS OF CANCER FOR WOMEN IN THE UNITED STATES: 2011 ESTIMATES

Cancer	Number of New Cases	Percentage of Cases
Breast	230,480	30%
Lung and bronchus	106,070	14%
Colon and rectum	69,360	9%
Uterine corpus	46,470	6%
Thyroid	36,550	5%
Non-Hodgkin lymphoma	30,300	4%
Melanoma of the skin	30,220	4%
Kidney and renal pelvis	23,800	3%
Ovary	21,990	3%
Pancreas	21,980	3%

Source: American Cancer Society (2011, p. 10).

TABLE 1.4. CANCER INCIDENCE AND MORTALITY STATISTICS FOR CHILDREN
AGED 19 YEARS AND YOUNGER

Cancer	Incidence	Mortality
Leukemia	8.6	1.2
Brain and other nervous system	3.3	0.7
Soft tissue	1.0	0.1
Non-Hodgkin lymphoma	0.9	0.1
Kidney and renal pelvis	0.8	0.1
Bone and joint	0.7	0.1
Hodgkin's lymphoma	0.5	0.0

Source: National Cancer Institute SEER Cancer Statistics Review, 1975–2003, 2006.

Rates are per 100,000 and are age-adjusted to the 2000 US standard population.

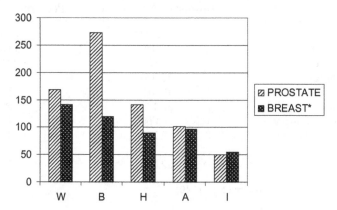

FIGURE 1.1. A comparison of the U.S. incidence rates for prostate cancer and breast cancer across five different ethnic groups. *Female only; **Per 100,000, age adjusted. W = Whites; B = African Americans; H = Hispanics; A = Asians and Pacific Islanders; I = American Indians and Alaskan Natives. *Source*: American Cancer Society (2006, p. 32).

In general, cancer risk increases with age, with the highest incidence occurring in people over age 65. Childhood cancers are relatively rare and account for less than 1% of all new cancer diagnoses. By far the most common childhood cancer is acute leukemia, which accounts for 34% of all pediatric cancers. See Table 1.4 for a listing of the most frequent forms of childhood cancer.

In each major ethnic group, prostate and breast cancers are by far the most common forms of malignancy. However, as shown by the cancer statistics from 2006, the incidence rates of these two cancers varied per ethnic group. (See Fig. 1.1.) African Americans have the highest overall cancer rates, while Native Americans (including Alaskan Natives) have the lowest cancer rates.

Cancer incidence rates also vary per geographic region. The states with the highest cancer incidence rates in 2011 (between 40,000 and 163,000 new cases) were California, Florida, Georgia, Illinois, Michigan, New Jersey, New York, North Carolina, Ohio, Pennsylvania, and Texas. The states with the lowest overall cancer rates in 2011 were Alaska, District of Columbia, North Dakota, Vermont, and Wyoming.

1.1.2. CANCER-RELATED MORTALITY AND SURVIVAL IN THE UNITED STATES

As shown in Table 1.5, cancer remains one of the leading causes of death in the United States (behind heart disease). Despite the relative rarity of cancer in children, it is one of the most common causes of death in this age group as well. Table 1.4 provides the cancer mortality rates for specific childhood cancers. For adults aged 25–44, deaths from cancer are more frequent than any other diseases, but rank below accidents and violent deaths (homicides and suicides).

It is encouraging to note that over the past two decades, more people are surviving their cancer diagnoses. The upward trend in cancer survival rates is partially due to the ability to detect cancers at earlier, more treatable stages. The greatest declines in mortality rates have been among women and individuals less than 65 years old. Specific mortality rates depend upon the site of cancer, how advanced the cancer is at diagnosis, and how amenable

TABLE 1.5. TEN LEADING CAUSES OF DEATH FOR TWO SPECIFIC AGE GROUPS AND FOR ALL AGES (IN DECREASING ORDER OF FREQUENCY)

Ages 5–14	Ages 25–44	All ages
Accidents	Accidents	Heart disease
Cancer	Homicide	Cancer
Congenital anomalies	Suicide	Stroke
Homicide	Cancer	COPD
Suicide	Heart disease	Accidents
Heart disease	Congenital anomalies	Diabetes
COPD	Stroke	Alzheimer's disease
Benign tumors	Influenza and pneumonia	Influenza and pneumonia
Influenza and pneumonia	HIV/AIDS	Chronic liver disease
Stroke	COPD	Septicemia

Source: National Vital Statistics, Estimated Rates for 2004, Reports Vol. 54 (19).

COPD, chronic obstructive pulmonary disease.

TABLE 1.6. U.S. CANCER MORTALITY RATES BY SITE AND GENDER:
2011 ESTIMATES

	Cancer	Number of Cases (%)
Men	Lung and bronchus	85,600 (28)
	Prostate	33,720 (11)
	Colon and rectum	25,250 (8)
	Pancreas	19,360 (6)
	Liver and intrahepatic bile duct	13,260 (4)
	Leukemia	12,740 (4)
	Esophagus	11,910 (4)
	Urinary bladder	10,670 (4)
	Non-Hodgkin lymphoma	9,750 (3)
	Kidney and renal pelvis	8,270 (3)
Women	Lung and bronchus	71,340 (26)
	Breast	39,520 (15)
	Colon and rectum	24,130 (9)
	Pancreas	18,300 (7)
	Ovary	15,460 (5)
	Non-Hodgkin lymphoma	9,570 (4)
	Leukemia	9,040 (3)
	Uterine Corpus	8,120 (3)
	Liver and intrahepatic bile duct	6,330 (2)
	Brain and other nervous system	5,670 (2)

Source: American Cancer Society (2011, p. 10).

the cancer is to treatment. As shown in Table 1.6, the highest number of cancer deaths in 2011 were from lung cancer, followed by prostate cancer in men and breast cancer in women.

One commonly used marker in oncology is the 5-year relative survival rate. This refers to the likelihood that a cancer patient will be alive (with or without disease) 5 years postdiagnosis, after adjusting for normal life expectancy. It is estimated that the overall 5-year survival rate for cancer is 68%. Because of this, genetic counselors will increasingly encounter clients who have personal histories of cancer. In fact, over 11 million Americans are cancer survivors and this figure continues to rise.

Table 1.7 lists the 1999–2006 5-year survival rates for specific cancers. Skin melanoma and breast, prostate, testis, and thyroid cancers had greater than 90% survival rates, while the survival rates for esophageal, liver/bile duct, lung/bronchus, and pancreatic cancer were less than 20%.

Cancer survival rates also differ among ethnic groups. African American men have the highest rates of cancer deaths and Asian women have the lowest rates. Table 1.8 compares 5-year survival rates for Caucasian Americans with African Americans, which reveals that African Americans

TABLE 1.7. THE 5-YEAR RELATIVE SURVIVAL RATES FOR SELECTED
CANCERS

Cancer	% for All Stages
Prostate	99.8
Thyroid	96.6
Melanoma (skin)	91.6
Breast	88.2
Cervix	73.3
Kidney	64.6
Colon and rectum	64.1
Ovary	44.6
Stomach	23.2
Lung and bronchus	15.3
Liver	9.0
Pancreas	4.6

Source: American Cancer Society (2006, p. 17).

Rates are adjusted for normal life expectancy and are based on cases diagnosed between 1995 and 2001, followed through 2002.

TABLE 1.8. A COMPARISON OF THE 5-YEAR RELATIVE SURVIVAL RATES* (%) BY RACE IN THE UNITED STATES FOR TWO PERIODS OF TIME: 1975–1977 AND 1999–2006

	Caucasians (%)		African Americans (%)	
	1975–1977	1999–2006	1975–1977	1999–2006
All cancers	51	69	40	59
Breast	76	91	62	78
Colon	52	67	47	55
Lung	13	17	12	13
Melanoma (skin)	83	93	60	74
Ovary	37	45	43	37
Prostate	70	100	61	97
Thyroid	93	98	91	95
Uterine corpus	89	86	61	61

Source: American Cancer Society (2011, p. 18).

*Survival rates are adjusted for normal life expectancy and are based on cases diagnosed in the SEER 9 areas from 1975 to 1977 and 1999 to 2006, and followed through 2007.

have poorer survival rates for almost all of the common cancers. Despite tremendous advances in cancer detection, prevention, and treatment, there remains a wide gap in the accessibility and uptake of services within certain population groups. Rather than focusing on ethnicity or race, many sociologists argue that the most important determinant of cancer risk is poverty, which is linked with inadequate health insurance, limited access to medical services, and an increased prevalence of known risk factors.

1.1.3. GLOBAL INCIDENCE OF CANCER

Over 11 million new cases of cancer were diagnosed worldwide in 2008. The World Health Organization predicts that this figure could increase to over 15 million annual new cases of cancer by the year 2020. Table 1.9 lists the most common cancers diagnosed throughout the world in 2008. Lung cancer topped the list, accounting for approximately 1.6 million new cases and 1.4 million deaths. For men worldwide, the most common forms of cancer in 2008 were lung and bronchus cancer, prostate cancer, and colorectal cancer. For women worldwide, the most common cancers in 2008 were breast cancer, colorectal cancer, and cervical cancer. The cancers with the highest mortality rates around the world were lung/bronchus, liver, stomach, colon/rectum, and esophageal cancers for men and breast, lung and bronchus, colon/ rectum, cervix uteri, and stomach cancers for women.

The risk of being diagnosed with cancer was highest in Australia, followed by North America and European countries. The countries with the lowest cancer rates were Afghanistan, Egypt, and India. (See Table 1.10.) Table 1.11 lists the countries with the highest cancer mortality rates.

Industrialized countries tend to have higher rates of cancer than developing countries, because cancer, for the most part, is a disease of old age. A comparison of the most common causes of death for industrialized and

TABLE 1.9. MOST COMMON FORMS OF CANCER FOR MEN AND WOMEN WORLDWIDE

	Cancer
Men	Lung and bronchus
	Prostate
	Colon and rectum
	Stomach
	Liver
Women	Breast
	Colon and rectum
	Cervix uteri
	Lung and bronchus
	Stomach

Source: Jemal et al. (2011).

TABLE 1.10. COUNTRIES WITH THE HIGHEST AND LOWEST INCIDENCE RATES OF CANCER

Highest Rates[a]	Lowest Rates[b]
Australia	Afghanistan
Belgium	Egypt
Croatia	India
France	Middle East (except Israel, Syria, and the Arab Republic)
Hungary	Northern Africa
Israel	Namibia
Luxembourg	Panama
New Zealand	Southeastern Asia
United States	
Uruguay	

Source: Mackay et al. (2006).

[a] 15% and higher risk of getting cancer before age 65.

[b] 5–7.4% risk of getting cancer before age 65.

TABLE 1.11. COUNTRIES WITH THE HIGHEST CANCER MORTALITY RATES

Rank	Country	Rate[a]
1	The Netherlands	433
2	Italy	418
3	Hungary	411
4	Luxembourg	410
5	Slovakia	405
6	Ireland	358
7	Czech Republic	335
8	New Zealand	327
9	United States	322
10	Australia	299
11	Norway	289
12	France	286
13	Austria	280
14	Sweden	268
15	Finland	255
16	United Kingdom	254

Source: Organization for Economic Cooperation and Development (OECD) 2004. Health Statistics: Death from cancer by country. http://www.nationmaster.com/graph/hea_dea_fro_ can–health–death–from–cancer.

[a] Per 100,000 for the year 2000.

TABLE 1.12. LEADING CAUSES OF DEATH IN LOW INDUSTRIALIZED AND
DEVELOPING COUNTRIES (IN DECREASING ORDER OF FREQUENCY)

Industrialized Counties	Developing Counties
Heart disease	Heart disease
Stroke	Stroke
Lung cancer	Lower respiratory infections
Lower respiratory infections	HIV/AIDS
COPD	Perinatal conditions
Colon and rectum cancers	COPD
Alzheimer's disease	Diarrhea
Diabetes mellitus	Tuberculosis
Breast cancer	Malaria
Stomach cancer	Motor vehicle accidents

Source: Lopez et al. (2006).

COPD, chronic obstructive pulmonary disease.

developing countries is shown in Table 1.12. Although people in developing countries have a greater chance of dying from an infectious disease than their counterparts in developed countries, cancer has become a major public health concern for all nations. In fact, the World Health Organization estimates that more than 70% of all cancer deaths in 2008 occurred in low- and middle-income countries. This is because developing countries have fewer resources for cancer detection and treatment and the types of cancer that occur (e.g., lung, stomach, liver, and esophageal) tend to be more difficult to treat.

It is important to be aware of the specific population rates of cancer when considering the likelihood of an inherited etiology. For example, the occurrence of breast cancer in three female relatives living in Japan or China is much more striking than three affected relatives in the United States or Canada. Conversely, a family history of gastric cancer, while rare in North America, is much more commonplace in Asia.

1.2. CANCER ETIOLOGY

In 1883, Sir Percival Potts in London noted that young boys who worked as chimney sweeps developed scrotal cancer at higher than usual rates. This was the first documented report linking an environmental exposure to cancer development. More than a century later, numerous factors in our environment are known or suspected to cause cancer.

In the majority of cases, it is a combination of factors that leads to cancer development. At this time, the interaction between genetic and environmental risk factors remains poorly understood. For example, the extent to which

TABLE 1.13. THE ESTIMATED AMOUNT OF CANCER CASES ATTRIBUTED TO
SPECIFIC RISK FACTORS

Risk Factors	Cases (%)
Diet	35
Tobacco use	30
Hereditary factors	5–10
Occupational exposures	5
Radiation	1–2
Viruses	1–2
Miscellaneous	16–23

Source: Offit (1998, p. 34).

lifestyle changes can modify the cancer risk in individuals with inherited predispositions to cancer is unclear.

Hereditary factors are the primary underlying source of cancer in only a small percentage of cases. About 65% of cancers are thought to be due to either dietary factors or tobacco exposure (see Table 1.13). Other factors are also important contributors in the occurrence of specific malignancies. To calculate a client's cancer risk, genetic counselors may need to consider nonhereditary factors, such as lifestyle, medical conditions, occupational exposures, ethnicity, and geographic region.

1.2.1. NONMODIFIABLE RISK FACTORS

Everyone is at risk for developing cancer at some point in their lives and the most significant risk factors are, for the most part, beyond our control. Table 1.14 lists the major nonmodifiable risk factors described below.

1.2.1.1. Aging

Age is probably the most significant predictor of cancer risk, with people over age 65 having the highest risks. This is likely due to the aging process, which results in increased genetic errors during cell mitosis and a less effective immune response.

1.2.1.2. Ethnicity or Race

Rates of specific cancers vary substantially by ethnic group. For example, melanoma and other cutaneous skin cancers are highest in fair-skinned people of European origin and lowest in dark-skinned people of African

TABLE 1.14. MAJOR MODIFIABLE AND NONMODIFIABLE CANCER RISK FACTORS

Nonmodifiable Factors	Modifiable Factors
Aging	Tobacco use
Ethnicity or race	Alcohol use
Hereditary	Unhealthy diet
Gender	Obesity
Chronic medical conditions	Physical inactivity
Chromosomal anomalies	Infectious agents
	Ultraviolet radiation
	Ionizing radiation
	Occupational exposures
	Environmental pollution
	Medicinal drugs
	Food contaminants

Source: Mackay et al. (2006), American Cancer Society, The Cancer Atlas, pp. 24–25.

origin. According to Judith Mackay and colleagues, the rate of skin melanoma in Australia (with a predominance of English descendents) is 51 in 100,000 compared with 2 in 100,000 in Zimbabwe, which also lies near the equator, but has mainly African descendents (2006, p. 36).

1.2.1.3. Heredity

It is estimated that 5–10% of cancers are due to an inherited gene mutation or deletion. However, a much higher proportion of cancers (perhaps 30–40%) may be due to moderately penetrant cancer susceptibility genes coupled with exposures to carcinogens.

1.2.1.4. Gender

Cancer risks are typically higher in men than in women. Drs. Zahm and Fraumeni (1995) postulate that the higher rates of cancer in men might be explained by their higher rates of tobacco and alcohol use, which are linked with a variety of malignancies. Exceptions are thyroid cancer and gallbladder cancer, both of which occur more frequently in women, which suggest hormonal triggers.

1.2.1.5. Chronic Medical Conditions

Some chronic diseases or medical conditions can, over time, lead to certain forms of cancer. One such condition is colitis, which is a series of inflammations in the colon that is associated with a 30% lifetime risk of colorectal cancer. There are also conditions which can be triggered by the same mechanisms that lead to malignancy, such as the increased rate of diabetes in families with familial pancreatic cancer.

1.2.1.6. Chromosomal Anomalies

Individuals with Down syndrome (trisomy 21), Klinefelter syndrome, and Turner syndrome have increased risks for developing specific forms of cancer. Children with Down syndrome have a 10–20-fold increased risk to develop acute lymphoblastic leukemia (ALL) as well as an increased risk of acute myeloid leukemia and a rare form of leukemia termed acute megakaryocytic leukemia. Males with Klinefelter syndrome (47, XXY) are known to be at higher risk of breast cancer and extragonadal germ cell tumors and they may also have higher risks of non-Hodgkin lymphoma and lung cancer. Females with Turner syndrome (45, X0) are at increased risk for developing Wilms' tumor, leukemia, gonadal tumors, neurogenic tumors, and if they take unopposed estrogen, uterine cancer.

1.2.2. MODIFIABLE RISK FACTORS

Carcinogens are identified on the basis of epidemiology studies or by testing in animals. The term carcinogen refers to an exposure that can increase the incidence of malignant tumors. Carcinogens rarely cause cancer at all times under all circumstances. For example, spending a few weeks painting the exterior of your house does not increase your risk of cancer; in contrast, professional house painters are at a decidedly increased risk of cancer due to chronic exposures to airborne carcinogens. The actual level of cancer risk depends on the carcinogenic potential of the agent as well as the intensity and duration of the exposure. Figure 1.2 illustrates the variety of carcinogenic potential in animal studies based on the amount and timing of specific exposures.

The study of potential carcinogens in humans is hampered by many inherent difficulties. Allan Okey et al. (2005) list the following challenges to identifying human carcinogens:

- The time interval between exposure to a potentially carcinogenic agent and the detection of a tumor may be 10–20 years. The long latency period in humans makes it difficult to link tumors with particular exposures.
- It is often difficult to quantify the level of exposures to specific agents, especially if it has occurred many years earlier. Most exposures do not leave any long-term traces of contamination with which to measure.

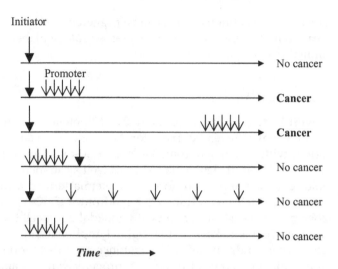

FIGURE 1.2. Outcome of various sequences of experimental exposure to initiating agents and promoting agents in mouse skin. Source: Okey et al. (2005, p. 27). Reproduced with permission from McGraw-Hill.

- Humans are exposed to a variety of chemicals and other agents over their lifetime. These complex exposures may influence the carcinogenic effects and can confound attempts to attribute a tumor to a particular agent.
- People may have very different susceptibilities to cancer despite similar exposures. This may make it difficult to ascertain the true carcinogenicity of a particular agent.
- Proving statistical causality requires an extremely large population group unless the agent has an extraordinarily high tumor potential. Establishing causality of agents that have low or moderate carcinogenic potential will be more difficult.

The United States-based National Toxicology Agency and the International Agency for Research on Cancer (IARC) both publish annual lists of known and suspected human carcinogens. The major cancer-causing agents are presented in the succeeding sections.

1.2.2.1. Tobacco Use

It is estimated that one in five cancer deaths are caused by cigarettes, cigars, and smokeless tobacco (chewing tobacco or snuff). Tobacco smoke contains about 4000 substances, more than 50 of which are known or suspected to cause cancer in humans. Secondhand exposure to tobacco, termed passive smoking, has also been determined to be carcinogenic. Acute myeloid leukemias and malignancies in the following organs have been directly linked to tobacco use: nasopharynx, nasal cavity and paranasal sinuses, lip, pharynx, uterus, cervix, kidney, lung, larynx, oral cavity, esophagus, bladder, stomach, and pancreas. The American Cancer Society estimates that a staggering 80% of lung cancers in men and 50% of lung cancers in women are directly related to tobacco exposure.

1.2.2.2. Alcohol Use

Heavy use of alcohol is linked to increased rates of cancer in the oral cavity, esophagus, colon, liver, and upper respiratory tract. Moderate use of alcohol is associated with an increased risk of breast cancer.

1.2.2.3. Unhealthy Diet

It is estimated that 30% of cancers in developed countries are due to a "Western diet," that is, a diet that is high in saturated fats and low in fruits and vegetables. The Western diet increases the risk of breast, colon, prostate, and esophageal cancers. In developing countries, salt-preserved foods can cause stomach cancer, Chinese-style salted fish can cause nasopharynx cancer, and repetitive ingestion of very hot drinks and food can cause cancers of the oral cavity, pharynx, and esophagus.

1.2.2.4. Obesity

Obesity is a significant cancer risk factor in developed countries and is linked to an unhealthy diet and physical inactivity (a triad known as the Western lifestyle). Obesity, defined as a body mass index (BMI) over 30.0, has been associated with an increased risk of endometrial, kidney, gallbladder, and breast cancers.

1.2.2.5. Physical Inactivity

A sedentary lifestyle is associated with an increased risk of colon cancer. In women, a lack of exercise may also increase the risk of breast cancer.

1.2.2.6. Infectious Agents

About 18% of cancers worldwide are caused by an infectious agent. In developing countries, approximately one in four cancers are caused by a bacterial, viral, or parasitic infection. Table 1.15 provides a list of the most common infectious agents that cause specific types of cancer. The most significant infectious agents are *Helicobacter pylori* (stomach cancer), human

TABLE 1.15. INFECTIOUS AGENTS KNOWN OR SUSPECTED TO BE CARCINOGENIC TO HUMANS

Agent	Type of Cancer
Viruses	
Epstein-Barr	Lymphoma, Hodgkin's disease, stomach
Hepatitis B	Liver
Hepatitis C	Liver
Human immunodeficiency virus (HIV)	Kaposi sarcoma, lymphoma, cervix
Human papilloma	Cervix, penis, anus, vulva, vagina, mouth, oropharynx
Human T-cell lymphotropic, type 1	Adult T-cell leukemia and lymphoma
Human herpes, virus 8	Kaposi sarcoma
Bacteria	
Helicobacter pylori (H. pylori)	Stomach
Parasites	
Schistosomes (flat worms)	Bladder
Opisthorchis viverrini (liver flukes)	Bile duct

Source: National Toxicology Program, Department of Health and Human Services (2011).

papillomaviruses (cervical cancer), and the hepatitis B and C viruses (liver cancer).

1.2.2.7. Ultraviolet Radiation

The main source of ultraviolet radiation is sunlight, although another source is radon, which is a gas produced from decaying uranium. Levels of radon, which is naturally emitted from rocks and soil, vary greatly around the globe. For urban dwellers, radon levels are generally highest in the basement and are often associated with poor ventilation. Long-term exposures to sunlight and other forms of ultraviolet radiation (including sunlamps and tanning beds) increase the risks of skin, lip, and lung cancer. The risk of skin cancer is higher in people with pale skin and/or if exposure occurs in childhood.

1.2.2.8. Ionizing Radiation

Excessive exposure to ionizing radiation, such as repeated X-rays and radiation therapy, is associated with increased rates of leukemia, bone cancer, and other solid tumors. (See Section 2.3.2 for more information about radiation therapy.)

1.2.2.9. Occupational Exposures

Between 2% and 4% of cancer cases are attributed to occupational exposures (see Table 1.16). Exposures to carcinogenic particles and gases can lead to a variety of cancer types, although lung cancer is the most common. Many of these carcinogens require moderate to high levels of exposure over a specified length of time. Exposures to carcinogens occur in a variety of jobs, from X-ray technicians to dry cleaners. Two of the most hazardous professions in terms of cancer risks are manufacturing and mining:

- *Manufacturing*—Factory workers can be exposed to a variety of carcinogenic agents, usually airborne. For example, workers in the dye industry are exposed to aromatic amines, benzidine, and napthylamine, and therefore have higher risks of mesothelioma and cancers of the lung, nasal passages, and sinuses. Manufacturers of shoes, hardwood floors, and furniture have documented increased risks of cancer, particularly lung cancer.

TABLE 1.16. OCCUPATIONAL AND EXPOSURE CIRCUMSTANCES KNOWN OR SUSPECTED TO BE CARCINOGENIC TO HUMANS

Known to be carcinogenic
Aluminum production
Arsenic in drinking water
Auramine, manufacture of
Boot and shoe, manufacture and repair
Coal gasification
Coke production/Coke oven emissions
Furniture and cabinet making
Hematite mining
Involuntary smoking
Iron and steel founding
Isopropanol manufacture
Magenta
Painter, occupation as
Rubber industry
Strong inorganic acid mists containing sulfuric acid
Sunlamps or sun beds
Tobacco smoking
Suspected to be carcinogenic
Art glass, glass containers, and pressed ware
Cobalt metal with tungsten carbide
Hairdresser or barber
Petroleum refining

Source: National Toxicology Program, Department of Health and Human Services (2011).

- *Mining*—Miners are continually exposed to air that is chock-full of minerals and dust. This can include arsenic, radon, polycylic hydro-carbons, and hematite. Miners are at increased risk for developing lymphoma and cancer of the skin, lung, liver, and nasal sinus.

1.2.2.10. Environmental Pollution

About 1–4% of cancer cases are caused by pollution of the air, water, and soil. This is a more serious problem in urbanized countries than in developing countries.

1.2.2.11. Medicinal Drugs

In the 1950s, expectant mothers were given a new drug called diethylstilbestrol (DES) to prevent miscarriage. Twenty years later, it was recognized that women exposed to DES in the womb (so-called DES daughters) have higher rates of vaginal and cervical cancers. Estrogen is a key ingredient in birth control pills and hormone replacement therapy, but is associated with increased risks of both endometrial and breast cancer. Certain medications may also be carcinogenic. For example, alkylating agents, which are used for chemotherapy, can lead to increased risks of leukemia. (See Chapter 2, Section 2.3.3.1 for more information about alkylating agents.)

1.2.2.12. Food Contaminants

A small proportion of cancers are due to food contaminants. These contaminants can be naturally occurring, such as aflatoxins, or man made, such as polychlorinated biphenyls (PCBs). Aflatoxins, which are by-products of *Aspergillus* fungus, are commonly found in grains and legumes and can cause liver cancer. PCBs, which are commercially produced chemical mixtures, seldom degrade fully and are now widespread through the aquatic food chain because of toxic dumping in rivers and oceans prior to 1977. Human ingestion of high levels of PCBs can cause multiple problems, including liver cancer. Other sources of food contaminants are pesticide sprays, bacteria, and food additives.

1.3. CASE EXAMPLES

Case 1: "Everyone in my old neighborhood has gotten cancer."

Monica, a counselor with 10 years' experience in cancer genetics, greeted her first client of the afternoon and smiled at the woman's colorful macaroni necklace, the result of an earlier kindergarten luncheon with her grandson.

The woman, Joan Smith, age 67, had recently moved from a small town in Maine to southern Massachusetts to be nearer to her daughter and four grandchildren. In fact, her main motivation for the genetic counseling visit was to clarify their possible risks of cancer.

Joan had been diagnosed with estrogen and progesterone (ER/PR)-positive breast cancer at age 60, 1 year after her twin sister had been diagnosed with ductal carcinoma *in situ*. Their mother also had breast cancer at age 72, but had recently celebrated her 90th birthday. No one else in this large family had been diagnosed with breast or ovarian cancer. The family was of French Canadian and Irish ancestry.

After completing the family history, Monica explained how frequently breast cancer occurred in the general population and reassured her client that the pattern of breast cancer in her family was unlikely to be indicative of a strong underlying inherited factor (e.g., a *BRCA1* or *BRCA2* mutation). She then asked Joan if she agreed with this assessment.

Joan (who had an annoying habit of calling everyone "dear," but was sweet-natured enough to get away with it) was relieved to learn she didn't need the genetic test that her doctor had badgered her about. However, she did raise another concern.

Pulling out a well-worn manila envelope, Joan began handing newspaper clippings to the genetic counselor. "I'm not concerned about that breast cancer gene, dear, but I am really worried about my family's risks of cancer because of where we grew up. I saw a movie once where this factory dumped chemicals into a nearby river and people got cancer from drinking contaminated water. Did you see the film?" She looked expectantly at the genetic counselor, who admitted that she had seen the film *Erin Brokovich*.

"Well dear, that got me worrying about my family, because everyone in my old neighborhood has gotten cancer! First, there's the neighbor in the house next door to me on the left who died from prostate cancer—here is his obituary. And then the next-door neighbor on my right got lung cancer—here is her obituary. Two doors down from us, Mr. Smith and his wife both had colon cancer a few years back; he died but she didn't. In the house on the corner, the family had a son who died from a brain tumor in his thirties; they had moved away by then but he had grown up in the neighborhood. The neighbors across the street lost a daughter to breast cancer and I recently learned that one of their sons has testicular cancer—or is it prostate cancer?— in his fifties. Then there are the breast cancer cases in our family. Isn't that a lot of cancer on one street?!"

Monica looked down at the stack of newspaper clippings sitting in her lap, then up at Joan's anxious face. She agreed that a lot of cancer had occurred on her street, but gently reminded her that collectively, cancer was a common disease. She reviewed the family history with Joan, noting that the cancers were varied, with most cases occurring over the age of 50. In addition, the one paper mill in the client's town had not been active for several decades.

Monica explained that exposures to carcinogens, such as contaminated drinking water, often caused clusters of similar types of cancer at younger than usual ages. The genetic counselor then said that she did not think the pattern of cancer in Joan's old neighborhood represented a true cancer cluster, but said she understood why the client had been concerned. Monica also encouraged the client to contact the Department of Public Health in Maine if she felt the situation warranted further scrutiny. Joan said that the conversation was "a load off her mind" and decided not to pursue it further.

Case 1 wrap-up: This case describes genetic counseling strategies for dealing with a possible (albeit unlikely) environmental cluster of cancer.

Case 2: "Yes, I know why people in my family get cancer. It's from the [fill in the blank]."

Deena, a recent genetic counseling graduate in her first job, still found it intimidating to provide "group" counseling, but allowed herself a brief moment of satisfaction at how smoothly the session was going. She had just finished collecting an extensive family history that cataloged four generations of breast and ovarian cancer in the Riske family. The three adult sisters, their mother, and a maternal aunt had all chimed in with information, which made it a chaotic process, but had allowed the counselor to see them interact together. The mother had undergone radical mastectomies in her thirties because of bilateral breast cancer and was the best candidate for testing, but all of the women seemed eager to gain control over the disease that had claimed so many of their relatives.

As a way of transitioning the discussion to genetic testing, Deena asked her clients if they knew why so many female relatives had developed cancer. Anticipating the response that cancer was clearly running through their family, the counselor began mentally preparing her mini lecture on the *BRCA1/2* genes and logistics of testing. The mother's answer was so unexpected, Deena asked her to repeat it, wondering if she had heard her correctly.

"Yes, I know why people in my family get cancer. It's from the cheese," said the mother emphatically. The other women in the family all nodded in agreement.

"The cheese ...?" asked the genetic counselor in a puzzled voice.

"My family is originally from Wisconsin and they were dairy farmers. They ate a lot of cheese. All kinds of cheese—Gouda, cheddar, Edam, Brie, Monterey Jack. My sisters and I grew up eating cheese with every meal and I admit that I also fed my kids a lot of cheese."

"We all did," interjected the maternal aunt with a nod. "Good for growing bones, that's what we were always told."

One of the sisters leaned forward and asked, "Maybe the type of cheese makes a difference; remember that Aunt Louise only ate cheddar." The family immediately began going through the family tree cataloging the average daily consumption of cheese (and which types) each female relative had eaten prior to developing cancer.

Unsure of how to steer the conversation back to genetics without seeming rude, Deena waited until there was a lull in the conversation.

"Anyway I've told my daughters to limit how much cheese they eat, but is there anything else they should be doing?" concluded the mother.

Deena saw her opening and grabbed it. "You know, it's hard to point to one risk factor and say with certainty that it's the culprit, it's the cause of cancer. In general, breast cancer and ovarian cancers are caused by a combination of factors. It could be that your family has more than one risk factor. The factor that increases breast and ovarian cancer risk by the greatest amount is not diet, but rather family history or genetic susceptibility."

Deena went on to discuss the *BRCA1* and *BRCA2* genes. She'd never convince the family that the cheese consumption did not partially cause their cancers, but did get them to realize they might also have an inherited risk.

Case 2 wrap-up: This case describes ways to discuss inherited factors while being respectful of the family's theories for why cancer occurred.

1.4. FURTHER READING

American Cancer Society. 2006. Cancer Facts & Figures 2006. American Cancer Society, Atlanta, GA. http://www.cancer.org/Research/CancerFactsFigures/CancerFactsFigures/cancer-facts-figures-2006.

American Cancer Society. 2011. Cancer Facts & Figures 2011. American Cancer Society, Atlanta, GA. http://www.cancer.org/Research/CancerFactsFigures/CancerFactsFigures/cancer-facts-figures-2011.

Gould, SJ. 2004. The median isn't the message. Ceylon Med J 49:139–140.

Jemal, A, Bray, F, Center, MM, et al. 2011. Global cancer statistics. CA: A Cancer Journal for Clinicians 61:69–90.

Lopez, AD, Mathers, CD, Ezzati, M, et al. 2006. Systematic analysis of population health data. Lancet 367:1747–1757.

Mackay, J, Jemal, A, Lee, NC, and Parkin, DM. 2006. The Cancer Atlas. American Cancer Society, Atlanta, GA.

McLaughlin, J, and Gallinger, S. 2005. Cancer epidemiology. In Tannock, I, Hill, RP, Bristow, RG, and Harrington, L (eds), The Basic Science of Oncology, 4th edition. McGraw-Hill Co, New York, 4–24.

Minino, AM, Heron, MP, and Smith, BL (eds). 2006. Deaths: Preliminary Data for 2004. National Vital Statistics Report. National Center for Health Statistics. Hyattsville, MD, vol. 54, no. 19.

National Toxicology Program, Department of Health and Human Services. 2011. The Report on Carcinogens (RoC), 12th edition. http://ntp.niehs.nih.gov/go/roc12.

Offit, K. 1998. Clinical Cancer Genetics: Risk Counseling and Management. John Wiley & Sons, New York.

Okey, AB, Harper, PA, Grant, DM, et al. 2005. Chemical and radiation carcinogenesis. In Tannock, I, Hill, RP, Bristow, RG, and Harrington, L (eds), The Basic Science of Oncology, 4th edition. McGraw-Hill Co, New York, 25–48.

Richardson, CD. 2005. Viruses and cancer. In Tannock, I, Hill, RP, Bristow, RG, and Harrington, L (eds), The Basic Science of Oncology, 4th edition. McGraw-Hill Co, New York, 100–122.

Ries, LAG, Harkins, D, Krapcho, M (eds). 2006. SEER Cancer Statistics Review, 1975–2003, National Cancer Institute, Bethesda, MD. http:seer.cancer.gov/csr975_2003/.

Zahm, SH, and Fraumeni, JF, Jr. 1995. Racial, ethnic, and gender variations in cancer risk: considerations for future epidemiologic research. Environ Health Perspect 103 (Suppl 8):283–286.

Cancer Detection and Treatment

> We must stop speaking of cancer in whispers, as if it is something shameful. For when it is brought out into the brilliant light of day it seems to shrink, to pull back, to diminish. Above all, know this: Cancer is a beatable, treatable, survivable disease.
>
> *(Girard, 2004, p. 3)*

A cancer genetic counseling session often begins with hearing the client's cancer story: the symptoms that led to the suspicion of cancer, the way in which the diagnosis was made, and the subsequent treatment regimen. This chapter describes the process of making a cancer diagnosis, the system used to classify tumors, and the current strategies for cancer treatment.

2.1. The Diagnosis of Cancer

This section provides the information necessary to understanding a cancer diagnosis, from how cancer is diagnosed to the nomenclature used to describe the tumor.

2.1.1. Cancer Detection

A diagnosis of cancer often begins with a worrisome symptom or problem on a medical intake or screening test. For example, a physical exam may

Counseling About Cancer, Third Edition. Katherine A. Schneider.
© 2012 Wiley-Blackwell. Published 2012 by John Wiley & Sons, Inc.

reveal swollen lymph glands or unusual tenderness. A routine screening test, such as a colonoscopy, cervical Pap smear, or blood test, may identify the presence of atypical cells or an unusually high number of cells. For example, a blood specimen that shows a dramatically high count of "blasts" (immature white blood cells) in a young child may point to the presence of acute lymphoblastic leukemia.

In many cases, the patients have noticed warning signs of cancer (see Table 2.1). They may note a new worrisome physical finding, such as a breast lump or they have health problems that are not abating over time (such as a persistent cough) or even getting worse (such as gastrointestinal upset).

People are more likely to experience symptoms or warning signs if their tumor:

- is pressing on neighboring tissue and causes pain
- is interfering with the functioning of normal tissue
- has invaded the blood vessels to cause abnormal bleeding
- has grown large enough to be seen or palpated

A malignant tumor can be present for months, even years, before it is detected. The reasons why cancer detection can be so difficult are presented in the succeeding sections.

2.1.1.1. Lack of Warning Signs

There may be no physical symptoms that signal the presence of early-stage cancer. Observable signs of cancer are more likely to be noticed as the cancer progresses. Unfortunately, this means that the hallmarks of cancer, such as a lump, bleeding, or pain, often indicate a malignancy that is already in an intermediate or advanced stage.

TABLE 2.1. COMMON WARNING SIGNS OF CANCER

- Fatigue, fever, or pain
- Change in bowel or bladder function
- Sores that do not heal
- White patches in the mouth or on the tongue
- Unusual bleeding or discharge
- Thickening or lump in breast or other part of the body
- Indigestion or trouble swallowing
- Skin changes, especially to a wart or mole
- Nagging cough or hoarseness

Source: American Cancer Society (2010).

2.1.1.2. Imperfect Screening Methods

To be effective, screening tests need to be easily performed, affordable, and accurate in detecting disease cases while limiting the number of falsely positive tests. The cancers must be detectable at early (more curable) stages and must occur at a frequency that justifies population screening. For example, the Pap smear is an effective screening test for cervical cancer, because it is a fairly common disease and early diagnosis has been shown to make a significant difference in survival. In contrast, it is no longer recommended that smokers obtain annual chest X-rays because detecting lung tumors by X-ray rather than waiting until symptoms develop does not seem to alter lung cancer mortality rates. Screening tests for less common forms of cancer, such as retinoblastoma, are offered only to children known to be at high risk, both because it is a rare disease and screening occurs under general anesthesia, which carries its own risks.

2.1.1.3. Elusive Premalignant Cells

Few organs can be readily and repeatedly sampled, which makes it difficult to monitor the organs for malignant or (even better) premalignant cells. At this point, only a few screening tests reliably detect premalignant cells, with the Pap smear (which identifies abnormal cells of the cervix) being one of the best examples.

2.1.2. MAKING THE DIAGNOSIS OF CANCER

The workup for cancer typically begins when other more likely explanations have been ruled out. For example, the differential diagnosis of frequent headaches includes vision problems, allergies, and stress. More serious possibilities, such as a brain tumor or neurological problem, are less likely to be entertained at the outset because of their relative rarity. Unfortunately, a common complaint among members of families with hereditary cancer syndromes is that signs of cancer were initially ignored or downplayed by their providers.

The method by which the cancer will be identified depends on the tumor type (see Table 2.2). The presence of cancer may be suggested by physical exam, imaging studies, specialized blood tests (tumor markers, chromosome studies), or invasive procedures. Biopsy is required to make a definitive diagnosis. For example, the diagnosis of renal cell carcinoma may start with an abnormal urine test and an ultrasound of the kidneys, but it is the biopsy and subsequent pathologic analysis that will make the diagnosis.

TABLE 2.2. EXAMPLES OF MEDICAL TESTS THAT CAN LOOK FOR EVIDENCE OF CANCER

- Physical examination
- Blood tests
- Fluid tests
- Stool tests
- Imaging tests
- Endoscopy
- Cytology
- Biopsy

Source: Dollinger et al. (2002).

TABLE 2.3. A LIST OF COMMONLY ORDERED TUMOR MARKERS

Tumor Marker	Cancer Being Screened
Alphafetoprotein	Liver, testis
CA 15-3/CA 27-29	Breast
CA 19-9	Colon, pancreas, stomach, liver
CA 125	Ovary, uterus
Human chorionic gonadotropin (HCG)	Testis, ovary, lung
IgA, IgG, IgM	Myeloma
Prostate-specific antigen (PSA)	Prostate
Carcinoembryonic antigen (CEA)	Colon, rectum, lung, breast, pancreas

Source: Dollinger et al. (2002).

Tumor marker tests look for the presence of proteins in the bloodstream that can be produced by specific tumors. (See Table 2.3.) The higher the level of proteins detected, the more worrisome it is that the person might have an active tumor. A few of the tumor marker tests are accurate enough to be used for screening, such as the alpha-fetoprotein (AFP) test for liver cancer. However, tumor markers are mainly used to look for evidence of recurrent disease.

Individuals will be referred to a medical oncologist either when the suspicion of cancer has been raised or following the initial diagnosis. As with most medical specialties, clinical oncology is divided into many subspecialties. Other members of the cancer care team include surgeons, radiologists, radiation oncologists, pathologists, and mental health professionals; the care of individuals with cancer requires a multidisciplinary team.

Cancer can be a high-burden disease on both patients and their families. Learning that one has cancer can engender feelings of shock, anger, intense sadness, and extreme anxiety. As patients enter cancer treatment, they often need to make major adjustments in terms of their family responsibilities and workload. At many cancer centers, patients and their families have the opportunity to meet with a social worker or psychologist. Patient support groups may also be helpful.

2.1.3. CANCER TERMINOLOGY

It is not naming as such that is pejorative or damning, but the name "cancer." As long as a particular disease is treated as an evil, invincible predator, not just a disease, most people with cancer will indeed be demoralized by learning what disease they have. The solution is hardly to stop telling cancer patients the truth, but to rectify the conception of the disease, to de-mythicize it.

(Sontag, 1977, p. 7)

Hippocrates named the hard gray tumor tissue that extends into normal tissue "Carcinoma" for its crablike appearance. The Latin word for crab is *cancer*, which continues to be used to describe all carcinomas and melanomas.

The terminology used to describe specific tumors can be daunting and it may be helpful to consider how these names are derived. Tumor nomenclature provides information about where in the body and in what type of tissue and cell the cancer originated.

2.1.3.1. Site of Origin

The medical term for a tumor is a neoplasm, which literally means new growth. Neoplasms can develop in almost every tissue of the body. The name of a neoplasm will first indicate the site in the body where the tumor has originated. As examples, a hepatocellular carcinoma is a liver cancer and a rhabdomyosarcoma is a tumor of the striated muscle.

2.1.3.2. Tissue Type

The rationale underlying the name and classification of tumors can be found in embryology (see Table 2.4). In the early embryo there are three layers of germ cells termed the ectoderm, the mesoderm, and the endoderm.

TABLE 2.4. EMBRYONIC ORIGINS OF TISSUE DETERMINES TUMOR TYPE

Embryonic Tissue	Tissue	Cancer
Ectoderm	Skin, nervous system	Carcinoma
Endoderm	Lining of internal organs	Carcinoma
Mesoderm	Bone, muscle, blood, lymphatic system	Leukemia, lymphoma, carcinoma

Source: Pierce and Damjanov (2006).

- *Ectoderm*—The ectoderm forms the outer layer of cells that comprise the skin and nervous system.
- *Mesoderm*—The mesoderm forms the middle layer of cells that are the connecting and supporting tissues of the body, such as bone, muscle, and blood.
- *Endoderm*—The endoderm forms the inner layers of cells and gives rise to the epithelial lining of the internal organs, such as the liver, stomach, and lungs.

The type of tissue in which the neoplasm has occurred—as well as its embryological origin—will typically be indicated within the name of the tumor. The major types of malignant neoplasms are carcinomas, sarcomas, leukemias and lymphomas, melanomas, and neuroectodermal tumors.

- *Carcinomas*—Carcinomas occur in the epithelial cells covering the surface of the body and lining the internal organs. (See Table 2.5.) Carcinomas account for about 90% of all cancer. Carcinomas occur in one of three embryologic types of cells: the outer layer of ectodermal cells (e.g., basel cell carcinomas), the middle layer of mesodermal cells (e.g., testicular carcinomas), or the inner layer of endodermal cells (e.g., lung carcinomas). Adenocarcinomas arise in organs with glands and squamous cell carcinomas arise from cells lining body cavities.

TABLE 2.5. SELECTED LIST OF CARCINOMAS BY ORGAN SYSTEM

Tissue Type	Tumor Type
Anus	Squamous cell
Breast	Ductal, lobular, medullary, comedo, colloid, papillary
Cervix	Squamous cell
Colon/rectum	Adeno-
Endometrium	Squamous cell
Gallbladder	Adeno-
Larynx	Squamous cell
Liver	Cholangio-, hemangio-, hepatocellular
Lung	Adeno-, squamous cell, small cell, large cell
Oral cavity (lip, tongue, mouth)	Squamous cell
Ovary	Adeno-, chorio-, yolk sac
Pancreas	Duct cell adeno-
Prostate	Adeno-
Stomach	Adeno-
Testis	Chorio-, embryonal, yolk sac

Source: National Cancer Institute (2011).

- *Sarcomas*—Sarcomas occur in tissues of mesodermal origin and are the rarest form of neoplasm. Sarcomas are solid tumors occurring in connective and supporting tissues, such as muscle or bone. (See Table 2.6.)

- *Leukemias and lymphomas*—Leukemias and lymphomas are cancers occurring in the lymph glands or bone marrow, which generates all of the cells of the circulatory or lymphatic systems. Leukemias and lymphomas comprise about 8% of all cancer. (See Table 2.7.) Leukemias (which literally mean "white blood") and lymphomas are sometimes referred to as liquid tumors in order to differentiate them from carcinomas, sarcomas, and melanomas, which are collectively termed solid tumors.

- *Melanomas*—Melenomas arise from the pigmented ectodermal cells of the skin and retina of the eye.

TABLE 2.6. SELECTED LIST OF SARCOMAS BY ORGAN SYSTEM

Tissue Type	Tumor Type
Blood vessels	Hemangiosarcoma, Kaposi's sarcoma
Fibrous tissue	Fibrosarcoma
Fat	Liposarcoma
Bone	Osteosarcoma and Ewing's sarcoma
Cartilage	Chondrosarcoma
Stomach	Leiomyosarcoma
Smooth muscle	Leiomyosarcoma
Striated muscle	Rhabdomyosarcoma
Nerve cells	Neurofibrosarcoma

Source: National Cancer Institute (2011).

TABLE 2.7. SELECTED LIST OF LEUKEMIAS AND LYMPHOMAS BY ORGAN SYSTEM

Tissue Type	Tumor Type
Blood cells (all)	Chronic myelogenous leukemia
Erythrocytes	Acute erythrocytic leukemia
Granulocytes	Acute myelo-, acute promyelocytic leukemia
Lymphocytes	Acute lymphocytic and chronic lymphocytic leukemia, Hodgkin's, non-Hodgkin's
Monocytes	Acute monocytic leukemia
Megakaryocytes	Acute megakaryocytic leukemia
Stomach	Lymphoma

Source: National Cancer Institute (2011).

- *Neuroectodermal tumors*—As the name implies, neuroectodermal tumors arise from ectodermal cells in the central and peripheral nervous system. Examples include gliomas, neuroblastomas, and schwannomas.

2.1.3.3. Cell Type

The name of a tumor will often describe the type of cell that has transformed into a cancer cell. Solid tumors can arise from adenomatous cells that are glandular or ductal, or from squamous cells that are flat. Tumors containing cells with features of both glandular and squamous cells may be called adeno-squamous carcinomas. Leukemias can arise from any of the various cells derived from myeloid or lymphoid lineages. Lymphomas occur in lymphocytes or macrophages, which are two types of cells present in the lymphatic system. Organs of the body are generally composed of more than one type of cell. Therefore, it is important to realize that more than one type of tumor can arise within the same organ.

2.1.3.4. Exceptions

Not all tumors are classified by these cell and tissue types. For example, cancers that resemble embryonic tissue are called blastomas. Examples include neuroblastomas and retinoblastomas. Another exception are teratomas, which arise in tissues derived from all three germ cell layers. To further complicate matters, some tumors have been named after the physicians who first described them. These include Ewing sarcoma, Hodgkin disease, Kaposi sarcoma and Wilms' tumor.

2.1.4. PRIMARY CANCER OR RECURRENCE

Your client explains that her mother was successfully treated for osteosarcoma at age 9 and was well until age 53 when she was diagnosed and treated for invasive breast cancer. Two years later she was found to have liver cancer and died at 56.

In deciphering a pattern of cancer in the family, it is important to determine whether a malignancy represents a primary cancer or is a recurrence of the initial tumor. In the above scenario, the mother's primary cancer is osteosarcoma, her breast cancer is a second primary, and the liver cancer most likely represents metastatic disease.

2.1.4.1. Primary Cancer

A newly arisen tumor is considered a primary tumor. Individuals can develop more than one primary cancer, although this is uncommon. These second (or third) primaries may occur as a consequence of treating the initial cancer.

For example, women with Hodgkin disease who are treated with radiation to the chest have higher rates of breast cancer. Multiple primary cancers are also more likely in those with hereditary cancer syndromes. For example, one individual referred to our center reported an uncle with Lynch syndrome who had developed a total of nine separate primaries!

2.1.4.2. Recurrence

A recurrence is the reappearance of cancer cells, either in the site of origin (local recurrence) or elsewhere in the body (systematic recurrence or distant metastasis). Recurrent cancer cells will demonstrate features that are consistent with the original tumor.

2.2. TUMOR CLASSIFICATION

The tumor classification system helps dictate treatment regimens, predict prognosis, and provide a systematic approach that can be universally recognized and understood. Tumors are assessed for malignant properties or potential and, if malignant, are graded and staged.

2.2.1. BENIGN OR MALIGNANT

The word "tumor" conjures up an image of cancer, yet not all tumors are cancerous. Thus, a lipoma (benign tumor of fat cells) may not be clinically significant, while a liposarcoma (malignant tumor of fat cells) represents a serious cancerous tumor. One of the initial steps in cancer diagnosis is to send a tumor specimen to a pathologist, who will determine if the tumor has any malignant properties.

There are several differences between benign and malignant tumors. The most significant difference is that benign tumors do not spread to other sites of the body while all malignant tumors have at least some metastatic potential. Benign tumors tend to be slow growing and innocuous. They are usually enclosed in a fibrous capsule and do not metastasize. Malignant tumors, in contrast, can proliferate rapidly and will, over time, spread to neighboring or distant tissues.

Despite the name, "benign" tumors are not always innocuous and can in fact cause significant risks of morbidity and mortality due to the following factors presented in the succeeding sections.

2.2.1.1. Location and Size

As a benign tumor grows, it may press against the normal surrounding tissue. This compression of the normal cell parenchyma can cause the normal cells to atrophy due to insufficient blood supply. In some sites of the body, there is sufficient space to tolerate a benign tumor. One example is the female uterus, in which fibroid tumors can grow to be quite large. In other sites, notably the brain and spine, there is little room for expansion and even moderately sized tumors can cause significant morbidity and mortality.

2.2.1.2. Excretion of Hormones

Benign tumors typically resemble their normal cell counterparts, which can be problematic if the cell type is hormone secreting. The benign tumor, not constrained by normal cell regulatory systems, may begin to produce additional amounts of hormones. Although benign tumors are generally less efficient at hormone production than normal cells, the sheer volume of tumor cells can result in massive—and toxic—levels of hormone being produced. For example, a pheochromocytoma is a benign tumor of the adrenal gland that produces the hormone epinephrine that triggers the "fight or flight" response. Excess levels of epinephrine caused by the pheochromocytoma can result in alarmingly high blood pressure and, if untreated, the danger of stroke or myocardial infarction.

In some cases, a benign tumor can be considered a precancerous tumor, that is, a tumor with malignant potential. Cells proceed through multiple steps before reaching a malignant state and some benign tumors may actually be malignant precursors. This has been shown to be the case for several types of cancer, such as pigmented moles (nevi) that can evolve into malignant melanoma and adenomas of the colon, which can eventually transform into adenocarcinomas.

Note that benign tumors typically end in the suffix *-oma*, which means "a tumor of" without the preceding "carcin" or "sarc". Examples are meningioma and glioma (two types of brain tumors). There are exceptions to this nomenclature, notably melanoma, which is a highly malignant skin cancer. *In situ* tumors are early stage malignant tumors (see Section 5.1.4 for a description of *in situ* breast cancers).

2.2.2. TUMOR GRADING

Once a tumor has been identified as malignant, a pathologist then determines the aggressiveness of the tumor cells by grading the tumor. Tumors are graded on their degree of malignancy on a scale of either 1 to 3 or 1 to 4, with 3 (or 4) being the most advanced, that is, worst. (See Table 2.8.) Grade 3 or 4 tumors are often associated with the poorest prognosis, although the truest indicator of prognosis is the extent of cancer spread, which involves staging the cancer (see Section 2.2.3).

Tumor grading involves analyzing the histological appearances and biological properties of the tumor in order to determine the extent to which the tumor resembles normal tissue. Histology is the study of the structure and

TABLE 2.8. HISTOLOGICAL GRADES OF TUMORS

GX	Grade cannot be assessed
G1	Well differentiated
G2	Moderately differentiated
G3	Poorly differentiated
G4	Undifferentiated

Source: National Cancer Institute at the National Institutes of Health. FactSheet: Tumor Grade. http://www.cancer.gov/cancertopics/factsheet/detection/tumor-grade, p. 2.

composition of cells, tissues, and organs. A tumor that shows only subtle differences from normal tissue will be considered low grade (well-differentiated), while a tumor that bears little or no resemblance to its normal counterpart is of high grade (poorly differentiated).

Tumor grading is also based on the degree of cell differentiation that is present. Cell differentiation is the process by which newly formed (immature) cells evolve into different kinds of mature cells. For example, myeloid progenitor cells in the bone marrow are immature blood cells, which will then differentiate into platelets, erythrocytes, leukocytes. The majority of cells in normal tissue are differentiated, in contrast to cancers in which the cells are less differentiated. Characterizing the differentiated cells in a tumor may help identify its site of origin. Tumors are graded on whether their cells appear well differentiated, moderately differentiated, or poorly differentiated. (See example in Fig. 2.1.)

Tumors containing a few atypical cells are considered to be dysplastic, which is a premalignant state. Low-grade (well-differentiated) tumors tend to be slow-growing and less aggressive, while higher grade (moderately or poorly differentiated) tumors tend to be fast-growing and more aggressive with a greater potential to metastasize. Tumors with a complete loss of normal differentiation are described as being anaplastic. Metastatic cancers of unknown primary are tumors that are metastatic at diagnosis and have unidentifiable sites of origin.

It is important to realize that the specific criteria used to grade a tumor are far from exact. Accurately grading a tumor depends upon the pathologist's skills and expertise. In cases of rare and/or unusual tumors, it may be useful to have the tumor slides reviewed by a second pathologist.

2.2.3. CLINICAL STAGING

The natural course of a malignancy is to grow and spread to other organs of the body. The purpose of clinical staging is to determine the extent of disease progression in a specific patient, to estimate prognosis, and help determine the best treatment plan. Clinical staging also provides a common set of criteria for oncologists and other medical specialists and provides a system for grouping patients in research treatment trials.

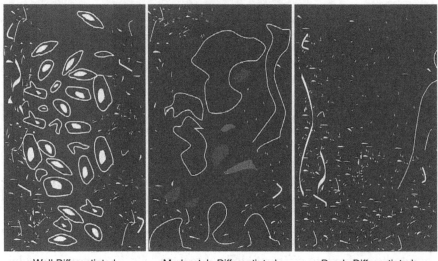

| Well Differentiated | Moderately Differentiated | Poorly Differentiated |

FIGURE 2.1. Cellular differentiation. The differences between a well-differentiated tumor cell (left), a moderately differentiated cell (middle), and a poorly differentiated cell (right) are shown. Adapted from: Pfeifer, J, and Wick, M. 1991. The Pathologic Evaluation of neoplastic diseases. In Amer. Cancer Society Textbook of Clinical Oncology. Holleb, A, Fink, D, and Murphy, G. (eds), ACS. Atlanta, Georgia, p. 11.

The clinical staging system most commonly used worldwide is the TNM system. The TNM system was developed by the American Joint Committee on Cancer Staging (AJCCS) and the International Union Against Cancer (IUAC) in an effort to standardize the staging criterion. The premise of staging is that cancers of the same site and histology will follow similar patterns of disease progression and will respond similarly to the same treatment regimens. Staging occurs after the initial assessment of the tumor and serves as a snapshot of the tumor prior to treatment. As treatment progresses, the tumor may be restaged as necessary.

The TNM system classifies cancer into Stages 0–IV, with Stage IV disease being the most advanced. Staging is made by assessing the size of the primary lesion, degree of invasion, and presence or absence of lymph node involvement or distant metastases. The more advanced the cancer, the higher each variable is graded. The three variables are specifically defined as:

- T—The extent of the primary tumor. This category considers the overall size and appearance of the tumor. Tumors are classified as being Tis (*in situ*), T1, T2, T3, or T4. *In situ* tumors are those that are confined to the cells lining the organ. Carcinomas and melanomas are the only cancers with an *in situ* stage. T4 tumors have invaded into tissues around the organ of origin.

TABLE 2.9. TNM CANCER STAGING OF MEDULLARY THYROID CARCINOMA

Stage I	T1 N0 M0
Stage II	T2 N0 M0 or T3 N0 M0
Stage III	T1 N1a M0 or T2 N1a M0 or T3 N1a M0
Stage IVA	T4a N0 M0 or T4a N1a M0 or T1 N1b M0 or T2 N1b M0 or T3 N1b M0 or T4a N1b M0
Stage IVB	T4b Any N M0
Stage IVC	Any T Any N M1

T (Primary Tumor): T1 = Tumor ≤2 cm; T2 = Tumor >1 cm but not >2 cm; T3 = Tumor >4 cm limited to thyroid or any tumor with minimal extrathyroid extension; T4a = tumor of any size extending beyond thyroid capsule to invade subcutaneous soft tissues, larynx, trachea, esophagus, or recurrent laryngeal nerve; T4b = tumor invades prevertebral fascia or encases carotid artery or mediastinal vessels. N (Regional lymph nodes): N0 = no regional lymph node metastasis; N1 = Regional lymph node metastasis; N1a = Metastasis to Level VI (pretracheal, paratracheal, and prelaryngeal/Delphian lymph nodes); N1b = Metastasis to unilateral, bilateral, or contralateral cervical (Levels I, II, III, IV, or V) or retropharyngeal or superior mediastinal lymph nodes (Level VII). M (Distant metastases): M0 = No distant metastases; M1 = Distant metastases.

Source: American Joint Committee on Cancer (2010), pp. 114–115.

- N—The extent of lymph node involvement. This is a strong predictor of systemic involvement. The lymph nodes are the gateway to the lymphatic or circulatory systems. Nodes can be classified as N0, N1, N2, or N3.

- M—The extent of distant metastases. Distant metastases are either absent (M0) or present (M1). The presence of distant metastases indicates an advanced stage of cancer.

The specific criteria used to define each variable in the TNM system depend upon the organ involved. Table 2.9 describes the TNM system for medullary thyroid carcinoma. Note that a particular stage of cancer can be composed of different TNM combinations.

Staging is an integral part of diagnosis and is performed for every tumor type. Because malignancies vary greatly across different organs and tissues, not all cancers are staged using the TNM system. In these cases, other classification systems have been developed. Examples include lymphomas, leukemias, and tumors of the central nervous system.

2.2.4. GENETIC ANALYSIS OF THE TUMOR

Cancer is a disease of "genes gone amok." Tumor histology is sometimes supplemented with a type of genetic analysis to further characterize the tumor and perhaps suggest additional therapies. These increasingly sophisticated genetic analyses include chromosome and targeted molecular studies.

2.2.4.1. Chromosome Studies

A cytogenetic analysis can identify major changes in the overall number or structure of a person's chromosomes. The normal human karyotype typically consists of 23 pairs of chromosomes—22 pairs of autosomes and one pair of sex chromosomes (46, XX for female and 46, XY for male). The karyotype of a tumor may be markedly different from the person's inherited set of genetic information (germline karyotype). Cytogenetic analysis can detect aneuplodies in which there are entire chromosomes that are missing (monosomies) or extra (trisomies). This analysis can also reveal partial deletions and duplications, as well as translocations in which segments of two genes have exchanged places.

Tumor nomenclature typically lists the karyotype with each aberrant chromosome listed in ascending order together with its structural abnormality, if appropriate. For example, a tumor in a male patient which contains an extra copy of chromosomes 10 and 17, a partial deletion of the short arm of chromosome 1, and a translocation of the long arms of chromosomes 18 and 20 could be written as: 48XY, del(1) (p12), +10, +17, t (18;20) (q21;q22).

2.2.4.2. Molecular Studies

Molecular studies provide a closer analysis of targeted gene segments or DNA nucleotides. Here are a few examples of molecular studies:

- *DNA sequencing*—Sequencing or reading the genetic code of a specific gene remains the gold standard for detection of a specific DNA substitution, insertion, or deletion. This strategy, which is generally automated, involves amplification of a particular gene's exons (coded regions) and exon/intron junctions and labeling each of the four types of nucleotides with different dyes. This process results in a series of wavy signal peaks that can be compared to a normal control. A mutation in one copy of the gene pair will result in two separate signals rather than the normal single signal. (See the example in Fig. 2.2.)
- *Southern blotting*—This strategy remains a standard method to analyze DNA structure. It involves isolating DNA and using restriction enzymes to chop the DNA into smaller fragments. These DNA fragments are then run on a gel, with the smaller fragments moving down the gel quicker than the larger fragments. The resulting bands can then to be compared to normal controls to reveal a large gene rearrangement or deletion.
- *Fluorescence* in situ *hybridization* (FISH)—This strategy is used to quickly detect specific translocations or chromosomal abnormalities. It involves labeling a specific cluster of DNA base pairs with a fluorescent tag, which can then be seen under the microscope.

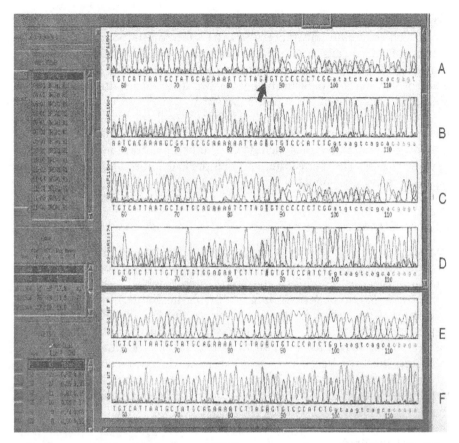

FIGURE 2.2. Automated fluorescent DNA sequence of a portion of exon 2 of the *BRCA1* gene. The cursor in frame A signifies the location of the first of two deleted bases. From this point downstream (to the right), there is a difference in sequence between the DNA strands as seen by direction. Frames C and D are repeat experiments of lanes A and B. Frames E and F depict the consensus ("normal") sequence; note the consistent peak heights and single signals at each position. (Courtesy of Dr. Brian Ward, Myriad Genetic Laboratories, Inc. Printed with permission from Offit, 1998, p. 249).

2.3. CANCER TREATMENT

With a diagnosis of cancer, patients and their families are thrust into a world with its own vocabulary and complicated treatment decisions. There are two overall aims of cancer treatment: to prolong life with radical therapy and to relieve suffering with palliative care.

A tumor is composed of a patchwork of cell populations and thus typically requires a variety of treatment modalities to eradicate it. It is important to recognize that clinical cure from cancer is defined as the absence of any detectable evidence of disease rather than the elimination of every single cancer cell (generally an impossible feat). Oncologists hope to reduce the number of cancer cells to a negligible amount that will not cause any significant symptoms or problems over the person's remaining life span. The treatment of cancer is a delicate balancing act to eradicate the tumor while limiting the amount of harm to the patient.

The treatment of cancer is divided into local therapies and systemic therapies. Local therapies include surgery, radiation, cryotherapy, and laser therapy. Systemic therapies include chemotherapy, hormonal therapy, and biologic agents. The succeeding sections present information on the major types of cancer treatments.

2.3.1. SURGERY

Surgical resection (removal) is the most effective strategy for treating localized disease and is the preferred strategy for eradicating solid tumors. The aim of surgery is to remove the entire tumor, which generally requires removing a margin of surrounding healthy tissue. Surgical resection is most successful if the tumor is slow growing, confined to a single organ, and can be removed without compromising any vital organs. Surgical risks include the small possibility of death related to the procedure or anesthesia, infection, short- or long-term disabilities, and disfigurement. The possible adverse effects of surgery are influenced by many factors, including the location of the tumor, extent of the surgery, and general health and age of the patient. Patients are usually given radiation treatments and/or chemotherapy either prior to surgery (neoadjuvant therapy) or following surgery (adjuvant therapy).

There are four major types of surgery used in treat cancer, presented in the succeeding sections.

2.3.1.1. Initial Diagnostic Surgery

The main purpose of the initial surgical procedure is to assess the extent of cancer that is present. In some cases, surgery can help determine where the cancer has originated. Surgical procedures, such as a biopsy, lymph node dissection, or laporoscopy, may also clarify the need for additional surgeries or other adjuvant treatments.

2.3.1.2. Radical Surgery

Radical surgery is used to completely eradicate the tumor and reduce the risk of local spread. This procedure may involve removing a fair amount of healthy tissue and can cause significant morbidity.

2.3.1.3. Conservative Surgery

In conservative surgery, only the tumor and a small margin of surrounding healthy tissue are removed. Thus, it is a far less extensive procedure than radical surgery, but typically requires adjuvant radiation and chemotherapy.

2.3.1.4. Palliative Surgery

The purpose of palliative surgery is to reduce pain or symptoms, caused by advanced disease rather than trying to eradicate the cancer. For example, a spinal cord tumor can cause difficulty walking and excruciating pain; debulking the tumor (removing part of it) may alleviate symptoms or restore organ function. In most cases, the relief of pain or other symptoms from palliative surgery is only temporary.

2.3.1.5. Other Surgical Procedures

Additional surgical procedures include the placement of a port catheter or pump to more easily administer chemotherapy and cosmetic reconstruction following cancer treatment.

2.3.2. RADIATION THERAPY

The aim of radiation therapy is to destroy tumor cells within the field being radiated. Radiation therapy is considered localized therapy and can be used to treat most solid tumors. Radiation therapy can be used prior to or instead of surgery to shrink tumors or after surgery to destroy remaining local cancer cells. Chemotherapy often follows a course of radiation therapy. Radiation can also be used to shrink inoperable tumors or for palliative care to relieve symptoms.

Radiation therapy involves targeting selected doses of ionizing radiation to the tumor site. The field of radiation can be compared to the beam of a flashlight. The radiation beam will be strongest at the center of the targeted site, but the "scatter" beam can also inflict damage to cells. This is actually a key benefit of radiation therapy because it can destroy cancer cells that have begun to spread locally. Tumor cells outside the field of radiation will not be affected, so radiation therapy is not an effective strategy for cancers that have metastasized.

How does radiation therapy work? The ionizing radiation deposits packets of energy into the cell, which causes DNA double-strand breaks and results in programmed cell death and/or blocked proliferation. Cells will either die immediately upon exposure or when they later attempt to undergo mitosis. Cancer cells that are actively dividing at the time of the radiation exposure are most vulnerable to radiation; higher doses of radiation are needed to destroy quiescent cells (ones that are not actively dividing) and slowly growing tumors with infrequent cell divisions. The radiation energy molecules are often delivered into the cells via the oxygen transport system. Thus, oxygen-poor tumors have some protection against radiation and require higher doses of radiation.

Radiation doses used to be measured in rads but are currently measured in units of Gray (Gy); a centiGray (cGy) is equivalent to a rad. Radiation therapy is typically given daily for 5–8 weeks as a series of daily doses of about 200 cGy. The daily dosages and total radiation exposure will differ depending on the tumor's location and size and the patient's tolerance of the treatments.

The effectiveness of radiation therapy depends largely on the tumor type and the sensitivity to radiation. One large dose of radiation is more effective than multiple small doses, which give cancer cells a chance to regrow, but it is also more toxic to normal tissue. Only a proportion of cancer cells are destroyed by a single dose of radiation. For example, if a single radiation dose kills 99% of a tumor that consists of 1 million cells, that translates to 10,000 tumor cells that remain.

Unfortunately, a proportion of normal cells within the field of radiation are also destroyed by the exposure to radiation. This is the major downside of radiation therapy and the toxicity must be monitored throughout the course of treatment. To determine the optimal radiation dose, radiation oncologists will consider the radiation sensitivity of the tumor, the bulk of disease, and the maximum amount of radiation that will be tolerated by the normal tissue. Normal cells generally recover faster than their malignant counterparts. Since normal stem cells infrequently divide, they are generally less vulnerable to radiation damage.

The side effects of radiation depend on the anatomic site being radiated. This includes hair loss if the radiation is to the head, diarrhea and cystitis if it is to the pelvic area. Radiation may also cause fatigue, redness of the skin, or scarring of the tissues. Long-term effects can include cataracts (irradiated eyes) and sterility (irradiated gonads). The lungs, liver, kidneys, and heart are also sensitive to radiation damage. These late responses can manifest months or years after the conclusion of treatment.

Radiation therapy in children can cause damage to bone and soft tissues, leading to reduced growth or deformity. Radiation therapy can also cause a second cancer, most commonly leukemia, or lymphoma, or if irradiated, breast cancer, thyroid cancer, or sarcomas.

2.3.3. Chemotherapy

Chemotherapy is systemic therapy that has the capability of destroying cancer cells throughout the body. Most drugs are given intravenously, but some are administered orally. The aims of chemotherapy are to further increase the chance that the tumor is eradicated and to prevent or delay metastases or to palliate symptoms. Because it is so difficult to detect micro-metastases, individuals will often be given adjuvant chemotherapy as a precautionary measure.

Chemotherapy can effectively destroy actively dividing cells, but is much less effective against quiescent (nondividing) cells. A course of chemotherapy can consist of a single drug, but often involves a combination of drugs. The efficacy of a particular drug depends on the inherent tumor sensitivity and its absorption, metabolism, distribution through the tumor, and excretion out of the body. Most chemotherapy agents target cells that are in particular mitotic phases; however, the use of multiple drugs in combinations allows all phases of the cell cycle to be targeted. If chemotherapy is being given for advanced stage cancer, then the regimen of drugs may need to be altered during the course of treatment, because the remaining tumor cells may have become resistant to the agents that have previously been used.

The properties of the tumor will determine the chemotherapeutic regimen. For example, in some cases, antimetabolites will be given to inhibit the formation of new blood vessels in order to starve the tumor. In other cases, drugs may be given to actually improve the tumor's blood vessels so that the chemotherapeutic agents can gain better access to the entire population of tumor cells. Chemotherapy can also be given for pain relief or to stabilize bodily functions.

The total number of chemotherapy courses administered will depend on the goal of therapy as well as the drug's effectiveness and toxicity. Typically, each course is spaced out in 1–3-week intervals in order to give the normal cell population a chance to recover.

Common side effects of chemotherapy include the loss of all body hair and the erosion of the mucosa of the gastrointestinal tract, leading to mouth sores, ulcers, and other digestive problems. Most types of chemotherapy cause bone marrow toxicity, leading to a decrease in white cells, platelets, or red cells. A drop in white blood cells temporarily increases the risk of infection. Most types of chemotherapy cause bone marrow toxicity, leading to a decrease in neutrophils or platelet production, which temporarily compromises the patient's immune system. Chemotherapy drugs can also cause permanent damage to nonrenewing tissues, including the heart and nervous system, and can cause sterility and, in women, temporary or permanent premature menopause.

Because of the cumulative toxicities, it is not possible for patients to remain indefinitely on chemotherapy. Most drugs have a narrow therapeutic index and individual variability or tolerance is not well understood. The emerging field of pharmacogenomics holds great promise in being able to better predict the individual metabolic responses and potential risk of serious side effects.

The first clinical use of chemotherapy was in 1942, when highly toxic nitrogen mustard was used to treat lymphoma. Today, there are numerous chemotherapeutic agents available, and chemotherapy regimens are increasingly designed to target a genetic tumor type. Types of chemotherapy include those in the succeeding sections.

2.3.3.1. Cytoxic Agents

Cytotoxic drugs include antimetabolites, alkylating agents, anti-tumor antibodies, and vinca alkaloids. Antimetabolites (e.g., 5-fluorouracil) work by blocking DNA transcription or by getting incorporated into DNA. Alkylating agents (e.g., adriamycin) directly damage the DNA, and vinca alkaloid agents (e.g., vincristine) damage the mitotic spindle. Cytotoxic drugs target dividing cells, which explains their effect on hair follicles, GI mucosa, and bone marrow.

2.3.3.2. Hormonal Agents

Steroid and nonsteroid hormones are actively involved in cellular proliferation and differentiation. Many tumors are sensitive to hormones, including cancers of the prostate, breast, endometruim, thyroid, ovary, and kidney. These types of tumors have surface hormonal receptors that can be targeted by hormonal therapy. Hormone (or trophic) therapy aims to shrink tumors by reducing the amount of available hormone and/or by inhibiting the binding of the hormone to the receptor. These agents can be used to treat advanced cancer or can increase the likelihood of cure if given after or with chemotherapy. Tamoxifen is an example of an antihormonal agent that successfully reduces breast cancer recurrences. One advantage to hormonal agents is that they rarely cause organ toxicity.

2.3.4. STEM CELL TRANSPLANTATION

Hematologic stem cells have the ability to differentiate into all the different types of mature cells in the circulatory and lymphatic systems. Since the major dose-limiting toxicity of chemotherapy is bone marrow suppression, obtaining stem cells prior to chemotherapy can permit the administration of higher doses of chemotherapy than would otherwise be possible. Stem cells can then be given back to regenerate the bone marrow and potentially rejuvenate a compromised immune system.

Bone marrow transplantation can be performed for curative or palliation purposes. There are many potential complications of transplantation, including infection, bleeding, mouth sores, hair loss, and, rarely, a complete rejection of the transplanted cells (graft rejection). In allogenic transplants, there is also the risk of an exuberant immune response mounted against the person's own body cells by the foreign stem cells, which is termed "graft versus host disease."

The three main sources of stem cells are the bone marrow, peripheral blood, and the umbilical cord. Most transplants performed today use peripheral blood because the cells are easier to obtain and the immune system recovers faster than with the more conventional bone marrow transplant. Stem cells are obtained from peripheral blood by artificially stimulating stem cell growth in the bone marrow by the use of growth factors. This causes the crowded bone marrow to release some of the stem cells into the bloodstream. These cells are then removed from the bloodstream through a process called apheresis. The stem cells are then returned to the patient following high-dose chemotherapy and/or radiation treatments.

While the umbilical cord is rich with stem cells, the overall small quantity of cells makes it impractical for use in adults. However, a family at high risk for childhood cancers may want to store their newborn's cord blood in case the baby (or a sibling) later develops cancer.

The two major types of bone marrow transplants are described below.

- *Allogeneic transplant*—In an allogeneic transplant, the transplanted stem cells are from a donor who shares similar human leukocyte antigens (HLAs). The HLA-matched donor is typically a sibling or parent. If there are no matches among family members, donor registries can be searched. Such registries have increased the number of potential matched donors, although minority ethnic groups remain underrepresented. Cancer patients who undergo allogeneic transplants face problems with rejection of the stem cells and either acute or chronic graft-versus-host disease. Allogeneic transplants have been successfully used to treat leukemias and lymphomas. As an aside, allogeneic transplants are also used to treat other genetic conditions, including severe combined immune deficiency syndrome and sickle cell disease.

- *Autologous transplant*—In an autologous transplant, the patient's own stem cells are removed and then returned to the patient after he or she has been given chemotherapy and/or radiation. The transplanted stem cells have been spared the exposure to the toxic treatments and can be returned to the patient without fear of graft-versus-host disease. Autologous transplants are performed for many types of hematologic and solid tumors, especially in children, although its efficacy in treating solid tumors in adults remains unproven.

2.3.5. Additional Cancer Therapies

Other cancer therapies include laser therapy, cryotherapy, gene therapy, immunotherapy, and retinoid agents.

2.3.5.1. Laser Therapy

This type of therapy is an effort to burn or vaporize the tumor. The laser beam, which emits an intense heat, is aimed directly at the tumor. Although laser therapy can be more precise than radiation in the area that is targeted, it cannot be used to target large areas. However, it is a very useful tool in removing solid tumors that are obstructing a passageway in the body and for treating several types of cancer, including that of the skin, esophagus, colon, rectum, and stomach.

2.3.5.2. Cryotherapy

This type of therapy uses extreme cold to freeze the tumor and interrupt its growth process. It is also useful in relieving pain and reducing swelling. In cryosurgery, the liquid nitrogen is poured into probes that have been inserted into the tumor until it has reached freezing temperatures. This form of therapy is being used to treat several types of solid tumors, especially cancers of the liver and prostate.

2.3.5.3. Gene Therapy

Although gene therapy continues to represent the hope of the future, it is slow to make its way into clinical care. Gene therapy involves inserting a specific cancer gene into a viral vector and injecting it into the tumor so that it can impact the tumor's genome. This strategy works best if a specific gene is targeted, such as the *MYC* oncogene in order to block transcription of the gene or the *TP53* tumor suppressor gene to reestablish the body's normal apoptosis pathway. Since it is not possible to inject the cancer gene into every tumor cell, this strategy also relies on a so-called bystander effect, which occurs when the death of one cancer cell triggers surrounding cells to implode.

2.3.5.4. Immunotherapy

The immune system may not always recognize a tumor as a threat because its cells are native to the body rather than foreign substances. Immunotherapy agents are typically purified proteins that bind to receptor molecules to stimulate the body's immune response against the tumor. This can be done by stimulating the population of T cells, which destroy foreign cells, and/or B cells, which make antibodies targeted toward specific foreign substances. These biological agents also encourage cellular differentiation, which impairs the tumor's ability to grow. Examples include interferon-alpha, which is used in the treatment of melanoma, hairy cell, and myelogenous leukemia; and interleukin-2, which is used to treat metastatic renal cell carcinoma. Short-term side effects include fatigue and flu-like symptoms.

2.3.5.5. Retinoid Agents

All-trans retinoic acid induces differentiation of epithelial cells, thus impairing the tumor's ability to grow. Retinoic acid has been found to be quite effective in treating a few types of cancer, including basal cell carcinomas, bladder cancer, and promyelocytic leukemia. Side effects include soreness of the skin, general malaise, and liver toxicity.

2.4. FURTHER READING

American Cancer Society. 2010. Signs and symptoms of cancer. http://www.cancer.org/cancer/cancerbasics/signs-and-symptoms-of-cancer.

American Cancer Society. 2011. Learn about Cancer: Find information and resources for a specific cancer topic. http://www.cancer.org/cancer/index.

American Joint Committee on Cancer. 2010. Cancer Staging Handbook, 7th edition. Springer, New York.

Boyer, MJ, and Tannock, IF. 2005. Cellular and molecular basis of drug treatment for cancer. In Tannock, IF, Hill, RP, Bristow, RG, and Harrington, L (eds), The Basic Science of Oncology, 4th edition. McGraw Hill, New York, 349–375.

Bristow, RG, and Hill, RP. 2005. Molecular and cellular basis of radiotherapy. In Tannock, IF, Hill, RP, Bristow, RG, and Harrington, L (eds), The Basic Science of Oncology, 4th edition. McGraw Hill, New York, 261–321.

Dollinger, M, Rosenbaum, EH, Tempero, M, Mulvihill, SJ, Ljung, BM, and Morita, ET. 2002. How cancer is diagnosed. In Dollinger, M, Rosenbaum, RH, Termpero, M, and Mulvihill, SJ (eds), Everyone's Guide to Cancer Therapy, 4th edition. Andrews McMeel Publishing, Kansas City, MO, 17–30.

Girard, V. 2004. Confronting the bully. In There's No Place Like Hope: A Guide to Beating Cancer in Mind-Sized Bites. Compendium Inc., Lynnwood, WA, 1–3.

National Cancer Institute. 2011. A to Z List of Cancers. The Website of the National Cancer Institute. http://www.cancer.gov/cancertopics/types/alphalist.

Offit, K. 1998. Laboratory methods of cancer genetic testing. In Clinical Cancer Genetics. Wiley & Sons Inc., New York, 240–253.

Parchment, RE. 2006. Oncology: the difficult task of eradicating caricatures of normal tissue renewal in the human patient. In McKinnell, RG, Parchment, RE, Perantoni, AO, Damjanov, I, and Barry Pierce, G (eds), The Biological Basis of Cancer, 2nd edition. Cambridge University Press, New York, 307–354.

Pierce, GB, and Damjanov, I. 2006. The pathology of cancer. In McKinnell, RG, Parchment, RE, Perantoni, AO, Damjanov, I, and Barry Pierce, G (eds), The Biological Basis of Cancer, 2nd edition. Cambridge University Press, New York, 14–50.

Schultz, WA. 2004. Cancer diagnosis. In Molecular Biology of Human Cancers. An Advanced Student's Textbook. Springer, The Netherlands, 427–447.

Sontag, S. 1977. Illness as Metaphor. Farrar, Straus, & Giroux, New York.

CANCER BIOLOGY

Over the past decade, a great change has occurred in how we think about cancer. Where once we viewed cancer as an unfathomed black box, now we have pried open the box and cast in the first dim light. Where once we thought of cancer as a bewildering variety of diseases with causes too numerous to count, now we are on the track of a single unifying explanation for how most or all cancers might arise. The track is paved with cells.

(Bishop, 2003, p. 135)

3.1. THE MALIGNANT CELL

The process by which a normal cell becomes malignant can be summed up as cell replication gone awry. This section provides an overview of the acquired features and functional properties of cancer cells.

3.1.1. FEATURES OF MALIGNANT CELLS

Cancer cells are anatomically and biochemically altered from normal cells (see Table 3.1). These differences are outlined in the succeeding sections.

3.1.1.1. Anatomical Features

The most obvious anatomic difference is that cancer cells have abnormal shapes and sizes as compared to their normal counterparts. In cancer cells,

Counseling About Cancer, Third Edition. Katherine A. Schneider.
© 2012 Wiley-Blackwell. Published 2012 by John Wiley & Sons, Inc.

TABLE 3.1. THE HALLMARKS OF CANCER

- Self-sufficiency in growth factor
- Insensitivity to antigrowth signals
- Evasion of apoptosis
- Limitless replicative potential
- Sustained angiogenesis
- Tissue invasion and metastases

Source: Hanahan and Weinberg (2011).

changes are present in each major component of the cell, from the genetic content of the nucleus to the hormone receptors in the outer cytoplasm. While normal populations of cells are characteristically homogeneous, tumors consist of heterogeneous clusters of oddly shaped cells.

3.1.1.2. Biochemical Features

Cancer cells have different biochemical requirements than normal cells, allowing them to have enhanced abilities to proliferate and survive. For example, cancer cells require lower concentrations of growth factors to replicate than normal cells. There are also biochemical features that are lost or gained within the cancer cells themselves, including the loss of fibronectin (a protein important for cell-to-cell adhesion) and the gained ability to produce their own growth factors.

3.1.1.3. Genetic Features

Tumor cells contain markedly abnormal and unstable karyotypes, which include alterations in the number and structure of both individual genes and entire chromosomes. Genetic aneuploidy is common, as are all types of chromosomal translocations, breakages, and other structural rearrangements. As illustrated in Figure 3.1, mutations in the three types of cancer predisposition genes—oncogenes, tumor suppressor genes, and mismatch repair genes—target different aspects of the cell cycle. While our inherited or constitutional genome remains standard across all normal cells, the genetic makeup of a tumor varies widely from cell to cell. Thus, tumor cells will proliferate and gain metastatic potential at varying rates and will have differing sensitivities to chemotherapy or radiation.

3.1.2. FUNCTIONAL PROPERTIES OF CANCER CELLS

A hallmark of cancer is the derailment of tightly regulated cellular processes, such as differentiation, proliferation, and programmed cell death. Cancer cells almost always shed normal cellular traits that are limiting

Cell Cycle

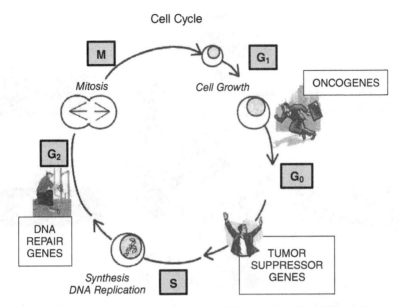

FIGURE 3.1. The cell cycle and placement of major cancer predisposition genes. These gene types are oncogenes, tumor suppressor genes, and DNA repair genes. See the text for further description of these cancer predisposition genes. Source: Offit (1998, p. 40, reprinted with permission).

and acquire traits that are useful to their survival and potential for growth. The major biological capabilities acquired by cancer cells are shown in Figure 3.2, and some of these properties are presented in the succeeding sections.

3.1.2.1. Lose Differentiation

Terminally differentiated cells have been programmed to have specific structures and functions and do not divide again under normal circumstances. Differentiation is one of the cellular mechanisms of halting or limiting cell growth. Losing the characteristics of a normal mature cell is termed dedifferentiation. Dedifferentiation occurs when a mature cell loses its normal phenotype due to somatic genetic changes that have occurred during replication. After puberty, the rate of normal cell division slows down and is merely required to maintain the size and function of the tissue. When normal cells are called upon to divide, one cell stays undifferentiated for the purposes of future growth and all the rest differentiate into mature cells. This is a very different composition from tumors, in which half the cells may remain undifferentiated.

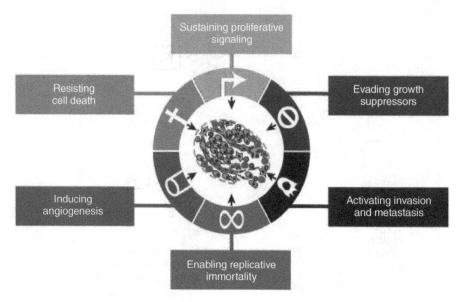

FIGURE 3.2. This figure illustrates the revised hallmarks of cancer. These biological properties are the ones that cancer cells acquire in order to thrive. Reprinted from *Hallmarks of Cancer: The Next Generation*, Douglas Hanahan and Robert A. Weinberg, Copyright 2011, with permission from Elsevier.

3.1.2.2. Gain Proliferative Abilities

Cell proliferation is the process by which new cells are generated. Fully differentiated cells do not ever replicate, while some less differentiated cells go through a preset number of growth cycles over their lifespan. The average human cell goes through 60–80 divisions before losing the ability to proliferate. For normal cells to proliferate, several requirements must be met, including the presence of sufficient growth factors and appropriate anchoring of the cell. The direct result of the genetic changes that occur in cancer cells is increased proliferation. Cancer cells divide with greater frequency and for a greater number of growth cycles than their normal counterparts. Cancer cells also become hypersensitive to the cellular growth signals, allowing them to maximally reproduce, and as the cancer cells mature, they acquire the ability to proliferate independent of the tissue's normal growth signals.

3.1.2.3. Bypass Cell Cycle Checkpoints

The purpose of the G1 and G2 checkpoints in the cell cycle is to check for DNA replication errors and to mark the aberrant cells which either need to be repaired or destroyed. In cancer cells, the genes responsible for halting mitosis may be mutated. This allows the cells to bypass these checkpoints and retain their damaged DNA content.

3.1.2.4. Dismantle DNA Repair

Cancer cells may continue to halt at the G1 and G2 checkpoints, but the problem may lie with the genes responsible for repairing the replication errors. Thus, the checkpoints may be rendered ineffective by faulty DNA repair genes. This allows the cells to survive and replicate further despite the presence of numerous DNA errors.

3.1.2.5. Achieve Immortality

Programmed cell death is termed apoptosis. Apoptosis constitutes an important mechanism for tissues to control the number of growth cycles per cell. Apoptosis serves many purposes, such as shaping tissues during development, eliminating hyperreactive immune cells, destroying cells infected by viruses, and maintaining the homeostasis of tissues. Normal cells undergo apoptosis either at a designated time or when perceived as damaged. Another safety mechanism of the tissue is replicative senescence, which allows the cell to live, but cuts off its ability to proliferate. Tumor cells that are able to dismantle or bypass these safety mechanisms become "immortal." Immortalized cells have greatly expanded life spans and rarely lose their proliferative ability.

3.1.2.6. Undergo Angiogenesis

A small-sized tumor, less than 2 mm, is usually able to sustain itself with nutrients siphoned off from the surrounding tissue. However, anything larger than a few cell layers will require its own food source. In response to this need, tumors undergo a process termed angiogenesis. Angiogenesis involves the differentiation of specific cells into capillaries that can bring blood, that is, nutrients, directly to the tumor. The tumor either builds a new network of capillaries or grows alongside the existing blood vessels to divert the blood supply that was meant for the normal surrounding tissue. Angiogenesis can also occur in noncancer cells to aid the healing of wounds or severe inflammation. Tissues—normal or tumor—that do not have a sufficient blood supply may contain large areas of necrosis (dead tissue).

3.1.2.7. Exhibit Altered Metabolism

A tumor's perpetual growth takes increased energy (analogous to teenage boys!). Tumor cells adapt to this need by manufacturing an increased number of enzymes used for growth signaling and biosynthesis. The surge of metabolism and increase of discarded waste products may also impact the metabolism of neighboring normal cells.

3.1.2.8. Display Genomic Instability

The abnormal structure and number of genes and chromosomes in a cancer cell may confer increased potential for growth and survival but also renders it quite unstable. Tumor populations are a mosaic patchwork of cells with differing genetic, metabolic, and functional properties. Thus, a tumor is never truly in a state of perfect balance or homeostasis. There are constant changes in the functional properties of the tumor as it grows and adapts to its environment, with advantages given to cells, which are the best at proliferating and surviving under adverse conditions.

3.1.2.9. Display Abnormal Cellular Signaling

There are over 6000 genes whose primary purpose is to relay messages to and from the different components of cells and tissues. The purpose of these signaling networks is to properly maintain each tissue in perfect balance (homeostasis). These signaling genes are sensitive to the physical environment and needs of the cell and will modify signals accordingly. The signaling networks rely on the unique configurations of a cell's surface receptors to determine if incoming messages should either be ignored or retrieved and relayed to the next cell downstream in the signaling system. Cancer cells present altered surface receptors that can confuse the signaling cells and derail the normal communications of the cellular pathways. In fact, mutations in tumor cells tend to target all aspects of the signaling networks. Cancer cells may also generate their own signaling system that allows them to function independently, and further confuses the surrounding normal cells, which keep adjusting their biochemical commands in reaction to the tumor's erratic growth.

3.1.2.10. Acquire Movement

Normal cells outside the circulatory or lymphatic systems tend to stay permanently fixed in one spot. The normal cells are kept in place by several cellular mechanisms, including a fixed adhesion to neighboring cells. The loss of this adhesion and the gain of locomotion are the first steps toward migration and metastasis.

3.2. CARCINOGENESIS

A cell goes through multiple steps en route to becoming a fully malignant cell. The development of a tumor begins with a single cancer cell somewhere in the body, which multiplies and creates a small colony of cells within the same tissue. Further genetic changes occur within this colony of abnormal cells, leading to cells with enhanced growth potential and other special features, such as mobility and expanded life spans. The phases of carcinogenesis may be completed rapidly or may take a decade or more. Some precancerous cells regress back to normal states or remain in precancerous states indefinitely; in others, the progression to full malignancy seems inevitable.

3.2.1. STAGES OF CARCINOGENESIS

The phases of carcinogenesis are termed initiation, promotion, progression, and metastasis. These phases are illustrated in Figure 3.3.

3.2.1.1. Initiation

The first stage of carcinogenesis is termed initiation. Typically, the initial event of carcinogenesis is the occurrence of a genetic mutation within a single cell, which leads to abnormal proliferation. Only cells with the ability to replicate, such as progenitor cells and stem cells, are at risk for becoming premalignant cells. The initiating mutation may be inherited in the germline, but most occur somatically. Somatic mutations occur because of a random error during mitosis or because of exposure to carcinogens termed initiators or initiating agents. When a carcinogen interacts with DNA, it creates an altered nucleotide, which is termed an adduct. Similar to a virus, the adduct inserts itself into the normal strand of DNA, potentially beginning the malignant cascade. The time span from this initial carcinogenic exposure to a detectable tumor can take several years; this is also referred to as the latency period. Two examples of initiating agents are tobacco and radiation. An initiated cell is a malignant stem cell that, given the right environment, has the potential of seeding a fully malignant tumor. Therefore, initiated cells do not appear different from their normal counterparts and will only transform into fully malignant cells under certain conditions. Initiated cells are permanently altered; however, they do not always progress to a malignant tumor. Some initiated cells will be destroyed prior to proliferation and others will remain fixed in an abnormal but nonneoplastic state.

3.2.1.2. Promotion

Promotion is the second phase of carcinogenesis. Within this stage, cells acquire a selective growth advantage, which leads to a rapid growth of abnormal cells and the formation of a small, benign tumor population. This period of rapid growth can occur because of a random error during cell division or exposure to certain carcinogens termed promoters or promoting agents. Hormones and dietary fat are two examples of promoters. Exposure to these types of promoter agents stimulates the growth of the initiated cells,

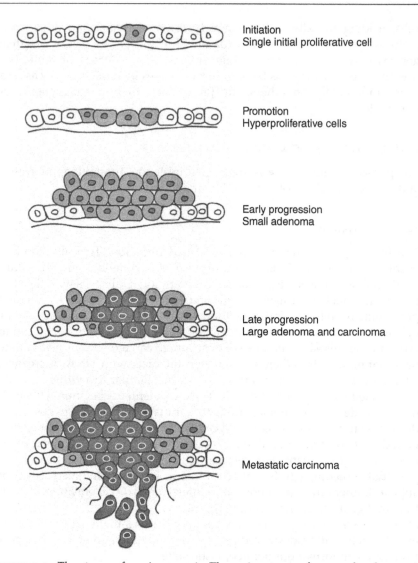

Initiation
Single initial proliferative cell

Promotion
Hyperproliferative cells

Early progression
Small adenoma

Late progression
Large adenoma and carcinoma

Metastatic carcinoma

FIGURE 3.3. The stages of carcinogenesis. The major stages of cancer development are termed initiation, promotion, progression, and metastasis. Note that the process begins with a single mutated cell (the lightly shaded cell) and ends with many fully carcinogenic cells (darkly shaded cells) breaking away from the tumor and traveling to other sites of the body. Source: Cooper, G. 1992. Elements of Human Cancer. Jones and Bartlett, Bouton, p. 23.

but it is an epigenetic effect in that it alters the phenotype rather than the genotype of the cell. Therefore, the carcinogenic process is still reversible at this point. If the exposure to the promoting agent is removed, then the cells will cease their growth and begin to die out. However, cells that continue to mutate and divide will continue on the carcinogenic pathway.

3.2.1.3. Progression

Progression designates the stage at which the situation goes from bad to worse. During this stage, genetic mutations continue to occur, allowing the cells in the tumor to gain or lose certain characteristics with the outcome that the tumor can now function completely independently from the host tissue. Progression is triggered by additional exposures to carcinogens, as well as spontaneous mutations within the increasingly abnormal and unstable genomes of the cancer cells. Genetic changes at this stage are irreversible and occur in a haphazard manner, giving the tumor its heterogeneous cluster of cell types. As the tumor continues to grow, certain mutated cells can be selected to proliferate depending on the needs of the tumor within its current environment. For example, a small subpopulation of cells that do not require hormones to replicate may eventually outgrow the cells that are hormone dependent. While tumor growth is stochastic rather than calculated, it does seem to follow a Darwinian survival of the fittest philosophy. Eventually, the tumor will consist of a population of fully malignant tumor cells, which display a vastly increased proliferative ability, an autonomous source of nutrition, a variety of abnormal karyotypes with unusual deletions and rear-rangements, and metastatic potential.

3.2.1.4. Invasion and Metastasis

Malignant cells undergo further genetic changes in order to gain the ability to invade surrounding tissues and set up distant tumor colonies (metasta-ses). The metastatic process involves multiple steps as listed in Table 3.2 and illustrated in Figure 3.4. First, the cells lose their adhesion to neighboring cells and gain the ability to move through locomotion. Then the cells invade the cell membrane, which gives them ample access to neighboring tissues and ultimately the circulatory or lymphatic system. This is why, regardless of the primary site of the cancer, blood samples and/or lymph nodes will be monitored during and after cancer treatment. Cancer cells enter the blood or lymphatic vessels, which is termed intravasation, and exit the vessels at other sites, which is termed extravasation. The specific route taken by a group of metastatic cells is specific and somewhat predictable depending on the type and location of the initial tumor. Metastatic cells usually seek "hos-pitable" tissues that are already equipped with microcapillary systems such as the liver, lung, kidney, and bone. However, cancer cells can potentially be

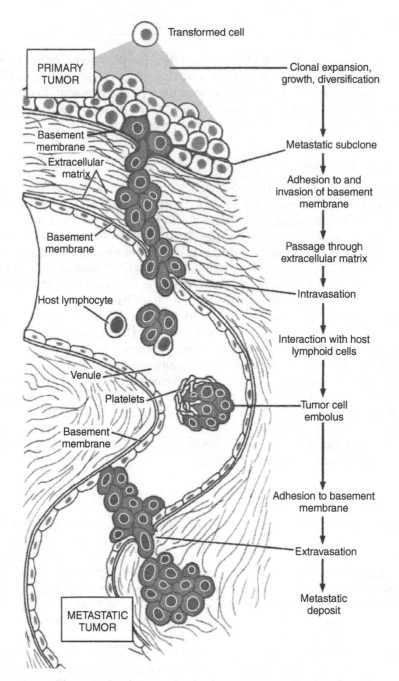

Transformed cell

PRIMARY
TUMOR

Basement
membrane

Extracellular
matrix

Basement
membrane

Host lymphocyte

Venule

Platelets

Basement
membrane

METASTATIC
TUMOR

Clonal expansion,
growth, diversification

Metastatic subclone

Adhesion to and
invasion of basement
membrane

Passage through
extracellular matrix

Intravasation

Interaction with host
lymphoid cells

Tumor cell
embolus

Adhesion to basement
membrane

Extravasation

Metastatic
deposit

FIGURE 3.4. The cascade of events that lead to metastasis. Reading from the top of the diagram to the bottom, the metastatic subclones (indicated with darkened cytoplasms and nuclei) bind to and disrupt the tissue's basement membrane and invade the extracellular matrix. The metastatic cells penetrate the vascular or lymphatic system (intravasation) and circulate until they adhere to the basement membrane of a vessel at a distant site. The metastatic cells then exit the vessel (extravasation) at a site where they form a metastatic colony. Source: McKinnell (2006, p. 55).

TABLE 3.2. THE METASTATIC CASCADE

- Detachment of cell
- Migration and mobility
- Breach of cell membrane
- Intravasation
- Extravasation
- Colonization

Source: McKinnell (2006).

carried to any site of the body. The final step of the metastatic cascade is termed colonization, which is when the cancer cells set up seeds or colonies in the new tissue. Some of these colonies will remain dormant for years, while others will immediately begin to grow. It is estimated that fewer than 1 out of 10,000 malignant cells successfully metastasize. However, this statistic is not comforting when considering that large primary tumors shed millions of cancer cells daily into the circulatory or lymphatic system. Metastasis is the main cause of cancer-related mortality. Unfortunately, it is estimated that about two-thirds of patients have signs of metastases when initially diagnosed.

3.2.2. KNUDSON'S MODEL OF RETINOBLASTOMA

In 1971, Alfred G. Knudson sought to describe cancer development in a way that explained both inherited and sporadic forms of retinoblastoma. His two-hit theory (illustrated in Fig. 3.5) explains that children with the inherited form of retinoblastoma are born with one working copy of the *RB* gene and one nonworking mutated copy. The retinal tumors occurs only if a second event or "hit" destroys the functional *RB* gene in any of the retinal cells. In contrast, children with the sporadic form of retinoblastoma are born with two functional *RB* genes, but develop the eye cancer after separate events knock out both *RB* alleles in a single retinal cell. This model explains why 9 out of 10 children with an inherited mutated *RB* gene eventually develop a retinoblastoma tumor, while the incidence of sporadic retinoblastoma tumors is about 1 in 20,000.

The Knudson two-hit hypothesis described cancer development as a process rather than as the result of a single event or exposure, and thus revolutionized our understanding of carcinogenesis. The two-hit model fits other neoplasms as well, but probably should be renamed the multiple-hit model, because as it turns out, most neoplasms require between two and seven separate hits to reach full metastatic potential.

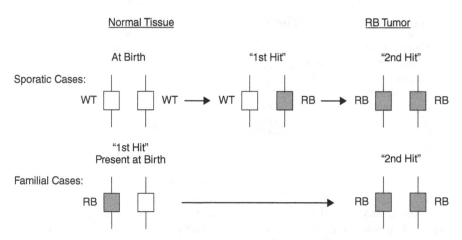

FIGURE 3.5. Knudson's two-hit model of carcinogenesis. This model demonstrates a mechanism that explains both sporadic and familial forms of retinoblastoma. WT = wild type; RB = mutation in *RB1* gene.

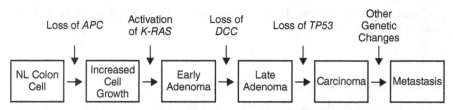

FIGURE 3.6. Vogelstein's multistep process of carcinogenesis. This model demonstrates the cascade of genetic events that need to occur for a normal (NL) colon cell to transform into a metastatic cancer cell. Source: Fearon, E, and Vogelstein, B. 1990. A genetic model for colorectal tumorigenesis. Cell 61: 759–767.

3.2.3. VOGELSTEIN'S MODEL OF COLON CANCER

The model of carcinogenesis in colorectal cancers, elegantly demonstrates that it is the combination of genetic events that leads to malignancy. (See Fig. 3.6.) The initial carcinogenic event may be a germline or somatic mutation in a tumor suppressor gene, such as the *APC* gene. Additional genetic mutations then lead to the activation of the *K-RAS* oncogene and loss of the *DCC* and *TP53* tumor suppressor genes. It is the accumulation of genetic events that is important; the exact order of genetic changes can vary. However, certain genetic changes occur more frequently as early events and other mutations as later events. This series of genetic changes corresponds to the development of adenomas (in early, intermediate, and late stages) and metastatic carcinoma. The ability to recognize whether genetic changes are indicative of early or advanced disease assists clinicians in staging and treating the malignancy.

3.3. ONCOGENES

The discovery of viral oncogenes in the 1960s provided the first evidence that specific genes could induce cancer. This section describes the normal cellular functions of proto-oncogenes and the processes that can trigger oncogene activation and lead to malignancy. The *RET* oncogene is described at the end of the section.

3.3.1. GENERAL DESCRIPTION OF ONCOGENES

Each tumor displays a characteristic subset of the nearly 100 oncogenes described to date. Oncogenes behave as dominant growth-promoting genes and thus, only one copy of the gene needs to be mutated in order to affect the cell's growth or expression. The activation of a single oncogene is not sufficient to cause cancer, although oncogenes do play an important role in tumorigenesis.

Oncogenes were originally studied in tumor viruses. This is reflected in their names, which are typically composed of three-letter acronyms referring to the type of cancer induced by the virus, or the species of animal the virus infects, or the scientist who first isolated the virus. For example, the *ABL* oncogene is named for the scientist Abelson and the cancer it induces (leukemia), while the *ras* oncogenes were first isolated from a rat sarcoma virus. Standard nomenclature for human oncogenes is written in italicized capital letters, while nonhuman oncogenes are written in italicized lowercase letters.

Oncogenes originate from normal cellular genes called proto-oncogenes. Although the name implies otherwise, the primary function of proto-oncogenes is not to give rise to oncogenes. Rather, protooncogenes play crucial roles in cell cycle regulation, cellular signal pathways, and DNA repair. Most proto-oncogenes are involved in the cell's signaling pathway. (See Fig. 3.7 for an illustration of this pathway.) Proto-oncogenes have remained highly conserved throughout evolution and appear to be crucial for normal tissue differentiation, particularly during embryogenesis.

In simplistic terms, the "sentry" proto-oncogenes recognize that certain external stimuli could be a threat to the cell and will initiate sending a warning message to the nucleus. The message is given to the nearest messenger gene, which hands it off to the next gene in line, and so on until the nucleus is reached. The nucleus will then evaluate the threat and decide whether to turn on or off appropriate genes in response. The response

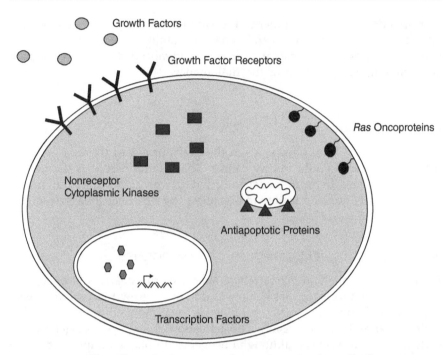

FIGURE 3.7. The role and placement of oncogenes in the cell. Oncogenes are involved in the cytoplasmic signaling pathway and in nuclear gene regulation. Types of oncogenes include growth factors and growth factor receptors, *ras* oncoproteins, nonreceptor cytoplasmic kinases, antiapoptotic proteins, and nuclear transcription factors. Source: Oster et al. (2005, p. 129). Reproduced with permission from McGraw-Hill.

messages from the nucleus are also relayed by messenger genes. A breakdown anywhere in the signaling pathway can therefore have major consequences for the function and integrity of the cell and its neighbors.

Proto-oncogenes are classified according to their function and location in the cell. The major types of protooncogenes are described below:

3.3.1.1. Growth Factors

The body has several specific growth factors that serve as intercellular signals for cell growth. Growth factors are secreted from the cell membrane. Examples of growth factor genes include *INT-1* and *SIS*. Mutations in these proto-oncogenes will stimulate adjacent cells to grow and will enable the genes to ignore signals to halt growth.

3.3.1.2. Growth Factor Receptors

The signal transduction pathway begins with the binding of growth factor to a receptor. Most growth factor receptors are tyrosine kinases that are located in the cytoplasm of the cell. Examples include *HER2/NEU*, *RET*, *MET*, and *ERBB-1*. Mutations in receptor genes can result in the overproduction of receptors, which in turn are extra sensitive to external stimuli. The cellular response to an overproduction of receptors is to divide into two cells; a process that will continue as long as the cells sense that extra receptors are present.

3.3.1.3. Nonreceptor Tyrosine Kinases

Certain proto-oncogenes act as intracellular messengers of growth signals. These genes are tyrosine kinases, which can be located in the cytoplasm or nucleus. Examples include the *SRC* and *ABL* genes. Mutated messenger genes can send false information to the nucleus that triggers a response of enhanced growth and proliferation.

3.3.1.4. Signal Transducers

Signal transducer proto-oncogenes act as intracellular messengers. These genes bind with guanosine-5′-triphosphate (GTP) and are present in the inner membrane of the cell. Aberrant genes lead to increased proliferation. Examples of signal transducer genes are the *RAS* genes (e.g., *K-RAS*, *H-RAS*); mutated *RAS* genes are found in about one-third of human cancers.

3.3.1.5. Cell Cycle Regulators

The cyclin-dependent proto-oncogenes (such as *CDK2* and *CDKN1A*) help initiate and sustain progression through the cell cycle. Many of these proto-oncogenes are negative regulators, thus ensuring important pauses during mitosis to assess the integrity of the genome and make DNA repairs as needed.

3.3.1.6. Nuclear Transcription Factors

At the end of the cellular signaling pathway are the nuclear factors, which can activate DNA replication or transcription. Nuclear transcription factors include *N-MYC*, *JUN*, and *FOS*. Mutated nuclear transcription factors can perpetuate cell growth indefinitely and are not dependent upon any extracellular factors.

3.3.2. ONCOGENE ACTIVATION

The transformation of a proto-oncogene to an oncogene is called activation. Oncogene activation leads to protein products that are overexpressed, overactive, deregulated, or mislocalized. Oncogene activation occurs more frequently at the progression stage of carcinogenesis than as an initiating event. The activation of a single oncogene is not typically sufficient to cause malignant transformation.

Oncogene activation more typically occurs at the somatic level than in the germline. In fact, there are very few examples of oncogenes that are activated in the germline (and are thus the basis of specific hereditary cancer syndromes). Examples include the *CDK4*, *KIT*, *MET*, and *RET* oncogenes (also see Table 3.3).

At the somatic level, there are several different mechanisms that can lead to oncogene activation, although some appear to be tumor specific. Oncogene activation can occur from the following, as presented in the succeeding sections.

3.3.2.1. Mutations

A simple error in cell replication can result in a hyperfunctional oncogene. These "gain-of-function" point mutations are the most common method of oncogene activation. For instance, the *RAS* oncogene in bladder carcinoma has been found to differ from its normal precursor by a single base pair change, which results in a single amino acid substitution. Splice mutations, which occur at the exon–intron junctions, can also result in altered or inefficient oncogene protein products.

3.3.2.2. Translocations and Inversions

Translocations and inversions can both result in oncogene activation by destroying or inactivating genes at the site of the chromosomal breaks. These types of chromosomal rearrangements appear to be a common cause of

TABLE 3.3. ONCOGENES ASSOCIATED WITH HEREDITARY CANCER SYNDROMES

Name	Gene Type	Syndrome
CDK4	Cell cycle regulator	Melanoma, cutaneous malignant
KIT	Tyrosine kinase	Gastrointestinal stromal tumors, familial
MET	Tyrosine kinase	Papillary renal cell carcinoma, familial
RET	Tyrosine kinase	Multiple Endocrine Neoplasia, type 2

Source: Lindor et al. (2008).

hematologic malignancies. For example, the *ABL* oncogene, located in chromosome 9, becomes activated when fused to the middle of a gene on chromosome 22 called *BCR* (named for *Breakpoint Cluster Region*). This rearrangement, known as the Philadelphia chromosome, makes a hybrid protein with growth-promoting properties, which predisposes cells to becoming leukemic. The Philadelphia chromosome is present in about 90% of chronic myelogenous leukemias. Translocations and inversions can be caused by exposures to certain carcinogens, such as radioactive iodine.

3.3.2.3. Insertions and Deletions

Frameshift mutations, such as insertions and deletions, can activate oncogenes by disrupting the normal coding region of the gene. This disruption can result in altering the gene's function and eventually destabilizing the gene.

3.3.2.4. Gene Amplification

Errors in replication or reproduction can also result in multiple copies of an oncogene. The presence of multiple oncogenes within a cell confers clonal advantage to the cell. Overexpression due to gene amplification is a common feature of many types of cancer. Neuroblastoma, for example, typically contains multiple copies of the *N-MYC* oncogene.

3.3.2.5. Aneuploidy and Polyploidy

The genome of a tumor often includes additional or missing copies of entire chromosomes, which will lead to a surplus or drought of multiple protein products. If the chromosome happens to contain a proto-oncogene, it will be affected accordingly.

3.3.2.6. Viral Insertion

Oncogenes were first discovered within viruses. In fact, all human oncogenes are thought to have viral counterparts. Because of the genetic similarities, viruses can insert themselves into the machinery of a human proto-oncogene and convert it into a viral oncogene. This has been reported to occur with DNA tumor viruses, such as Epstein–Barr virus and human papillomavirus and also retroviruses, such as HIV. Viral exposures have been implicated in about 5% of human cancers.

3.3.3. THE *RET* ONCOGENE

The underlying cause of Multiple Endocrine Neoplasia (MEN), types 2A and 2B, is a germline mutation in the *RET* oncogene. The mutated *RET* oncogene is dominantly inherited and individuals with MEN2A or 2B have increased risks for developing medullary thyroid carcinoma (MTC) and other endocrine tumors. (See Section 4.20 for features of MEN2A and MEN2B.) The *RET* proto-oncogene is one of the receptor genes in the signaling pathway. Specifically, it is a tyrosine kinase gene that encodes a receptor for GDNF (glial cell-derived neurotrophic factor).

The *RET* gene lies on chromosome 10q11.2 and is one of the few cancer susceptibility genes in which there appears to be clear genotype–phenotype correlation. As shown in Figure 3.8, specific *RET* mutations cause MEN2A or 2B, while other mutations lead to familial MTC or Hirschsprung's disease.

3.4. TUMOR SUPPRESSOR GENES

The majority of dominant hereditary cancer syndromes are due to a germline mutation in a tumor suppressor gene. This section describes tumor suppressor genes and their role in cancer development and ends with descriptions of the *TP53* gene and mismatch repair genes.

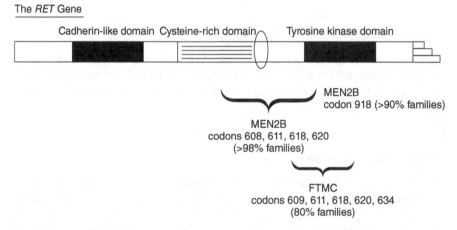

FIGURE 3.8. The phenotype–genotype correlations of germline *RET* mutations. As shown in this diagram, mutations in specific codons of the *RET* gene predict the resulting disease pattern. FMTC = familial medullary thyroid carcinoma. Reprinted from *Journal of Medical Genetics*, J.R. Hansford and L.M. Mulligan, vol. 37, p. 818, copyright 2000, with permission from BMJ Publishing Group Ltd.

3.4.1. GENERAL DESCRIPTION OF TUMOR SUPPRESSOR GENES

The overall purpose of tumor suppressor genes is to negatively regulate the growth of cells. Tumor suppressor genes encode proteins along a variety of signaling pathways that modulate cell growth, differentiation, and death (apoptosis). Over 30 tumor suppressor genes have now been characterized or cloned.

In contrast to oncogenes, it is the inactivation or loss of tumor suppressor genes that leads to cancer development. The presence of a single functional tumor suppressor gene appears sufficient to suppress unchecked growth. However, the loss of both alleles can result in deregulated growth and potential malignancy. Thus, tumor suppressor genes can be said to behave in both a dominant and recessive manner; dominant in terms of its inheritance pattern (genotype) and recessive at the cellular level (phenotype).

3.4.2. GATEKEEPERS, CARETAKERS, AND LANDSCAPERS

According to Drs. Vogelstein and Kinzler, there are three major categories of tumor suppressor genes:

- *Gatekeepers*—Gatekeeper genes are directly involved in some aspect of cell growth. Gatekeeper genes negatively regulate the cell's progression through the normal cycle of growth, differentiation, and apoptosis. In other words, these genes determine whether or when cells proceed through the cell cycle. In normal cells, gatekeeper genes counteract cellular growth and promote cellular death, which creates a counterbalance to proto-oncogenes, which encourage cellular growth. The inactivation of gatekeeper genes allows tumor cells to circumvent the normal cellular "checks and balances," which can lead to unrestricted growth, dedifferentiation, and immortality. Certain tumors can arise only if they dismantle specific gatekeeper genes. Examples of gatekeeper genes include the *APC*, *PTEN*, and *VHL* genes.

- *Caretakers*—Caretaker genes maintain the overall genomic stability of the cell. A mutation in a caretaker gene can increase the rate of mutated cells, which in turn can lead to activated oncogenes and inactivated gatekeeper tumor suppressor genes. In essence, caretaker genes protect the function of the gatekeeper genes. Caretaker genes affect the biology of the cell only indirectly by controlling the rate at which cells accumulate mutated genes. Caretaker genes are also termed genome maintenance genes because they are responsible for maintaining normal stasis of the cell. Examples of caretaker genes include the *MLH1* and *MSH2* genes.

TABLE 3.4. TUMOR SUPPRESSOR GENES ASSOCIATED WITH HEREDITARY CANCER SYNDROMES

Name	Type of Gene	Associated Syndrome
APC	Gatekeeper	Familial Adenomatous Polyposis
*BRCA1**	Caretaker	Hereditary Breast–Ovarian Cancer syndrome
*BRCA2**	Caretaker	Hereditary Breast–Ovarian Cancer syndrome
CDKN2A	Gatekeeper	Melanoma, cutaneous malignant
MLH1	Caretaker	Lynch syndrome
MSH2	Caretaker	Lynch syndrome
PTCH	Gatekeeper	Gorlin syndrome
PTEN	Gatekeeper	PTEN Hamartoma syndrome
*TP53**	Caretaker	Li–Fraumeni syndrome
VHL	Gatekeeper	von Hippel–Lindau syndrome

Source: Schultz (2005c); Oster et al. (2005).

*Also has some gatekeeper functions.

- *Landscapers*—Landscaper genes are ones that create cellular environments that are primed for the development of cancer. In other words, mutations in these types of genes foster environments that are conducive to unregulated cell growth. Examples include disruptions to the cell-to-cell or cell-to-extracellular matrices. Defects in landscaper genes do not appear to be the underlying causes of hereditary cancer syndromes, although they are likely to contribute to the development of both sporadic and hereditary cancers.

Table 3.4 lists examples of gatekeeper and caretaker genes that are associated with specific hereditary cancer syndromes. Note that a few of the tumor suppressor genes, notably *TP53*, *BRCA1*, and *BRCA2*, have both gatekeeper and caretaker characteristics.

3.4.3. TUMOR SUPPRESSOR GENE INACTIVATION

The inactivation of the initial tumor suppressor allele can occur at either the germline or somatic level. Inactivation of the second tumor suppressor allele always occurs at the somatic level. As described below, there are six major ways for the second allele to become inactivated.

3.4.3.1. Point Mutation or Deletion

A simple error in cell replication can cripple the tumor suppressor gene. These genetic errors are either simple substitutions (missense mutations) that impair the gene or frame-shift deletions that are always deleterious.

3.4.3.2. Chromosome Rearrangement

Translocations or insertions can also result in the inactivation of a tumor suppressor allele.

3.4.3.3. Mitotic Nondisjunction

Mitotic nondisjunction causes the loss of the entire chromosome containing the normal tumor suppressor gene. During mitosis, nondisjunction occurs, resulting in one daughter cell with three copies of a chromosome and one daughter cell with a single abnormal copy. The daughter cell, lacking a functional tumor suppressor gene, will divide further, leading to a small colony of abnormal cells.

3.4.3.4. Mitotic Recombination

Mitotic recombination leads to the loss of the normal tumor suppressor gene. Recombination between the maternal and paternal alleles, followed by mitosis, will lead to one daughter cell with both maternal alleles and one daughter cell with both paternal alleles. One cell, therefore, may have two abnormal tumor suppressor genes.

3.4.3.5. Gene Amplification

The overexpression of certain proteins can result in the inactivation of a tumor suppressor protein. For example, overexpression of certain proteins (such as mdm-2) can lead to the binding and subsequent inactivation of TP53 protein products.

3.4.3.6. Epigenetic Silencing

A tumor suppressor gene may be structurally sound, but may be silenced due to a problem with imprinting or methylation. This is typically due to abnormal DNA methylation (also see Section 3.5.2).

3.4.4. THE *TP53* TUMOR SUPPRESSOR GENE

The *TP53* gene has been termed "the guardian of the genome," because it controls the cell cycle, initiates apoptosis, and maintains the integrity of the genome. (See Fig. 3.9.) The *TP53* gene monitors the accumulation of DNA damage and mediates F1 cell cycle arrest so that DNA repair can be initiated. If the damaged cell is beyond repair, *TP53* will induce apoptosis. Dismantling the *TP53* regulatory system allows malignant cells to attain immortality. The loss of normal *TP53* protein also appears to lead to overall

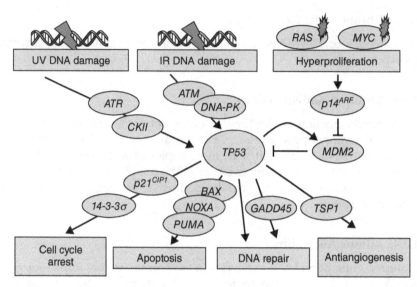

FIGURE 3.9. A sketch of the *TP53* network. Only a central part of the network is shown. Source: Schulz (2005c, p. 103). UV = ultraviolet; IR = infrared.

genomic instability. Over 50% of all tumors contain damaged or absent *TP53* genes—by far the most common genetic error that occurs in neoplasms. (As an aside, note that gene names are italicized; protein names are not.)

The *TP53* gene lies on chromosome 17p13 and its product is a 53-kd protein that binds in the nucleus. Normal cells express low levels of TP53 protein, while higher levels are present in damaged cells. When mutated, the *TP53* gene can act like a growth-promoting oncogene, thus conferring a clear advantage to the cell.

The *TP53* gene is a key regulatory factor, which initiates apoptosis in response to cellular stress and homeostatic needs of the cell. The lack of normal TP53 protein compromises the ability of a cell to react to cellular threats such as ultraviolet radiation, viral infection, or genomic damage.

3.4.5. MISMATCH REPAIR GENES

The major function of DNA repair genes is to identify and fix DNA nucleotide errors made during replication. This process has been compared to the spell-checker function on a computer. As illustrated in Figure 3.10, successful DNA repair requires multiple steps, including:

- Recognition of the sequence error
- Recruitment of the appropriate proteins

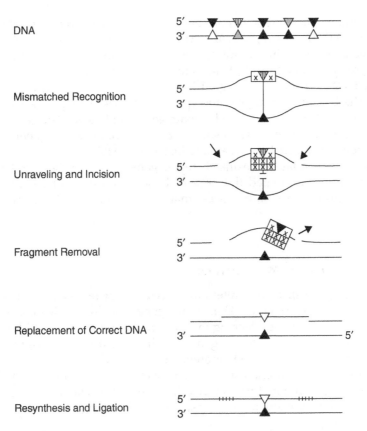

DNA

Mismatched Recognition

Unraveling and Incision

Fragment Removal

Replacement of Correct DNA

Resynthesis and Ligation

FIGURE 3.10. The DNA repair system. This illustration depicts the five major steps involved in DNA repair. (Also see the text.) Source: Squire, J, Whitmore, G, and Phillips, R. 1998. Genetic basis of cancer. In Tannock, I, and Hill, R. (eds), The Basic Science of Oncology. McGraw-Hill, New York, p. 66. Reproduced with permission from McGraw-Hill.

- Incision of the DNA and excision of the mistaken nucleotide(s)
- Resynthesis of the correct nucleotide(s)
- Reattachment of the DNA strand

Inactivation of any of the genes involved in the repair process will make the system less efficient, leading to the accumulation of DNA errors within a cell. Over time, this can result in the formation of a tumor. Therefore, DNA repair genes are in the family of caretaker genes. Examples of hereditary cancer syndromes associated with DNA repair genes include Fanconi Anemia, Lynch syndrome, and Xeroderma Pigmentosum.

Several mismatch repair genes have been implicated in Lynch syndrome including *MLH1*, *MSH2*, *MSH6*, *PMS1*, *PMS2*, and *TACSTD1*. Mismatch repair genes have the important function of correcting DNA errors that occur during replication. At multiple sites in the genome, there are sequences of repeated DNA nucleotides (e.g., TTTT or CACACA) called microsatellite DNA. These sequences appear susceptible to errors during DNA transcription. Cells with faulty mismatch repair genes will cause "stutters" in the microsatellite DNA and can result in greatly lengthened sequences. This phenomenon is termed microsatellite instability (MSI). The presence of MSI is suggestive of a faulty mismatch repair gene, although the correlation is not perfect. It is estimated that 90% of Lynch syndrome-related colorectal tumors demonstrate MSI, while less than 10% of sporadic colorectal tumors do so.

3.5. EPIGENETIC MECHANISMS

Epigenetic "gene silencing" refers to processes that render genes nonfunctional without disturbing the DNA of the gene. Therefore, if it were possible to repair or lift the gene silencing mechanism, then the gene would be functional. When tumor suppressor genes are the ones that are inappropriately silenced, then this can cause heightened cancer risks.

The two major mechanisms of gene silencing are genomic imprinting and methylation. It may turn out that these genetic mechanisms account for more hereditary cancers than intrinsic defects in oncogenes or tumor suppressor genes.

3.5.1. GENOMIC IMPRINTING

As demonstrated by genomic imprinting, the maternal and paternal copies of each gene and chromosome are required for normal development. In addition to having the full complement of 46 chromosomes, it is important to have an equal balance of maternal and paternal alleles. Thus, contrary to Mendel's theory, maternal and paternal alleles are not always equivalent, and two copies of an allele, without attention to parental origin, are not sufficient to assume normal function. An extreme example of this can be observed when an embryo is erroneously formed with two sets of paternally derived chromosomes or two sets of maternally derived chromosomes. A paternal-only genome results in the formation of a hydatidiform mole and a maternal-only genome forms a complete ovarian teratoma. Thus, an imbalance of maternal and paternal alleles has the potential of causing a neoplasm.

Genomic imprinting is an epigenetic modification of a specific parental allele of a gene or chromosome that leads to differential expression of the two alleles in the offspring's cells. In other words, this process silences one copy of each allele and, in many cases, the inactivation of an allele is not random but rather based on the allele's parent of origin and the specific needs of the tissue. The most important imprinting event occurs during embryogenesis when the allelic expression of different tissue types is "locked into place" by use of imprint organizing centers. Genomic imprinting is then maintained, at least in part, through a process termed methylation. Thus, normal genomic imprinting is a continuous, developmental process, not a single event.

The presence of two alleles derived from the same parent is termed uniparental disomy (UPD) and results in abnormal imprinting due to the excess of one allele and absence of the other. In paternal UPD, for example, the maternal alleles are lost (silenced) and the paternal alleles, which are duplicated, will be amplified. The majority of hereditary paragangliomas in the Netherlands are associated with paternal UPD involving the *SDHD* gene. Paternal UPD is also associated with some cases of Wilms' tumor, rhabdomyosarcoma, and osteosarcoma. Maternal UPD has been reported in cases of neuroblastoma and acute myelogenous leukemia.

Beckwith–Wiedemann syndrome (BWS) is a classic example of a genetic condition that can be caused by abnormal genomic imprinting. BWS is an overgrowth syndrome that is associated with increased risks of embryonic tumors. Various genomic imprinting errors can result in the BWS phenotype, including:

- Switched imprinting (the maternal allele is erroneously silenced, the paternal allele is erroneously activated)
- A rearrangement in the maternal allele, which disrupts the function of the normally activated genes
- Paternal UPD, which causes the overexpression of the paternal allele and loss of the maternal allele

3.5.2. DNA METHYLATION

The process of methylation effectively silences an allele of a gene or chromosome. DNA methylation is a carefully programmed process based on the potential of DNA methyl groups to act as a "fifth base pair." This fifth base pair can be formed and maintained at any cytosine–guanine (CpG) dinucleotide, effectively blocking or silencing the gene. DNA methylation generally occurs in the CpG islands of the genes. CpG islands are regions that have a high number and concentration of CpG dinucleotides. CpG islands are frequently present in the promoter region or first exon of the so-called housekeeping genes (including growth regulatory genes). It is estimated that 80% of CpG islands within genes are methylated.

During a person's lifetime, methylation can only be removed during the replication process or by enzymatic action. For example, overexpression of the enzyme methyltransferase can "flag" a gene for silencing. The methylation status of a particular gene is generally permanent and is somatically inherited. However, the pattern of methylated genes is reversed in many tumors.

Abnormal methylation can result in switching allele activation from the maternal to the paternal allele or vice versa, or can lead to the activation or silencing of both alleles. This process can lead to neoplastic growth if it has activated normally quiescent copies of growth-promoting genes or has silenced normally functional copies of tumor suppressor genes. For example, in Wilms' tumor, the maternal allele can be abnormally silenced (which results in the loss of two tumor suppressor genes, *H19* and *CDKN1C*) and/ or the paternal allele can be activated (which retains the advantageous growth factor, IGF2).

Specific tumors that have demonstrated abnormal methylation include colorectal cancers, Wilms' tumor, neuroblastoma, rhabdomyosarcoma, osteosarcoma, hepatoblastoma, and acute myelogenous leukemia. Colorectal tumors with MSI may have germline *MLH1* mutations if familial and promoter hypermethylation, and loss of expression of MLH1 protein if sporadic due to hypermethylation. Other genes that are sensitive to methylation include *RB1, VHL, TP16,* and possibly *BRCA1*.

The contribution of imprinting or methylation in the development of cancer is still poorly understood. Future research may demonstrate that epigenetic mechanisms play an important role in both heritable and non-heritable malignancies.

3.5.3. OTHER GENE-SILENCING MECHANISMS

Other mechanisms that can lead to inappropriate gene silencing are presented in the succeeding sections.

3.5.3.1. A Defect in the Imprint Organizing Center

Abnormal imprinting can result from a deletion or mutation in any of the genes that comprise one of the imprint organizing centers. This type of defect can cause a failure of the initial "locking in" regarding which parental-origin alleles are to be silenced.

3.5.3.2. Separation of the Imprint Organizing Center from Target Genes

In chromosome rearrangements, such as translocations, a gene might become separated from its imprint organizing center. This could lead to abnormal gene expression patterns.

3.5.3.3. The Loss of *Trans*-Acting Factors

Little is known about *trans*-acting factors except that they appear to play an important role in maintaining normal patterns of gene expression. Mutations in or loss of these *trans*-acting factors could result in relaxed or abnormal imprinting or methylation.

3.6. FURTHER READING

Bishop, JM. 2003. Opening the black box of cancer. In How to Win the Nobel Prize (An Unexpected Life in Science). Harvard University Press, Cambridge, MA, 133–180.

Fearon, ER. 1998. Tumor suppressor genes. In Vogelstein, B and Kinzler, KW (eds) The Genetic Basis of Cancer. McGraw-Hill, New York, 229–240.

Hanahan, D, and Weinberg, RA. 2000. The Hallmarks of Cancer. Cell 100:57–70.

Hanahan, D, and Weinberg, RA. 2011. Hallmarks of Cancer: The next generation. Cell 144:646–674.

Hansford, J, and Mulligan, L. 2000. Multiple endocrine neoplasia type 2 and RET: from neoplasia to neurogenesis. J Med Genet 37:818.

Kinzler, KW, and Vogelstein, B. 1997. Gatekeepers and caretakers. Nature 386:761–762.

Kinzler, K, and Vogelstein, B. 1998. Landscaping the cancer terrain. Science 280:1036–1037.

Lindor, NM, McMaster, ML, Lindor, CJ, et al. 2008. Concise handbook of familial cancer susceptibility syndromes—second edition. J Natl Cancer Inst Monogr 38:1–93.

McKinnell, RG. 2006. Invasion and metastasis. In McKinnell, RG, Parchment, RE, Perantoni, AO, Damjanov, I, and Pierce, GB (eds) The Biological Basis of Cancer, 2nd edition. Cambridge University Press, New York, 51–79.

Offit, K. 1998. Cancer as a genetic disorder. In Clinical Cancer Genetics. Wiley & Sons, New York, 39–65.

Oster, S, Penn, L, and Stambolis, V. 2005. Oncogenes and tumor supressor genes. In Tannock, IF, Hill, RP, Bristow, RG, and Harrington, L (eds), The Basic Science of Oncology, 4th edition. McGraw Hill, New York, 123–141.

Perantoni, AO. 2006. Cancer associated genes. In McKinnell, RG, Parchment, RE, Perantoni, AO, Damjanov, I, and Pierce, GB (eds), The Biological Basis of Cancer, 2nd edition. Cambridge University Press, New York, 145–194.

Schulz, WA. 2005a. An introduction to human cancers. In Molecular Biology of Human Cancer. Springer, Dordrecht, The Netherlands, 1–23.

Schulz, WA. 2005b. Cancer epigenetics. In Molecular Biology of Human Cancer. Springer. Springer, Dordrecht, The Netherlands, 167–191.

Schulz, WA. 2005c. Tumor suppressor genes. In Molecular Biology of Human Cancer. Springer, Dordrecht, The Netherlands, 91–111.

Weinburg, RA. 2007a. Cellular oncogenes. In The Biology of Cancer. Garland Science, New York, 91–118.

Weinburg, RA. 2007b. Tumor suppressor genes. In The Biology of Cancer. Garland Science, New York, 209–254.

Hereditary Cancer Syndromes

The ramifications of having one of these [inherited cancer] diseases are significant for both the patient and their family, with a high risk of developing a malignancy in many organs at an early age. Clinicians should be prepared to recognize and manage these diseases. This is not as simple as it sounds.

(C. Neal Ellis, Jr. 2004, p. v)

This chapter describes 36 hereditary syndromes in which cancer is a prominent feature. The syndromes are listed in alphabetical order and the references used to compile the disease entries are listed at the end of the chapter. Please refer to Appendix A for a list of syndromes classified by organ system.

4.1. Ataxia Telangiectasia

Frequency:	From 1 in 30,000 to 1 in 100,000 live births
	The frequency of heterozygote carriers is 0.2–1.0%
Inheritance:	Autosomal recessive
Genes:	*ATM* at 11q22.3
Gene test:	Clinically available

4.1.1. Cancer Risks of Ataxia Telangiectasia

Individuals with Ataxia telangiectasia (A-T) have 30–40% lifetime risks of cancer. Mortality from cancer is estimated at 15%. The most common malignancies are non-Hodgkin lymphoma (typically B cell) and leukemia (acute or chronic forms). Lymphomas and leukemias account for over 80% of the A-T-associated cancer diagnoses.

Other associated tumors are medulloblastomas, gliomas, gastric cancer, uterine cancer, basal cell carcinomas (BCCs), and possibly ovarian dysgerminomas. Female A-T mutation carriers appear to have increased risks of breast cancer. Radiation treatments are contraindicated given the frequency of chromosomal breakage in radiation exposed cells.

4.1.2. Diagnostic Criteria

Diagnosis of A-T is typically based on the presence of early-onset ataxia, oculocutaneous telangiectases, oculomotor apraxia, and immunodeficiency. Diagnostic tests include the alpha-fetoprotein test (95% have elevated levels), immunoblotting for ATM protein (90% have no detectable levels), karotype (15% have 7; 14 chromosome translocation), and radiosensitive DNA synthesis. Radiosensitive DNA synthesis analyzes the frequency of spontaneous chromosomal aberrations, particularly at T-cell and B-cell receptor sites. Such breakpoints may be seen in 10% of mitoses in individuals with A-T, making it a reliable test for the diagnosis of A-T. However, it is a less reliable screen for detecting heterozygous carriers. DNA sequencing of the *ATM* gene has a 95% success rate in detecting the specific mutation(s) in the family.

4.1.3. Clinical Features

A young child with A-T walks with an unsteady, lurching gait; a hallmark of the syndrome. Cerebellar ataxia, which occurs in early childhood, is present in 100% of cases and choreoathetosis and dystona are present in 90%. Most individuals with A-T are wheelchair bound by adolescence and many develop degenerate spinal muscular atrophy as they reach adulthood. Other features include slurred speech, disturbed eye movements (oculomotor apraxia), vision problems, endocrine dysfunction, immunodeficiency, vitiligo, café au lait spots, premature aging and graying of the hair, and telangiectasia. Telangiectases, which are red marks caused by the abnormal dilation of capillaries, typically develop by age 5 in skin exposed to the sun. Mental retardation and dementia are not typical features of A-T. Although affected individuals often live into their thirties, they rarely live past age 45. Infection is the number one cause of death for individuals with A-T.

4.1.4. SYNDROME SUBTYPES

- *A-T heterozygotes*—Female A-T heterozygote carriers appear to have a greater than twofold increased relative risk of breast cancer over women in the general population. A-T heterozygotes (men and women) may also be at increased risk for radiation-induced DNA damage, as well as leukemia, stomach cancer, and colon cancer.

4.1.5. RESOURCES FOR FAMILIES

- A-T Children's Project: http://www.atcp.org
- A-T Ease Foundation: http://www.ateasefoundation.org

4.2. AUTOIMMUNE LYMPHOPROLIFERATIVE SYNDROME (ALSO CANALE–SMITH SYNDROME)

Incidence:	Rare
Inheritance:	Autosomal dominant (AD)
Genes:	ALPS 0: *FAS* (TNFRSF6) at 10q24.1 (inheritance of two damaged *FAS* alleles)
	ALPS IA: *FAS* (TNFRSF6) at 10q24.1
	ALPS IB: *FASL* (FASLG, TNFSF6) at 1q23
	ALPS IIA: *CASP10* at 2q33-q34
	ALPS IIB: *CASP8* at 2q33-q34
	ALPS III: clinical features of ALPS but no detectable gene mutation
Gene test:	*FAS* and *CASP10* genes—clinically available
	FASL and *CASP8* genes—available on a research basis only

4.2.1. CANCER RISKS

Individuals with autoimmune lymphoproliferative syndrome (ALPS) have greatly increased risks of lymphoma. Straus et al. (2001) reported that, the risk of Hodgkin lymphoma was 51 times greater and the risks of non-Hodgkin T-cell and B-cell lymphomas were 14 times greater than for the general population. The average onset of cancer was 28 years. Other cancers in ALPS include carcinomas of the breast, liver, skin, thyroid, and tongue. Gliomas and adenomas of the breast and thyroid are also seen.

4.2.2. DIAGNOSTIC CRITERIA

The cardinal features of ALPS are autoimmune hemolytic anemia, thrombocytopenia, hypergammaglobulinemia, splenomegaly, and lymphadenopathy. Onset of symptoms almost always occurs during childhood. All individuals with ALPS contain an increased number of alpha/beta double-negative T cells in their white blood cells.

4.2.3. Clinical Features

Most individuals with ALPS have type IA. The average age of onset of symptoms is 5 years. Children with ALPS IA often present with markedly enlarged lymph nodes and spleen and may be aggressively worked up for cancer. The lymphadenopathy and splenomegaly are caused by the hemolytic anemia and thrombocytopenia. Affected individuals have an increased number of DNT (double-negative T cell) lymphocytes, which can lead to an abnormally heightened immune system response. This hyperimmune response can also trigger other autoimmune disorders, such as Guillain–Barre syndrome, lupus, arthritis, and panniculitis. However, there is great variability in the extent of clinical problems found in people with ALPS.

4.2.4. Syndrome Subtypes

- *ALPS IB, ALPS IIA, ALPS IIB, and ALPS III*—Individuals with these ALPS subtypes are thought to have clinical features similar to individuals with ALPS IA, although this has yet to be confirmed.
- *ALPS 0*—Children with ALPS, type 0 have inherited two damaged alleles of the *FAS* gene. The children are usually homozygous for a single mutation but can also be double heterozygotes. Children with ALPS 0 present at birth or shortly afterwards with severe lymphoproliferation and significant autoimmune disease and usually die in early childhood.

4.2.5. Resources for Families

- Learning about Autoimmune Lymphoproliferative syndrome: http://www.genome.gov/10001585
- Genetics Home Reference, ALPS: http://ghr.nlm.nih.gov/condition/autoimmune-lymphoproliferative-syndrome

4.3. Beckwith–Wiedemann Syndrome (Also Exomphalos Macroglossia Gigantism [EMG] Syndrome)

Frequency: 1 in 13,700
Inheritance: AD, though 85% of cases are sporadic
Genes: Imprinting errors of the Beckwith–Wiedemann syndrome (BWS) region at 11p15 includes the *IGF2*, *H19*, *CDKN1C*, *KVLQT1*, and *LIT1* genes
Gene test: Clinically available

4.3.1. CANCER RISKS

Children with BWS are estimated to have an 8% risk of malignancy. Malignancies associated with BWS typically occur by age 5 and tend to be tumors of embryonal origin. The most common malignancy is Wilms' tumor (WT), which accounts for 60% of cancers in children with BWS. Additional tumors seen in children with BWS include adrenocortical carcinoma, gonadoblastoma, hepatoblastoma, neuroblastoma (NB), and rhabdomyosarcoma. Children with mutations or imprinting errors involving the *IGF2* and *H19* genes seem to have higher cancer risks than children with other genetic errors.

Individuals with BWS may also develop various benign tumors, including hamartomas, myxomas, ganglioneuromas, adenomas, and breast fibroadenomas. Pituitary and pancreatic islet cell hyperplasia also occur.

4.3.2. DIAGNOSTIC CRITERIA

Children are diagnosed with BWS if they meet at least three (two major and one minor) criteria.

Shuman et al. (2005) list the following clinical criteria for BWS:

Major criteria of BWS:

- Positive family history
- Macrosomia (height and weight >97th percentile)
- Anterior linear earlobe creases/posterior helical ear pits
- Macrogloassia
- Omphalocele/umbilical hernia
- Visceromegaly involving one or more abdominal organs including liver, spleen, kidneys, adrenal glands, and pancreas
- Embryonal tumor (e.g., WT, hepatoblastoma, NB, rhabdomyosarcoma) in childhood
- Hemihyperplasia (asymmetric overgrowth of one or more regions of the body)
- Adrenocortical cytomegaly
- Renal abnormalities, including structural abnormalities, nephromegaly, and nephrocalcinosis
- Cleft palate (rare)

Minor criteria of BWS:

- Polyhydramnios
- Prematurity

- Neonatal hypoglycemia
- Facial nevus flammeus
- Hemangioma
- Characteristic facial features including midfacial hypoplasia and infraorbital creases
- Cardiomegaly, structural cardiac anomalies, cardiomyopathy (rare)
- Diastasis recti (abdominal separation)
- Advanced bone age
- Monozygotic twinning

4.3.3. CLINICAL FEATURES

BWS is an example of an overgrowth syndrome. It is characterized by exomphalos (umbilical hernia), macroglossia, gigantism, and adrenocortical cytomegaly. Renal anomalies and abdominal wall defects also occur. Affected individuals range from normal intelligence to moderate mental retardation and exhibit compulsive overeating as they become older. In terms of causes of BWS, there is a possible association with assisted reproductive technologies (ART) such as *in vitro* fertilization (IVF).

4.3.4. SYNDROME SUBTYPES

None.

4.3.5. RESOURCES FOR FAMILIES

- Beckwith-Wiedemann Children's Foundation: http://www.beckwith-wiedemannsyndrome.org
- Beckwith-Wiedemann Family Forum: http://www.beckwith-wiedemann.info

4.4. BIRT–HOGG–DUBÉ SYNDROME

Frequency: Rare
Inheritance: AD
Genes: *FLCN* at 17p11.2
Gene test: Clinically available

4.4.1. CANCER RISKS

Individuals with Birt–Hogg–Dubé syndrome (BHDS) have a sevenfold increased risk of developing kidney cancer compared to the general population. The average age of developing kidney cancer among people with BHDS is 48 years, and the renal tumors seem more likely to be bilateral, multifocal, and slow growing. The types of kidney tumors seen in people with BHDS include oncocytomas, oncocytic hybrid tumors, and renal cell carcinomas of the chromophobe, clear cell, and papillary sub-types. Other benign lesions associated with BHDS include perifollicular fibromas, fibrofolliculomas, trichodiscomas, acrochordons, and possibly lipomas, collagenomas, and colon polyps.

4.4.2. DIAGNOSTIC CRITERIA

The best strategy for diagnosing BHDS is to perform *FLCN* genetic testing. It is estimated that 85–90% of affected individuals will be found to have a detectable mutation via full gene sequencing. According to Dr. Jorge Toro (2008), individuals should undergo *FLCN* genetic analysis if they exhibit at least one of the following features:

- Five or more facial or truncal papules with at least one histologically confirmed fibrofolliculoma with or without a family history of BHDS.
- Facial papules histologically confirmed to be angiofibroma in an individual who does not fit the clinical criteria of tuberous sclerosis complex (TSC) or multiple endocrine neoplasia, type 1 (MEN1).
- Multiple and bilateral chromophobe, oncocytic, and/or hybrid renal tumors.
- A single oncocytic, chromophobe, or oncocytic hybrid renal tumor and a family history of renal cancer with any of the above renal cell tumor types.
- A family history of AD primary spontaneous pneumothorax without a history of smoking or chronic obstructive pulmonary disease (COPD).

4.4.3. CLINICAL FEATURES

The major triad of features in BHDS includes skin manifestations, pul-monary cysts and spontaneous pneumothorax, and renal tumors. The skin lesions include multiple benign lesions of the hair follicles (e.g., perifollicular fibromas, fibrofolliculomas, trichodiscomas) and acrochor-dons (skin tags), which typically develop between ages 30 and 50. Nearly all affected individuals will have at least one manifestation of BHDS, although the severity of lung and kidney problems is quite variable even within the same family. Individuals with BHDS are recommended to avoid cigarette smoking and high ambient pressures (which can trigger a pneumothorax).

4.4.4. SYNDROME SUBTYPES

None.

4.4.5. RESOURCES FOR FAMILIES

- Birt Hogg Dubé syndrome (Myrovytis Trust & BHD Family Alliance): http://www.bhdsyndrome.org

4.5. BLOOM SYNDROME

Frequency: Rare in the general population
                Frequency of heterozygotes among people of Ashkenazi Jewish ancestry is 1%
Inheritance: Autosomal recessive
Genes: *BLM* at 15q26.1
Gene test: Clinically available for the BLMAsh founder mutation in people of Ashkenazi Jewish descent. Research testing is available for other *BLM* mutations

4.5.1. CANCER RISKS

Cancer rates are greatly increased among individuals with Bloom syndrome (BS) and it is one of the most common causes of death for individuals with this syndrome. Children with BS have increased risks of lymphomas, acute leukemias, and WT. As children reach adolescence and early adulthood, the cancer risks expand to include malignancies of the breast, cervix, colon, esophagus, skin, larynx, lung, and stomach. Colon adenomas are also reported. Individuals with BS are at higher risks to develop multiple primaries and tend to develop cancer at earlier than typical ages. In the Bloom Syndrome Registry, the average age of cancer diagnosis was 25.9 years (range: 2–48 years) and the most common malignancy noted was colon cancer (Sanz and German, 2006). *BLM* mutation carriers may have higher risks of colon cancer.

4.5.2. DIAGNOSTIC CRITERIA

Diagnosis is based on the clinical features of growth deficiency with normal body proportion and sun-sensitive skin. Confirmatory laboratory testing involves looking at cultured peripheral blood lymphocytes for unusual chromosomal breakages and rearrangements as well as an increased rate of sister chromatid exchanges (SCE). Individuals with BS may have SCE rates that are 10-fold greater than the normal population.

A variety of *BLM* mutations and large deletions have been reported, including several founder mutations. Genetic testing for the founder mutation, BLMAsh, is often as part of a prenatal screening profile offered to couples of Ashkenazi Jewish ancestry. The BLMAsh founder mutation consists of a 6 bp del/7 bp ins frameshift mutation at nucleotide 2281.

4.5.3. CLINICAL FEATURES

BS is characterized by severe growth deficiency (but normal body proportion), sun-sensitive facial erythema/telangiectasia ("butterfly rash"), and characteristic facies that includes malar hypoplasia, nasal prominence, a small mandible, and dolichocephalic skull (Lindor et al., 2008). Affected individuals demonstrate hypersensitivity to sunlight and often have skin lesions or problems. Café-au-lait spots are also seen. They are highly susceptible to infection due to a severe immune defect with reduced gammaglobulin (IgA and IgM) levels and are at increased risks to develop diabetes, myelodysplasia, and chronic pulmonary disease. Survival past age 40 is rare. Females with BS have reduced fertility and males are sterile. Individuals with BS may have high-pitched voices and some form of learning disability.

4.5.4. SYNDROME SUBTYPES

None.

4.5.5. RESOURCES FOR FAMILIES

- Bloom's Syndrome Foundation: http://www.bloomssyndrome.org
- The Brandon Betts Blooms Syndrome support group (on Facebook): www.facebook.com

4.6. BLUE RUBBER BLEB NEVUS SYNDROME (ALSO TERMED BEAN SYNDROME)

Incidence:	Rare
Inheritance:	AD (although most cases are sporadic)
Genes:	Unknown; a few families have been localized to 9p
Gene test:	Not available

4.6.1. CANCER RISKS

Individuals with blue rubber bleb nevus syndrome (BRBNS) can develop multiple internal hemangiomas throughout the digestive tract. Hemangiomas can develop in other organs as well, including the eyes, pharynx, and uterus.

In early descriptions of BRBNS, childhood medulloblastoma was mentioned as a possible feature. However no additional cases of medullolastoma have been reported, which makes it questionable whether it is truly an associated feature of BRBNS.

4.6.2. Diagnostic Criteria

The diagnosis of BRBNS is based on the presence of the characteristic skin hemangiomas in combination with the internal hemangiomas, which are detected by imaging studies and endoscopy.

4.6.3. Clinical Features

All individuals with BRBNS seem to develop the characteristic raised skin lesions, which can be blue, green, or purple in color. Some people develop several of these vascular skin hemangiomas, while others develop hundreds of them. The shape and size of the hemangiomas vary greatly among affected individuals. The skin hemangiomas may be present at birth, but can continue to appear during childhood and adulthood.

Individuals with BRBNS also tend to develop internal hemangiomas. These internal hemangiomas can cause significant medical problems depending on their size and location. Complications associated with BRBNS include severe iron deficiency anemia, gastrointestinal (GI) bleeding, compromised breathing, and impaired vision.

4.6.4. Syndrome Subtypes

None.

4.6.5. Resources for Families

- Information about BRBNS from the National Organization of Rare Diseases: http://rarediseases.info.nih.gov/GARD/condition/5940/Blue_rubber_bleb_nevus.aspx
- Blue Rubber Bleb Nevus Support Group: http://www.experienceproject.com/groups/have-Blue-Rubber-Bleb-Nevus/89552

4.7. Breast–Ovarian Cancer Syndrome, Hereditary

Frequency:	1 in 800 in general population
	1 in 40 in people of Ashkenazi Jewish ancestry
Inheritance:	AD
Genes:	*BRCA1* at 17q21
	BRCA2 at 13q12.3
Gene test:	Clinically available

4.7.1. CANCER RISKS

Women with hereditary breast–ovarian cancer syndrome (HBOCS) have high lifetime risks of breast and ovarian cancer. A woman with a *BRCA1* mutation has an estimated 65% (51–75%) risk of invasive breast carcinomas and an estimated 39% (22–51%) risk of serous ovarian carcinomas. A woman with a *BRCA2* mutation has an estimated 45% (33–54%) risk of invasive breast carcinomas and an estimated 11% (4–18%) risk of serous ovarian carcinomas to age 70. Women with *BRCA1* mutations tend to develop breast cancer at younger ages than women with *BRCA2* mutations. The risk of contralateral breast cancer is also high for women with *BRCA1* or *BRCA2* mutations.

Women with *BRCA1* and *BRCA2* mutations are also at increased risk to develop ductal carcinoma *in situ* (DCIS), fallopian tube carcinoma, pancreatic cancer, and primary papillary serous carcinoma of the peritoneum. Although endometrial cancer is not a confirmed feature of HBOCS, it remains under review. Despite initial published data, the risk of colon cancer does not appear to be increased in families with *BRCA1* mutations. Lobular carcinoma *in situ* (LCIS) and mucinous or borderline ovarian tumors do not seem to be associated features of HBOCS.

Men with *BRCA1* and *BRCA2* mutations also have increased risks of cancer. The lifetime risk of breast cancer is about 1% for men with *BRCA1* mutations and between 6% and 7% for men with *BRCA2* mutations. Men with *BRCA1* and *BRCA2* mutations are also at increased risk to develop prostate cancer and pancreatic cancer.

Individuals with *BRCA2* mutations may also have small increased risks for developing cutaneous and ocular melanoma as well as gallbladder, bile duct, and stomach cancers.

4.7.2. DIAGNOSTIC CRITERIA

Individuals are identified as having HBOCS when they are found to have a deleterious mutation or large deletion in the *BRCA1* or *BRCA2* gene. *BRCA* mutations may account for about 2–5% of total breast cancer cases and 10–15% of ovarian cancer cases. The likelihood of finding a *BRCA* mutation increases if there are multiple cases of breast or ovarian cancer over at least two generations, early age of onset, bilateral disease, multiple primaries, male breast cancer, or Ashkenazi Jewish heritage. Three specific founder mutations have been identified in the Ashkenazi Jewish population, which are the 187delAG (also called 185delAG) and 5385insC (also called 5382insC) mutations in the *BRCA1* gene and the 6174delT mutation in the *BRCA2* gene. *BRCA1* and *BRCA2* mutations have been found in populations around the globe and founder mutations in other ethnic groups have been identified.

Individuals with personal or family histories that include pancreatic cancer or triple-negative medullary breast tumors also appear to have an increased likelihood of having a positive BRCA test result. If a mutation has not been identified in the family, testing should initially be offered to a family member who has had a BRCA-associated malignancy whenever possible.

4.7.3. CLINICAL FEATURES

HBOCS is characterized by the malignancies listed above. Families with HBOCS tend to exhibit patterns of cancer that include the following features: premenopausal breast cancer (under age 50); bilateral breast cancer; triple-negative hormone receptor breast cancer; male breast cancer; cancers of the ovary, pancreas, fallopian tube, and peritoneum; and multiple primaries (especially breast and ovarian cancer). (Also see Section 5.3.1 for additional information for HBOCS.)

4.7.4. SYNDROME SUBTYPES

- *BRCA1*—Women with *BRCA1* mutations have a higher risk of developing breast cancers that are premenopausal, triple hormone negative, and of the medullary subtype. *BRCA1*-related breast tumors tend to be fast growing and of high grade, making them difficult to treat. New clinical trials involving Poly (adenosine diphosphate [ADP]-ribose) Polymerase (PARP) inhibitors are encouraging in treating *BRCA1*-related tumors.
- *BRCA2*—There is no predominant breast cancer histology or subtype associated with *BRCA2* mutations. Women with mutations in the middle of the gene (DNA nucleotides 3035–6629) seem to have higher risks of ovarian cancer and lower risks of breast cancer than women with mutations at either end of the gene.
- *Double carrier of BRCA1 and BRCA2 mutations*—A small number of people carry both a *BRCA1* mutation and a *BRCA2* mutation. Interestingly, the risks of cancer in these individuals seem comparable to those with a single gene mutation. However, the risk of passing on the syndrome to offspring is 75% rather than 50%.
- *Biallelic BRCA1 mutations*—Inheriting homozygous or double heterozygous mutations in the *BRCA1* gene is thought to be incompatible with life and probably results in an early miscarriage.
- *Biallelic BRCA2 mutations*—Children who inherit homozygous or double heterozygous mutations in the *BRCA2* gene have Fanconi anemia (FA), type D_1, which is a chromosome breakage syndrome associated with severe anemia and hematologic malignancies. (See the section on FA for more detailed information.)

4.7.5. Resources for Families

- Facing Our Risks Empowered (FORCE): http://www.facingourrisk. org
- Previvors: Facing the breast cancer gene and making life-changing decisions. www.previvors.com

4.8. Carney Complex, Types I and II (Includes NAME Syndrome and LAMB Syndrome)

Frequency:	Rare
Inheritance:	AD
Genes:	Carney complex (CNC), type I: *PRKAR1A* at 17q22-q24
	CNC, type II: localized to 2p16
Gene test:	Clinically available

4.8.1. Cancer Risks

Individuals with CNC are at increased risk for developing multiple benign and malignant tumors. About 30% of males will develop testicular cancer, with most cases being either Leydig cell or large-cell calcifying Sertoli–Leydig cell tumors. Other associated malignancies include thyroid and pancreatic cancers and possibly also colorectal and ovarian cancers. Individuals with CNC typically develop an array of benign skin lesions including blue nevi, black–blue macules, café au lait spots, compound nevi, cutaneous myxomas, and lentigines. Spotty pigmentation is common. Over 70% of people with CNC develop cardiac myxomas. Other benign lesions associated with CNC include: breast adenomas and myxomas, myxoid uterine leiomyomas, osteo-chondromyxomas (of bone), pituitary adenomas, schwannomas, and thyroid adenomas.

4.8.2. Diagnostic Criteria

According to Lindor et al. (2008, p. 30), the diagnosis of CNC is based on the identification of at least two of the following features:

- Spotty skin pigmentation with a typical distribution (often vermillion border (erythema) of lips, conjunctiva and ocular canthi, vaginal or penile mucosa).
- Myxoma (cutaneous—often on the eyelid, external ear, nipple)
- Cardiac myxoma

- Breast myxomatosis or fat-suppressed magnetic resonance imaging (MRI) findings suggestive of this diagnosis

- Primary pigmented nodular adrenocortical disease (PPNAD) or paradoxical positive response of urinary glucocorticosteroids to dexamethasone administration during Liddle's diagnostic test for Cushing syndrome

- Acromegaly due to growth hormone (GH)-producing adenoma (somatotropinomas)

- Large-cell calcifying Sertoli cell tumor (LCCST) of testis or characteristic calcification on testicular ultrasonography

- Thyroid carcinoma or multiple hypoechoic nodules on thyroid ultrasonography in a young patient

- Psammomatous melanotic schwannoma

- Blue nevus, epithelioid blue nevus (multiple)

- Breast ductal adenoma (multiple) or mammary tumor with intraductal papilloma

- Osteochondromyxoma of bone (a histological diagnosis)

A person who meets only one of the above-listed criteria but has either a positive *PRKAR1A* gene test result or an affected first-degree relative also meets clinical criteria for CNC.

About half the families with CNC, type I have detectable mutations or deletions in the *PRKAR1A* gene. It is estimated that about 30% of children with CNC represent *de novo* cases.

4.8.3. CLINICAL FEATURES

CNC is the combination of two rare syndromes termed NAME syndrome and LAMB syndrome. The NAME syndrome acronym refers to nevi, atrial myxoma, myxoid neurofibromas, and ephelides (freckles) and the LAMB syndrome acronym refers to lentigines, atrial myxomas, mucocutaneous myxoma, and blue nevi syndrome.

The characteristic skin findings (listed above) may be present at birth, but tend to accumulate during adolescence. The average age of diagnosis of CNC is 20 years. The spotty pigmentation is often present on the face, eyelids, lips, glans penis, vulva, hands and feet, but does not typically involve the buccal mucosa (which is a hallmark feature of Peutz–Jeghers syndrome [PJS]). Individuals with CNC may have acromegaly (excess production of growth hormone).

Males with CNC appear to have an increased risk of infertility.

4.8.4. SYNDROME SUBTYPES

None.

4.8.5. RESOURCES FOR FAMILIES

- Information about CNC from the National Institutes of Health: http://rarediseases.info.nih.gov/gard/condition/1119/Carney-complex.aspx

- Patient's organization for Carney complex: www.inspire.com/groups/rare-disease/discussion/patients-organisation-for-carney-complex/

4.9. DIAMOND–BLACKFAN ANEMIA

Frequency:	5–7 cases per 1 million live births
Inheritance:	AD, 10–25% of cases are familial
	A few cases display possible autosomal recessive inheritance
Genes:	*RPL5* at 1p22.1
	RPL11 at 1p36.1-p35
	RPL35A at 3q29-qter
	RPS7 at 2p25
	RPS10 at 6p
	RPS17 at 15q
	RPS19 at 19q13
	RPS24 at 10q22-q23
	RPS26 at 12q
Gene tests:	Clinically available

4.9.1. CANCER RISKS

The cancer risks in Diamond–Blackfan anemia (DBA) are increased but are not well quantified. Children with DBA are at increased risk for developing leukemia.

4.9.2. DIAGNOSTIC CRITERIA

Diagnosis of DBA is based on the results of a CBC (complete blood count) that reveals hypoplastic anemia, normal leucocytes, and normal platelets. Affected individuals also have an increased number of chromosome break-ages. About 25% of children with DBA are caused by a mutation in the *RPS19* gene. An additional 20% of cases are thought to be due to mutations in the *RPS24*, *RPS17*, *RPL35A*, *RPL5*, *RPL11*, and *RPS7* genes. (It is unknown how many DBA cases are explained by mutations in the *RPS26* and *RPS10* genes.)

The *de novo* mutation rate in DBA is estimated to be between 55% and 60% so the majority of affected children will not have a significant family history of the disorder.

4.9.3. Clinical Features

DBA is characterized by congenital hypoplastic anemia. About 30–40% of affected children have congenital anomalies, including thumb and other hand abnormalities, cleft lip and/or palate, ventricular septal defects, kidney hypoplasia, short stature, and congenital glaucoma. Most children with DBA are diagnosed by 3 months of age and treated with steroids and transfusions. The risk of congenital malformations may be highest in children with *RPL5* or *RPL11* gene mutations.

4.9.4. Syndrome Subtypes

None.

4.9.5. Resources for Families

- Diamond-Blackfan Anemia Foundation, Inc: http://www.dbafound ation.org
- Diamond-Blackfan Anemia and You: http://www.diamondblack fananemia.com

4.10. Familial Adenomatous Polyposis (Also Attenuated FAP, Gardner's Syndrome, Turcot Syndrome, and Hereditary Desmoid Disease)

Frequency: From 1 in 6000 to 1 in 13,000 live births
Inheritance: AD
Genes: *APC* gene at 5q21
Gene test: Clinically available

4.10.1. Cancer Risks

Familial adenomatous polyposis (FAP) accounts for less than 1% of colon cancer cases. All affected individuals will develop colon cancer unless the colon is surgically removed (colectomy). The average age of colon cancer is 39 years, although 7% of cases develop before age 21. There is about a 4–12% risk of developing cancer of the small intestine (duodenum), especially at the site of the ampulla of Vater, which joins the small and large intestines.

The risk of pancreatic cancer is 2%, as is the risk of nonmedullary thyroid cancer. Children with FAP have about a 0.6% risk of developing hepatoblastoma between infancy and age 6. There is also an increased risk of brain tumors. Most of the FAP-associated brain tumors are medulloblastomas, although gliomas and ependymomas have also been reported. Individuals with FAP also have increased risks for developing cancer of the rectum, bile duct, and stomach. The risk of FAP-associated gastric cancer is higher in Japan than in other parts of the world.

The hallmark feature of FAP is polyposis, which is a carpeting of the colon and rectum with a hundred to thousands of adenomatous polyps. These polyps can be flat, making them difficult to see on an endoscopic exam. In addition, most individuals with FAP develop adenomatous polyps elsewhere in the GI tract, such as in the small intestine, periampulla, or stomach. About 50% of individuals with FAP have fundic gland polyps in the stomach.

Desmoid tumors are benign clonal fibrous tumors that occur in the abdomen and are remarkably difficult to remove or treat. Desmoid tumors occur in about 8% of men and 15% of women with FAP, unless the individual has a first-degree relative with a desmoid, then the risk of an FAP-associated desmoid tumor increases to about 25% for both genders.

Other benign growths have also been reported in people with FAP, including jaw osteomas, adrenal adenomas, lipomas, and juvenile nasopharyngeal angiofibromas.

4.10.2. DIAGNOSTIC CRITERIA

The clinical criteria for classic FAP are:

- The development of greater than 100 adenomatous polyps prior to age 40.
- The development of fewer than 100 adenomatous polyps and a relative who has been diagnosed with FAP.

The clinical criteria for attenuated FAP are:

- The development of 10–99 adenomatous polyps.
- The development of greater than 100 adenomatous polyps over age 40.
- A personal history of colorectal cancer before age 60 and a family history of multiple adenomatous polyps.

APC genetic testing is recommended for people who meet criteria for classic or attenuated FAP. APC genetic testing can also be considered in people who have any of the other features, especially if they also have any colorectal polyps. Testing is offered to individuals who have a personal or family history of colorectal polyps plus the following:

- Osteomas or CHRPE (congenital hypertrophy of the retinal pigment epithelium)
- Abdominal desmoid tumor (desmoid tumors can also develop on one's limbs, hands or feet, but the extra-abdominal desmoid tumors do not appear to be associated with FAP)
- Hepatoblastoma, which is a rare childhood liver tumor

The vast majority (70–80%) of *APC* mutations result in protein truncation. About one-quarter of cases represent *de novo* mutations (thus, the family history may be negative). Mutations in the extreme ends of the *APC* gene (before codon 157 and after codon 1595) and at the splicesite of exon 9 are associated with attenuated FAP. Mutations between codons 1250 and 1464 seem to confer the most serious form of polyposis (>1000 polyps). Attard et al. (2007) have suggested that mutations in codons 679–1224 are associated with increased risks of brain tumors.

4.10.3. CLINICAL FEATURES

On average, colon adenomas appear by age 16 and these precancerous polyps may even occur at age 9 or 10. In addition to the malignant and benign tumors listed above, individuals with FAP can exhibit supernumerary or absent teeth dentigerous cysts associated with the crown of unerupted teeth, sebaceous or epidermoid cysts, and characteristic eye lesions termed CHRPE. (Also see Section 6.3.1 for additional information about FAP.)

4.10.4. SYNDROME SUBTYPES

- *Attenuated FAP*—The attenuated form of FAP is associated with fewer colorectal polyps that occur at older ages. This may make it difficult to distinguish from Lynch syndrome (nonpolyposis colorectal cancer). Individuals with attenuated FAP have increased risks of colon cancer, but the risks are well below 100%.
- *Deletion 5q22*—This microdeletion syndrome is associated with the features of classic FAP as well as mild to moderate mental retardation and other mild congenital abnormalities or dysmorphic features.
- *Gardner's syndrome*—Gardner's syndrome is characterized by polyposis and colorectal cancer plus extra-colonic features, such as sebaceous cysts, lipomas, desmoid tumors, and fibromas. Other features include epidermoid cysts, osteomas of the mandible, impacted teeth, or other dental problems and CHRPE. It is now recognized that almost all families with FAP have "extra-colonic" features.

- *I1307K mutation*—This mutation was discovered serendipitously and is estimated to be carried by 6% of the Ashkenazi Jewish population. Individuals with the I1307K mutation do not develop polyposis, but do have a twofold increased risk of colon cancer. This is interesting considering that other mutations in the same region of the gene lead to a more classic FAP phenotype. Genetic testing for the I1307K mutation is not routinely recommended.
- *Turcot syndrome*—Turcot syndrome is characterized by polyposis and other FAP-related malignancies plus brain tumors, particularly medulloblastomas.

4.10.5. RESOURCES FOR FAMILIES

- Desmoid Tumor Research Foundation: http://www.dtrf.org
- FAP Gene Support Group: www.fapgene.org.uk/yahoogroup.html
- FAP International Information Foundation: www.fapinfo.com/forum/index.php
- John's Hopkins guide for patients and families: FAP: www.macgn.org/cc_fap1.html

4.11. FANCONI ANEMIA

Frequency:	1 in 300 in the general population
	Carrier frequency is about 1 in 89 in people of Ashkenazi Jewish ancestry, 1 in 100 in people of black African descent, and 1 in 77 Afrikaners.
Inheritance:	Autosomal recessive except for *FANCB*, which is X-Linked recessive
Genes:	*FANCA* at 16q24.3
	FANCB (FAAP95) at Xp22.31
	FANCC at 9q22.3
	FANCD1 (BRCA2) at 13.q12.3
	FANCD2 at 3p25.3
	FANCE is 6p22-21
	FANCF at 11p15
	FANCG (XRCC9) at 9p13
	FANCI (KIAA1794) at 15q25-26
	FANCJ (BRIP1, BACH1) at 17q22
	FANCL (PHF9, FAAP43, POG) at 2p16.1
	FANCM (FAAP250, HEF) at 14q21.3
	FANCN (PALB2) at 16p12
	FANCO (RAD51C) at 17q22
	FANCP (SLX4) at 16p13
Gene test:	Clinically available

4.11.1. CANCER RISKS

Individuals with FA are at greatly increased risk of developing leukemia, usually acute myeloid leukemia. There is also a greatly increased risk of developing squamous cell carcinoma, hepatocellular cancer, and brain tumors. Women with FA have increased risks of developing cancers of the vulva and cervix.

Benign liver adenomas have been reported in people with FA.

4.11.2. DIAGNOSTIC CRITERIA

FA is diagnosed by assessing levels of chromosome breakage, which is not visible on a standard karyotype. Testing is performed by doing either a mitocycin C chromosome stress test or the DEB test (diepoxybutane). These tests will reliably detect homozygotes but not heterozygotes. About 25% of children with FA will not display any of the syndromic features. Any child with aplastic anemia should be worked up for possible FA.

About 65% of FA cases involve mutations in the *FANC-A* gene. However, a variety of founder mutations have been noted across the many FA genes. Of note, most cases of Fanconi Anemia, type C (FANC-C) are due to an Ashkenazi Jewish founder mutation termed IVS4 + 4A > T.

4.11.3. CLINICAL FEATURES

FA is typically diagnosed by age 8, because of aplastic anemia, and/or bone marrow failure. There is a wide variability of features among individuals with FA. Affected individuals may have a typical facies (small head, eyes, and mouth) as well as growth retardation, skin hyperpigmentation, café au lait spots, absent or abnormal thumbs, ear anomalies, skeletal deformities, heart defects, and renal malformations. Hyperinsulinemia and diabetes are also in FA. Individuals with FA may have hypogonadism and reduced fertility. The underlying problem in FA is the progressive pancytopenia and chromosome breakage that worsens with exposure to alkylating agents. The life expectancy for individuals with FA is about age 30.

4.11.4. SYNDROME SUBTYPES

• *FANCD1*—About 2% of FA cases have the *FANCD1* subtype, which is caused by inheriting two mutated *BRCA2* alleles. (Also see Breast–Ovarian Cancer syndrome in Section 4.7.) Children with this FA subtype seem to have a more severe manifestation of the syndrome and are generally diagnosed during infancy or early childhood due to congenital anomalies, failure to thrive, and severe anemia. The risk of cancer seems to be greater than 95% and typically occurs by age 5.

- *FA heterozygotes*—Women who carry one mutated allele of the *FANCD1* (*BRCA2*) gene have substantially increased risks of breast and ovarian cancer and male carriers also have some increased cancer risks. (Also see Section 4.7.) Women who carry one mutated allele of the *FANCN* (*PALB2*) gene also appear to have increased risks of breast cancer. At this time, it is not clear whether carriers of other FA subtypes have increased cancer risks.

4.11.5. Resources for Families

- Canadian Fanconi Anemia Research Fund: http://www.fanconi canada.org
- Fanconi Anemia Research Fund: http://www.fanconi.org
- Fanconi Anemia Support Group: www.mdjunction.com/fanconi-anemia

4.12. Gastric Cancer, Hereditary Diffuse

Frequency:	Unknown; probably rare
Inheritance:	AD
Genes:	*CDH1* at 16q22.1
Gene test:	Clinically available

4.12.1. Cancer Risks

In Hereditary Diffuse Gastric Cancer syndrome (HDGC), the risk of diffuse gastric cancer is about 67% for men and 83% for women. The average age of diagnosis is 38 years, with a range of 14–69 years. Diffuse gastric cancers (also termed signet ring carcinomas) are poorly differentiated adenocarcinomas that infiltrate the stomach wall, causing a thickening or bulging of the stomach wall rather than a more distinct tumor mass.

Women with HDGC also have an estimated 39% lifetime risk of lobular breast cancer. Cases of ductal breast cancer, signet ring colon cancer, and islet cell pancreatic cancer have also been reported in people with HDGC and may be part of the syndrome.

4.12.2. Diagnostic Criteria

Individuals meet clinical criteria for HDGC if they have at least one of the following features:

- Two or more documented cases of diffuse gastric cancer in first- or second-degree relatives with at least one diagnosis under age 50.
- Three or more cases of documented diffuse gastric cancer in first- or second-degree relatives regardless of age.

The above criteria were developed by the International Gastric Cancer Linkage Consortium. In addition to these clinical criteria, the following individuals may also wish to consider genetic testing to look for *CDH1* mutations:

- An individual with diffuse gastric cancer diagnosed <age 40 who does not live in a region with high general population risks (e.g., Japan, Korea).
- An individual who has developed both diffuse gastric cancer and lobular breast cancer.
- An individual who has one relative diagnosed with diffuse gastric cancer and another relative diagnosed with lobular breast cancer.
- An individual who has one relative diagnosed with diffuse gastric cancer and another relative diagnosed with signet ring colon cancer.

4.12.3. CLINICAL FEATURES

Individuals with diffuse gastric cancer tend to be younger and have a poorer prognosis than individuals with the more common intestinal-type of gastric adenocarcinomas. For this reason, at risk individuals may wish to consider prophylactic gastrectomy. Intestinal gastric adenocarcinomas, which do not appear in HDGC, are more likely to be caused by ulcers or the *Helicobacter pylori* infection.

About one-third of families meeting the clinical criteria for HDGC will be found to have detectable mutations in the *CDH1* gene. Most individuals with HDGC will have positive family histories; *de novo* mutations in the *CDH1* gene have not been reported and are assumed to be rare. (Also see Section 5.3.2 for additional information about HDGC syndrome.)

4.12.4. SYNDROME SUBTYPES

None.

4.12.5. RESOURCES FOR FAMILIES

- HDGC On-Line Support Group: http://groups.yahoo.com/group/HDGC/summary
- Be Strong Hearted: Chelcun Family Foundation for Stomach Cancer Research: http://www.bestronghearted.org
- No Stomach for Cancer: http://www.nostomachforcancer.org
- Stanford Medicine Cancer Institute: HDGC (CDH1): http://cancer.stanford.edu/patient_care/services/geneticcounseling/HDGC.html

4.13. GASTROINTESTINAL STROMAL TUMOR, FAMILIAL (ALSO MULTIPLE GI AUTONOMIC NERVE TUMORS)

Frequency:	Unknown, probably rare
Inheritance:	AD
Genes:	*KIT* at 4q11-q12
	PDGFRA at 4q12
	SDHB at 1p36.1-p35
	SDHC at 1q23.3
Gene test:	Available on research basis only

4.13.1. CANCER RISKS

The risk of developing a familial gastrointestinal stromal tumor (GIST) is estimated to be about 90% by age 70. However, this risk figure may prove to be an overestimation as it is based on a small number of families. Most GIST tumors are benign and slow growing, with only 10–30% being malignant at diagnosis.

Cases of melanoma have also been reported.

4.13.2. DIAGNOSTIC CRITERIA

At this time, there are no formally agreed-upon criteria for familial GIST syndrome. Individuals who are diagnosed with GIST tumors and have any positive family history of GISTs, abdominal tumors, or sarcomas may have familial GIST and should consider genetic testing. (Also see Hereditary Paraganglioma-Pheochromocytoma syndrome, Section 4 for more information about the *SDH* genes.)

4.13.3. CLINICAL FEATURES

Familial GIST was initially termed "familial intestinal neurofibromatosis." GISTs are sarcoma-like tumors that do not express the typical muscular Schwann cell markers. GISTs develop in the mesenchymal cells that regulate the muscular contractions responsible for moving food through the digestive tract. About 70% of GIST tumors occur in the stomach, 20% occur in the small intestine, and the remainder are scattered elsewhere in the digestive tract, such as the esophagus, colon, and rectum. Familial GISTs are diagnosed at a median age of 48 years with a range of 29–77 years. In comparison, the average age of developing a sporadic GIST is 67 years.

About two-thirds of individuals with *C-KIT* mutations have hyperpigmented spots on their fingers, toes, elbows, knees, anus, genital region, and/ or face.

Individuals with *PDGFRA* mutations may have notably larger-sized hands compared with other relatives.

4.13.4. SYNDROME SUBTYPES

None.

4.13.5. RESOURCES FOR FAMILIES

- GIST Support International: http://www.gistsupport.org
- The Life Raft Group: http://www.liferaftgroup.org

4.14. JUVENILE POLYPOSIS (INCLUDES HEREDITARY MIXED POLYPOSIS)

Frequency:	From 1 in 16,000 to 1 in 100,000 live births
Inheritance:	AD
Genes:	BMPRIA at 10q22.3
	SMAD4 at 18q21.1
	ENG at 9q34.1
Gene test:	Clinically available for the BMPR1A and SMAD4 genes; ENG gene testing is available on a research basis only

4.14.1. CANCER RISKS

The risk of colon cancer may be as high as 40% for people with juvenile polyposis syndrome (JPS). There is also an estimated 20% risk of cancer elsewhere in the GI tract, especially in the stomach, duodenum, and pancreas.

The pathognomonic feature of JPS is the presence of "juvenile" polyps. These characteristic hamartomatous polyps typically occur in the stomach, small intestine, colon, and/or rectum. People with JPS can also develop colorectal adenomatous polyps. Although the polyps often develop in childhood, the cancers more typically occur in adulthood.

4.14.2. DIAGNOSTIC CRITERIA

There are no formally accepted clinical criteria for individuals with JPS. Genetic testing for BMPRIA and SMAD4 mutations should be considered if any of the following criteria are met:

- An individual has three or more juvenile colorectal polyps
- An individual has multiple juvenile polyps throughout the GI tract
- An individual has one or more juvenile polyps plus a family history of JPS
- An individual who does not have additional features of PTEN Hamartoma syndrome (PHS) or PJS

About 25% of individuals with JPS are found to have a mutation in the *BMPRIA* gene and about 15–20% of cases are found to have a mutation in the *SMAD4* proto-oncogene. Mutations in the *ENG* gene have been reported in two children with early-onset JPS; however, at this point, the role of *ENG* mutations in the causation of JPS has not been firmly established.

4.14.3. CLINICAL FEATURES

JPS is associated with hamartomatous polyps in the colon, rectum, stomach, and small intestine. The number of polyps can range from a few to several hundred. Most people with JPS have developed at least one polyp by the time they are in their twenties. Individuals who have juvenile polyps throughout their digestive tract are said to have generalized juvenile polyposis while individuals who have juvenile polyps confined to the colon are said to have juvenile polyposis coli. The major problems for people with JPS are the anemia, bleeding, and pain caused by the size and number of GI polyps.

The majority of individuals with *SMAD4* mutations will also develop symptoms consistent with hereditary hemorrhagic telangiectasia (HHT). Individuals with combined JPS/HHT syndrome are at risk for developing features of both syndromes. The main features of HHT syndrome are the development of telangiectases and arteriovenous malformations (abnormal blood vessel formation) in the lungs, liver, and brain. Some affected children will have other associated anomalies, such as clubbing of the fingers or toes. (Also see Section 6.3.2 for additional information about JPS.)

4.14.4. SYNDROME SUBTYPES

- *Juvenile polyposis of infancy*—Children born with a 10q deletion of both the *PTEN* and *BMPR1A* genes are said to have juvenile polyposis of infancy. This contiguous gene deletion syndrome is typically diagnosed within the first few months of life. The syndrome is characterized by the numerous hamartomatous polyps scattered throughout the child's entire GI tract. This condition is considered the most severe form of JPS and affected children have a poor prognosis.
- *Hereditary mixed polyposis syndrome*—Individuals with hereditary mixed polyposis syndrome (HMPS) develop multiple colorectal polyps. These polyps are of various types, including juvenile polyps, adenomas, and hyperplastic lesions. Individuals with HMPS have increased risks of colorectal cancer, but these risks have not been quantified. At least one large family with HMPS has been found to carry a mutation in the *BMPRIA* gene, lending credence to the theory that HMPS is a form of juvenile polyposis.

4.14.5. RESOURCES FOR FAMILIES

- Juvenile Polyposis: A Guide for Patients and their Families: http://www.uihealthcare.com/topics/medicaldepartments/cancercenter/juvenilepolyposis/index.html
- Peutz-Jeghers syndrome and Juvenile Polyposis syndrome online supportgroup: www.geneticalliance.org/organization/peutz-jeghers-syndrome-online-support-group

4.15. LEIOMYOMATOSIS RENAL CELL CANCER, HEREDITARY

Frequency: Unknown, probably rare
Inheritance: AD
Gene: *FH* at 1q42.1
Gene test: Clinically available

4.15.1. CANCER RISKS

Individuals with hereditary leiomyomatosis renal cell cancer (HLRCC) have a 10–16% risk of developing renal cell carcinoma and the mean age of diagnosis is 44 years. Most cases of renal cancer are type II papillary carcinoma, but other types of renal cancer have been observed, including tubulopapillary carcinomas and collecting-duct carcinomas. Cases of uterine leiomyosarcoma and testicular Leydig cell tumors have also been reported.

Over 75% of individuals with HLRCC develop at least one of the characteristic skin lesions termed cutaneous leiomyomata. Almost all women with HLRCC will develop uterine leiomyomata (fibroids), typically between the ages of 20 and 35. People with HLRCC may also be at increased risk to develop adrenal adenomas and ovarian cystadenomas.

4.15.2. DIAGNOSTIC CRITERIA

There are no formally accepted clinical criteria for HLRCC. Diagnosis of HLRCC is generally based on testing the enzymatic levels of fumarate hydratase and/or genetic testing. It is estimated that 80% of individuals with HLRCC will be found to have detectable mutations in the fumarate hydratase (*FH*) gene. The following individuals warrant consideration of testing to rule out or confirm HLRCC:

- An individual who has multiple cutaneous leiomyomas with at least one histologically confirmed leiomyoma.
- An individual who has a single leiomyoma in the presence of a family history of HLRCC.
- An individual who has one or more tubulopapillary, collecting duct, or papillary type II renal tumors with or without a family history of HLRCC.

Since uterine fibroids are so prevalent in the general population, the presence of uterine leiomyomata is seldom useful in the diagnosis of HLRCC.

The FH mutation database (http://chromium.liacs.nl/LOVD2/SDH/home.php?select_db=FH) can be helpful in determing the clinical significance of *FH* mutations.

4.15.3. CLINICAL FEATURES

Many individuals with HLRCC develop at least one of the skin leiomyomas. These lesions are skin-colored or light brown papules that appear on the trunk and limbs and occasionally the face and genital area as well. On average, these cutaneous leiomyomas appear around age 25 (range 10–48 years) and the number of lesions can range from one to dozens. While not malignant, these lesions can be problematic because they are typically painful to the touch and quite sensitive to cold.

Almost all women with HLRCC develop one or more uterine leiomyomata, which is much younger than sporadic cases of fibroids. It is not uncommon for these women to develop multiple large-sized uterine fibroids that can cause pain, irregular or heavy menses, and may result in a hysterectomy at an unusually young age.

4.15.4. SYNDROME SUBTYPES

Biallelic *FH* gene mutations—Infants who are born with homozygous or compound heterozygous *FH* mutations have an autosomal recessive condition termed fumarate hydratase deficiency (FHD). This rare condition is characterized by brain malformations and severe neurologic abnormalities, which can include marked hypotonia, poor feeding, failure to thrive, and seizures. The prognosis is grim for children with FHD, although a few affected individuals have survived into adulthood.

4.15.5. RESOURCES FOR FAMILIES

- HLRCC FamilyAlliance: http://www.vhl.org/hlrcc
- HLRCC Online Support Community: http://www.inspire.com/groups/VHL-family-alliance/search/?query=hlrcc

4.16. LI–FRAUMENI SYNDROME

Frequency:	Possibly as high as 1 in 20,000
Inheritance:	AD
Genes:	*TP53* at 17p13
Gene test:	Clinically available

4.16.1. CANCER RISKS

The risk of cancer associated with Li–Fraumeni syndrome (LFS) is about 50% by age 30 and 90% by age 60. Gender affects the risks of cancer; women with LFS have at least 90% lifetime risks of cancer while men have lifetime cancer risks that are less than 70%.

The most common malignancies associated with LFS are: sarcomas of bone and soft tissue, breast cancer, brain tumors, and adrenocortical carcinomas. It is estimated that these core cancers account for most of the diagnoses in LFS. A rare pediatric brain tumor, termed choroid plexus carcinoma, is highly associated with germline *TP53* mutations.

The risk of multiple primary cancers is also increased in LFS and Li–Fraumeni like (LFL) families. It is estimated that cancer survivors with LFS have a 57% risk of developing a second cancer and about a 38% risks of developing a third cancer.

A number of other malignancies have also been reported in LFS and LFL families. These noncore cancers include colorectal cancer, endometrial cancer, esophageal cancer, gonadal germ cell tumors, leukemias, lymphomas, lung cancer, melanoma, nonmelanoma skin cancers, NB, ovarian cancer, pancreatic cancer, prostate cancer, stomach cancer, thyroid cancer, WT, and other kidney cancers.

Malignant phyllodes breast tumors and malignant triton tumors (a rare brain tumor) have been reported in families with LFS. To date, cases of Ewings sarcoma has not been reported in families with *TP53* mutations. Male breast cancer seems to be uncommon.

4.16.2. DIAGNOSTIC CRITERIA

The diagnosis of LFS is based on a review of the pattern of cancer in the family. Clinical criteria for classic LFS and LFL syndrome are listed in Table 4.1. The diagnosis of LFS is confirmed by the presence of a *TP53* mutation

TABLE 4.1. DIAGNOSTIC CRITERIA FOR CLASSIC LI–FRAUMENI SYNDROME (LFS) AND LI–FRAUMENI-LIKE (LFL) SYNDROMES

The criteria for LFS syndrome are:
- Proband with sarcoma <45 years, and
- First-degree relative with any cancer <45 years, and
- First- or second-degree relative with any cancer <45 years or sarcoma at any age

The criteria for LFL syndrome are:
- Proband with any childhood cancer or sarcoma, brain tumor, or adrenocortical tumor <45 years, and
- First- or second-degree relatives with typical LFS cancer at any age,[a] and
- First- or second-degree relative with any cancer <60 years

Source: Li and Fraumeni (1969); Birch et al. (1994).

[a]Typical LFS cancers are: soft tissue sarcomas, bone sarcomas, breast cancer, adrenocortical carcinoma, brain tumors, and leukemia.

or deletion. Although a few families with LFS have been found to carry *CHK2* mutations, *CHK2* is not considered to be a major causal gene of LFS. The following individuals may be candidates for *TP53* genetic testing:

- Any individual whose personal and family history meets criteria for LFS or LFL syndrome (see Table 4.1). About 70% of LFS families and 8–22% of LFL families will be found to have *TP53* mutations. Individuals who meet criteria for classic LFS syndrome but test negative by sequence analysis should also be tested for *TP53* genomic rearrangements, testing that has recently become clinically available.

- Any individual who meets Chompret's criteria for *TP53* testing (described below). The likelihood of a positive *TP53* result is about 20% in individuals who meet Chompret's criteria, which are:
  - A proband who has a tumor before age 36 from the narrow LFS tumor spectrum (soft tissue sarcoma, osteosarcoma, brain tumor, premenopausal breast cancer, or adrenocortical carcinoma) and has at least one first- or second-degree relative with an LFS tumor (except breast cancer if the proband is affected with breast cancer) before 46 years or with multiple tumors.
  - A proband with multiple tumors, two of which belong to the narrow LFS tumor spectrum and the first of which occurred before 36 years of age.
  - A proband with adrenal cortical carcinoma (ACC) at any age, irrespective of the family history.

- Any individual who has a personal history of ACC, regardless of family history. The likelihood of a positive *TP53* result is about 80% for individuals with childhood ACC. Individuals with adult-onset ACC also have increased risks of having *TP53* mutations, especially if the diagnosis of ACC occurred under age 50. Since *de novo* cases have been reported, it is suggested that all individuals with ACCs be offered *TP53* testing even if there are no other cases of cancer in the family.

- Any individual who has a personal history of a rare brain tumor termed choroid plexus carcinoma, regardless of family history. Children who are diagnosed with choroid plexus carcinomas have very high probabilities of having germline *TP53* mutations. Since *de novo* cases have been reported, it is suggested that all children with choroid plexus carcinomas be offered *TP53* testing even if there are no other cases of cancer in the family.

- Any woman who has a personal history of very early-onset breast cancer (<age 30) and has tested negative for *BRCA1* and *BRCA2* mutations. Woman with very early-onset breast cancer have small increased risks of having *TP53* mutations, especially if there are any other features of LFS or LFL syndrome in the family.

4.16.3. CLINICAL FEATURES

Individuals with LFS have extraordinarily high risks of developing a diverse array of malignancies, both in childhood and in adulthood. Ages of onset are skewed to younger ages, with half of the cases occurring before age 30 and lifetime risks of cancer, especially for women, are as high as 90%. Lifetime cancer risks are higher for women than men because of the high breast cancer risks among female *TP53* mutation carriers. Male breast cancer is not a feature of LFS.

All types of bone and soft tissue sarcomas have been seen in families with LFS with the exception of Ewings' sarcoma, which is not an associated feature.

Cancer survivors with LFS have high risks of developing additional primary cancers. The risk of a second primary tumor may be as high as 57% and the risk of a third primary tumor may be as high as 38%. Radiation exposure appears to increase the risks of additional malignancies and individuals with LFS are recommended to avoid excessive radiation exposure whenever possible.

Families with LFS exhibit evidence of genetic anticipation, with cancers occurring more frequently and at younger ages over subsequent generations. A few genetic modifiers have been identified in LFS families, including shortened telomere length and a specific marker in the *MDM2* gene that works closely with the *TP53* gene. (See Section 5.3.3 for additional information about LFS.)

4.16.4. SYNDROME SUBTYPES

- *LFL syndrome*—It is recognized that some families with *TP53* mutations will not meet classic LFS criteria due to the lack of sarcoma diagnoses, small family size, or possible genetic modifiers. LFL families who test positive for *TP53* mutations should be given the same cancer risk information as families who meet classic LFS criteria. LFL families who test negative for *TP53* mutations may or may not actually have the syndrome. Some families will turn out to have different syndromes and some may not have an underlying hereditary cancer syndrome.

- *TP53* entire gene deletion—Children who are born with chromosome 17p deletions may have developmental delay and other medical issue. It is unclear whether these children have increased cancer risks.

4.16.5. RESOURCES FOR FAMILIES

- LFS online support group: http://www.mdjunction.com/li-fraumeni-syndrome
- LFS information: http://ghr.nlm.nih.gov/condition/li-fraumeni-syndrome

4.17. Lynch Syndrome (Also Termed HNPCC)

Frequency: 2–3% of all colon cancer cases
Inheritance: AD
Genes: *MLH1* at 3p21.3
                  MSH2 at 2p21-22
                  MSH6 at 2p16
                  MSH3 at 5q11-q12
                  PMS1 at 2q31-q33
                  PMS2 at 7p22
                  TACSTD1 at 2p21
Gene test: Clinically available for the *MSH6, MSH2, MLH1, PMS2,*
                  and *TACSTD1* genes
                  Analyses of the *MSH3* and *PMS1* genes are available on
                  a research basis only

4.17.1. Cancer Risks

Lynch syndrome confers a 70–80% lifetime risk of colorectal carcinomas. Individuals with *MLH1* or *MSH2* mutations appear to have the highest risks of colorectal cancer, which occurs at a mean age of 44 years. *MSH6* and *PMS2* mutations are associated with lower lifetime risks of colon cancer and the diagnoses tend to occur at older ages than with *MLH1* or *MSH2* mutations. All types of colorectal cancer are seen, including signet-ring cancers.

Individuals with Lynch syndrome have an 11–19% lifetime risk of intestinal-type gastric cancer with a mean age of diagnosis of 56 years. The risk of gastric cancer is even higher in countries with high general population risks of gastric cancer. In Japan, for example, the most frequent diagnosis in people with Lynch syndrome is stomach cancer, not colorectal cancer.

Women with Lynch syndrome have increased risks of both endometrial and ovarian cancers. The lifetime risk of endometrial cancer is 30–60% and the average age of onset is between 46 and 62 years. The lifetime risk of ovarian cancer is 9–12% and the mean age at diagnosis is 42 years. Various forms of ovarian cancers are seen in families with Lynch syndrome; however, borderline ovarian tumors are not a feature of Lynch syndrome.

Additional malignancies associated with Lynch syndrome include small bowel cancers, hepatobiliary cancers, and urinary tract cancers, which are typically transitional carcinomas of the ureter and renal pelvis. Pancreatic cancer is also thought to be associated with Lynch syndrome.

People with Lynch syndrome are also at higher risk for developing skin lesions such as sebaceous carcinomas, keratoacanthomas, and epitheliomas. Brain tumors (typically glioblastomas), can also occur as part of Lynch syndrome.

Increased risks of breast cancer, laryngeal cancer, and hematologic cancers have also been suggested in some Lynch syndrome families, but it remains unclear whether they are true features of the syndrome.

Individuals with Lynch syndrome have higher risks of developing adenomatous polyps in their colon and rectum. Lynch syndrome is also termed HNPCC syndrome to distinguish it from the rare syndromes that are associated with the development of greater than 100 polyps (polyposis).

4.17.2. DIAGNOSTIC CRITERIA

Individuals are clinically diagnosed with HNPCC if they meet the Amsterdam II criteria, which are as follows:

- Three or more family members, one of whom is a first-degree relative of the other two, with HNPCC-related cancers (defined as colorectal, endometrial, stomach, small intestinal, hepatobiliary, renal pelvic, or ureteral cancer)
- Two successive affected generations
- One or more of the HNPCC-related cancer diagnosed before age 50

Individuals who have personal and/or family histories consistent with HNPCC should always be offered genetic testing. Individuals who test positive for a mutation or deletion in the *MSH2, MLH1, MSH6,* or *PMS2* mismatch repair (MMR) gene are considered to have Lynch syndrome. It is estimated that 90% of families with Lynch syndrome will be found to have mutations or deletions in the *MSH2* or *MLH1* gene, 7% of families will have *MSH6* gene mutations, and less than 5% of families will have *PMS2* mutations. The roles of the *PMS1* and *MSH3* genes in the causation of Lynch syndrome are still being established and analysis of these two genes for clinical purposes is not recommended at this time.

The modified Bethesda Criteria help determine whether individuals have sufficient features of Lynch syndrome to warrant genetic testing, specifically the tumor analyses discussed below. The modified Bethesda Criteria recommends that the tumor genetic analyses be performed for individuals who meet any of the following criteria:

- Colorectal cancer diagnosed in an individual younger than age 50
- Presence of synchronous or metachronous colorectal, or other HNPCC-associated tumors, which includes colorectal, endometrial, gastric, ovarian, pancreatic, ureter and renal pelvis, biliary tract, and brain tumors (mainly glioblastomas), regardless of age.
- Colorectal cancer with the microsatellite instability (MSI)-high histology diagnosed in an individual younger than age 60.

- Colorectal cancer diagnosed in one or more first-degree relatives with an HNPCC-related tumor, with one cancer diagnosed before age 50.
- Colorectal cancer diagnosed in two or more first- or second-degree relatives of any age.

Individuals who meet Amsterdam or Bethesda criteria are recommended to have genetic testing. Analysis of the tumor is often an important part of the genetic workup and consists of the following two tests:

- *MSI*—The MSI test evaluates the level of instability that is present in the repetitive sequences of DNA nucleotides. This test is an indirect way of determining whether all of the MMR genes are functional. The possible results are:
  - *MSI high*—instability present in greater than 30% of cells tested
  - *MSI low*—instability noted in fewer than 30% of cells tested
  - *MSI stable*—no measurable instability in which none of the cells show instability

About 90% of inherited tumors are MSI high, so this is an excellent screening test for individuals who have a low or moderate likelihood of having Lynch syndrome. Conversely, MSI-high tumors are not always due to an inherited germline mutation in an MMR gene. The main somatic causes of MSI-high tumors are methylation and mutations in the *BRAF* gene. In addition, people with MSI-low or MSI-stable tumors still have a small risk of having Lynch syndrome. In particular, people with *MSH6* mutations have a higher likelihood of having MSI-low tumors. For this reason, it is recommended that the MSI test be done in conjunction with the immunohistochemistry (IHC) test.

- *IHC*—The IHC analysis looks for the absence or presence of protein expression for each of the MMR genes. This test typically checks for the following five MMR genes: *MLH1*, *MSH2*, *MSH6*, *PMS1*, and *PMS2*.

IHC results demonstrating a loss of protein expression increase the likelihood that the individual has a germline mutation or deletion in a specific MMR gene. This is especially true in tumors that are found to be MSI high. However, this is not always the case; methylated MMR genes also cause absent protein expression.

Unless there is a known mutation or deletion in the family, individuals with cancers suggestive of Lynch syndrome are recommended to have MSI and/or IHC testing. These tumor genetic analyses can be done in conjunction with DNA testing or can be used to determine whether DNA testing is warranted.

Analysis of a malignant colorectal tumor is more useful than testing tumors at other sites. Colorectal adenomas and sebaceous carcinomas or adenomas may also be tested, but the lesions need to be large enough to analyze. Colorectal adenomas are more likely to yield useful results if they exhibit high-grade dysplasia. However a negative MSI or IHC result on an adenoma does not always exclude the possibility of Lynch syndrome.

4.17.3. CLINICAL FEATURES

Individuals with Lynch syndrome have markedly increased risks of developing colorectal cancers. These tumors usually arise from colon polyps, although true polyposis is absent. These colon polyps may be flat adenomas, making them more difficult to detect on colonoscopy. In addition, the malignant transformation of a polyp can occur over a short period of time, making it imperative that at-risk individuals undergo annual colonoscopies even if prior exams were completely negative. (Also see Section 6.3.3 for more information.)

4.17.4. SYNDROME SUBTYPES

- *Constitutional mismatch repair-deficiency (CMMR-D) syndrome*— CMMR-D is caused by the inheritance of bi-allelic mutations or deletions of the *MSH2, MLH1,* or *PMS2* genes. This condition is autosomal recessive. Children with CMMR-D syndrome appear to have very high risks for developing malignancy and the cancers often occur in early childhood or adolescence. The risk of multiple primaries also seems to be increased. The major malignancies reported in this rare condition are: cancers of the colon, stomach and small intestine, leukemias, lymphomas, and brain tumors. The associated brain tumors are often gliomas or glioblastomas but many other types of brain tumors have been observed. Over 75% of children with CMMR-D syndrome develop one or more café au lait spots and some may initially be thought to have neurofibromatosis, type 1.
- *Muir–Torre syndrome*—People with Muir–Torre syndrome have all the features of Lynch syndrome plus they have higher risks of developing uncommon cancerous or precancerous lesions of the skin. These characteristic skin lesions include sebaceous adenomas and carcinomas, epitheliomas, and keratoacanthomas. Many families with the clinical manifestations of Muir–Torre syndrome are found to have mutations or deletions in the *MSH2* gene.

- *Turcot syndrome*—Individuals with colon cancer and brain tumors are said to have Turcot syndrome, although this terminology is less useful since the advent of molecular testing. People with the Turcot syndrome associated with Lynch syndrome have a 1–2% risk of developing brain tumors. Most of the Lynch syndrome related brain tumors are glioblastomas. Families with *PMS2* mutations may have higher risks of brain tumors compared to families with other mismatch repair gene mutations.

4.17.5. RESOURCES FOR FAMILIES

- Johns Hopkins Patient Booklet on HNPCC: http://www.macgn. org/cc_hnpcc1.html
- Lynch Syndrome International: www.lynchcancers.com
- HNPCC (Lynch syndrome) Online Support Group: http://health. dir.groups.yahoo.com/dir/1600061624

4.18. MELANOMA, CUTANEOUS MALIGNANT (INCLUDES FAMILIAL ATYPICAL MOLE-MALIGNANT MELANOMA SYNDROME, DYSPLASTIC NEVUS SYNDROME, AND MELANOMA–ASTROCYTOMA SYNDROME)

Frequency: Possibly 5–7% of melanoma cases
Inheritance: AD
Genes: CMM1: mapped to 1p36
               CMM2: *CDKN2A (TP16)* at 9p21
               CMM3: *CDK4* at 12q14
               CMM4: mapped to 1p22
Gene test: *CDKN2A* testing is clinically available.
               CDK4 testing is available on a limited clinical basis (if familial mutation has been identified).

4.18.1. CANCER RISKS

Individuals with Cutaneous Malignant Melanoma (CMM) syndrome, types 1–4 have high lifetime risks of developing multiple malignant melanomas. The risk of CMM for people with *CDKN2A* mutations is about 67% and the average age of diagnosis is 34 years. The lifetime risks of melanoma appear to be similar for people with *CDK4* mutations, although this is a less common gene finding and limited information is available about affected families.

People with CMM syndrome who live in areas with high sun exposure have higher rates of melanoma than those living in areas with low sun exposure. For example, people with CMM syndrome who live in Australia have greater than 90% risks of developing melanoma.

CDKN2A mutations are associated with increased risks of pancreatic cancer and breast cancer. The risk of pancreatic cancer with a CDKN2A mutation may be as high as 17%.

Some families with CMM syndrome have developed both cutaneous and ocular melanomas, although to date no CDKN2A mutations have been identified in this group. Astrocytomas have also been reported in a few families with CMM syndrome. Head and neck squamous cell carcinomas may also be a feature of CMM.

Individuals with CMM syndrome are often identifiable via clinical examination, because of their propensity for developing multiple dysplastic nevi (moles).

4.18.2. DIAGNOSTIC CRITERIA

The criteria for a "melanoma family" include the presence of three or more affected blood relatives located in regions of intense sun exposure and two or more affected blood relatives in less heavily sun-exposed areas.

The following individuals are more likely to have CDKN2A mutations:

- Individuals with 10—>100 dysplastic nevi of varied size, color, and outline, on their upper trunk and limbs
- Individuals with personal or family histories of melanoma, breast cancer, astrocytoma, and/or pancreatic cancer

An individual who has had multiple primary melanomas has a 10–15% chance of having a CDKN2A mutation. The likelihood of a CDKN2A mutation increases to 20–54% if two first-degree relatives have had melanoma, and increases to 45% if there is a personal or family history of both melanoma and pancreatic cancer. To date, mutations in the CDK4 oncogene have been reported in only a few families with CMM syndrome.

Genetic testing remains controversial because many families who meet clinical criteria for CMM syndrome will not be found to have detectable gene mutations. Even more disturbing, individuals who test negative for gene mutations known to be in their families still appear to have some increased risk of melanoma.

4.18.3. CLINICAL FEATURES

Melanomas are neoplasms of the melanocytes that can occur spontaneously or from a benign nevus (mole). Melanomas typically occur cutaneously (involving skin cells), but may also occur at other sites, such as the eye.

Individuals with CMM syndrome have greatly increased risks of developing multiple melanomas, particularly in areas of the body that are exposed to the ultraviolet light of the sun. Melanoma that has metastasized may also cause a severe form of night blindness termed melanoma-associated retinopathy.

4.18.4. SYNDROME SUBTYPES

None.

4.18.5. RESOURCES FOR FAMILIES

- Booklet on Moles and Dysplastic Nevi: http://www.cancer.gov/pdf/WYNTK/WYNTK_moles.pdf
- Melanoma Patients Australia: http://www.melanomapatients.org
- The Melanoma Patient's Information Page: http://www.mpip.org

4.19. MULTIPLE ENDOCRINE NEOPLASIA, TYPE 1 (ALSO WERMER SYNDROME)

Frequency: 1 in 5000–50,000 in the Caucasian population
Inheritance: AD
Genes: *MEN1* at 11q13
Gene test: Clinically available

4.19.1. CANCER RISKS

MEN1 is associated with increased risks of about 20 endocrine and nonendocrine tumors. Most of the tumors associated with MEN1 are benign, although they can still cause serious medical problems.

Individuals with MEN1 are at high risk for developing malignant islet cell tumors of the pancreas, including insulinomas. They are also at increased risk to develop carcinoid tumors, such as gastriomas. MEN1-related carcinoid tumors most frequently occur in the duodenum, but may also develop in the thymus, bronchus, or stomach. About half of affected individuals develop a carcinoid tumor.

Additional malignant tumors include GISTs, adrenocortical carcinomas, nonmedullary thyroid cancer, and peripheral sheath tumors (malignant schwannomas).

Associated benign tumors include pituitary, and adrenocortical adenomas, meningiomas, ependymomas, lipomas, leiomyomas, collagenomas, and skin lesions such as facial angiofibromas. Ovarian cancer and pheochromocytomas (PCCs) are possible features of MEN1.

4.19.2. DIAGNOSTIC CRITERIA

An individual who meets any of the following criteria is considered to have MEN1 syndrome:

- An individual who has been diagnosed with two endocrine tumors involving the parathyroid, pituitary gland, or GEP tract (gastro-entero-pancreatic tract, which includes the stomach, duodenum, pancreas, and intestinal tract).
- An individual who has been diagnosed with three or more tumors of the parathyroid, endocrine pancreas, pituitary gland, or adrenal gland, or a neuroendocrine carcinoid tumor.
- An individual who has been diagnosed with one endocrine tumor in the parathyroid, anterior pituitary or endocrine pancreas, and has a first-degree relative previously diagnosed with MEN1 syndrome.
- An individual who has one endocrine tumor in the parathyroid, anterior pituitary, or endocrine pancreas and has been found to carry a germline mutation in the *MEN1* gene.

About 80–90% of people with personal and family histories of MEN1 syndrome will be found to have detectable mutations or deletions in the *MEN1* gene. An individual with a personal history consistent with MEN1 but no family history of the disorder has a 65% likelihood of having an *MEN1* mutation. It is estimated that 10% of the *MEN1* mutations represent *de novo* mutations, which may explain the lack of affected relatives in some cases. However, individuals who have only one of the tumors associated with MEN1 syndrome and negative family histories rarely have *MEN1* gene mutations.

4.19.3. CLINICAL FEATURES

Most of the endocrine pancreas tumors are nonfunctioning, which means they do not secrete hormones (making them more difficult to detect). In fact, pancreatic cancer is the most common cause of death in people with MEN1, with almost half the cases being metastatic at the time of diagnosis. Even in the absence of malignant disease, the pancreas of a person with MEN1 typically exhibits some unusual and abnormal cell morphology. The carcinoid tumor may present as peptic ulcer disease.

MEN1 has variable expressivity and childhood onset is rare. Almost everyone with MEN1 develops parathyroid disease by age 50, 50–75% develop pancreatic disease, 30–55% develop pituitary disease, and 16% develop adrenal disease.

Carcinoid tumors, which are the second most common cause of death in MEN1, can cause Zollinger–Ellison syndrome, which is a peptic ulcer with or without chronic diarrhea. It is estimated that one-quarter of patients with Zollinger–Ellison syndrome have a germline mutation in the *MEN1* gene.

MEN1 is not associated with medullary thyroid carcinoma (MTC), which is a major feature of multiple endocrine neoplasia, type 2 (MEN2). Both MEN1 and MEN2 are associated with tumors of the parathyroid.

4.19.4. SYNDROME SUBTYPES

None.

4.19.5. RESOURCES FOR FAMILIES

- Association for Multiple Endocrine Neoplasia Disorders (AMEND): http://www.amend.org.uk
- Multiple Endocrine Neoplasia Support Group: http://www.mdjunction.com/multiple-endocrine-neoplasia

4.20. MULTIPLE ENDOCRINE NEOPLASIA, TYPE 2 (ALSO SIPPLE SYNDROME, FAMILIAL MEDULLARY THYROID CARCINOMA SYNDROME)

Frequency:	1 in 30,000 births
Inheritance:	AD
Genes:	*RET* at 10q11.2
Gene test:	Clinically available

4.20.1. CANCER RISKS

The risk of MTC is between 95% and 100% for individuals with MEN2. This rare form of thyroid cancer generally occurs before age 40 and may occur as young as age 3. Individuals with multiple endocrine neoplasia, type 2B (MEN2B) are at the greatest risk for developing MTCs in early childhood.

Individuals with multiple endocrine neoplasia, type 2A (MEN2A) or MEN2B have a 50% likelihood of developing at least one PCC. About 10% of the PCCs are malignant at the time of diagnosis.

Other associated tumors include parathyroid adenomas, GI tract ganglioneuromas, and mucosal neuromas. Papillary thyroid carcinomas have also been reported.

4.20.2. DIAGNOSTIC CRITERIA

The clinical criterion for MEN2A is:

- The diagnosis of two or more specific endocrine tumors (MTC, PCC, and/or parathyroid adenoma or hyperplasia) in a single individual or in close relatives.

The clinical criteria for MEN2B are:

- The diagnosis of MTC plus the presence of mucosal neuromas of the lips and tongue, medullated corneal nerve fibers, distinctive facies with enlarged lips, and a Marfanoid body habitus.

The clinical criterion for Familial Medullary Thyroid Carcinoma (FMTC) is:

- A family history that consists of four cases of MTC with an absence of PCC or parathyroid adenoma/hyperplasia.

Over 90% of individuals meeting clinical criteria for MEN2 will be found to have a germline mutation in the *RET* gene. About half of the MEN2B cases represent *de novo* cases, while this is true of less than 5% of MEN2A cases.

There is an on-line mutation database of *RET*, which can be accessed via: http://www.arup.utah.edu/database/MEN2/MEN2_welcome.

4.20.3. CLINICAL FEATURES

About 3–10% of all thyroid malignancies are of the medullary subtype. It is recommended that all individuals diagnosed with MTCs undergo *RET* testing, mainly to determine the risks of thyroid cancer for other relatives.

It is estimated that 25% of MTCs will have *RET* mutations.

4.20.4. SYNDROME SUBTYPES

- *MEN2A*—In MEN2A, individuals have a 95% risk of developing MTC, which usually occurs by early adulthood. Individuals with MEN2A also have a 50% risk of PCC, a 20–30% risk of parathyroid disease, and a 10–20% risk of hyperthyroidism. MEN2A is the most common subtype of MEN2.
- *MEN2B*—Individuals with MEN2B have nearly a 100% likelihood of developing MTC. The thyroid cancers often occur under age 10 and seem to be especially aggressive and difficult to treat. Similar to MEN2A, the risk of PCC in MEN2B is about 50%. Children with MEN2B may also have other distinctive physical characteristics, including enlarged lips and a Marfanoid habitus (tall with broad

chest and unusually long arms). Hyperthyroidism and parathyroid disease are uncommon in MEN2B.

- *FMTC*—By definition, individuals with FMTC have been diagnosed with MTC, but have not developed a PCC, hyperthyroidism, or parathyroid disease. The MTCs tend to occur after age 50 and are generally amenable to treatment. Papillary thyroid carcinomas have also been reported in families with FMTC.

4.20.5. Resources for Families

- Association for Multiple Endocrine Neoplasia Disorders: http://www.amend.org.uk
- Multiple Endocrine Neoplasia Support Group: http://www.mdjunction.com/multiple-endocrine-neoplasia

4.21. MYH-Associated Polyposis

Frequency:	1% of the general population is heterozygous carriers
Inheritance:	Autosomal recessive
Genes:	*MYH* at 1p32.1-p34.3
Gene test:	Clinically available

4.21.1. Cancer Risks

Individuals with MYH-associated polyposis (MAP) are at greatly increased risk to develop carcinomas of the colon, rectum, and small intestine. The lifetime risk for developing colorectal cancer may be as high as 80%. In one study conducted in the Netherlands, the average age of developing colorectal cancer was 45 years.

MAP is considered a polyposis syndrome and individuals typically develop multiple colon adenomas. However, not everyone will develop frank polyposis. About one-third of individuals with MAP will develop fewer than 100 colorectal polyps.

Individuals with MAP may also exhibit features often associated with FAP, including fundic gland polyps in the stomach, jaw osteomas, dental cysts, and CHRPE.

Additional associated features include sebaceous gland adenomas, duodenal adenomas, and pilomatricomas. Desmoid tumors may also be a feature of MAP.

4.21.2. Diagnostic Criteria

There are no formally agreed-upon clinical criteria for MAP syndrome. MAP can be considered in people who have developed more than 15 synchronous colorectal adenomas or have developed colorectal cancer under the age of 50.

Indications for *MYH* testing are based primarily on an individual's personal history of colorectal polyps and/or cancer. It is estimated that about 2% of colorectal cancer cases, which are MSI stable and diagnosed under age 50, are due to bi-allelic *MYH* mutations.

It is estimated that two specific mutations, Y165C and G382D, account for about 80% of *MYH* mutations in North America.

4.21.3. Clinical Features

MAP is a recessively inherited cancer syndrome. This means that individuals with MAP are more likely to have negative family histories or to have affected siblings rather than an affected parent. Carriers of bi-allelic *MYH* mutations will have MAP syndrome while carriers of one mutated *MYH* allele do not appear to have increased risks of cancer.

MAP is a newly described syndrome and information continues to be gathered regarding associated features and the lifetime risks of cancer. (Also see Section 6.3.4 for additional information about MAP syndrome.)

4.21.4. Syndrome Subtypes

None.

4.21.5. Resources for Families

- FAP International Information Foundation (Forum on MYH): http://www.fapinfo.com/forum/index.php
- Mt Sinai Hospital Familial GI Cancer Registry: http://www.mountsinai.on.ca/care/fgicr

4.22. Neuroblastoma, Familial

Prevalence:	About 1–3% of neuroblastoma cases
Inheritance:	AD
Gene:	*ALK* at 2p23
	PHOX2B at 4p12
Testing:	Clinically available

4.22.1. Cancer Risks

In familial neuroblastoma (NB), the risk of NB is about 55–65%, although there may be some lower penetrance families. NB is a malignant tumor of the central nervous system that occurs in childhood.

Ganglioneuroblastomas and ganglioneuromas have also been reported in children with *ALK* mutations.

4.22.2. DIAGNOSTIC CRITERIA

There are no set diagnostic criteria for familial NB. Families in which there are three cases of NB have the highest likelihood of testing positive for an *ALK* gene mutation. Genetic testing should be offered to children with NB who have a positive family history of NB, ganglioneuroblastoma, or ganglioneuroma. Children who are diagnosed with multifocal NB or have been diagnosed below 1 year of age may also be at increased risk to have germline *ALK* mutations.

Most familial NB cases are caused by a mutation in the *ALK* gene. To date, all of the germline *ALK* mutations have been in the tyrosine kinase domain (exons 21–28) of the gene.

Children with NB who also have features of other neural crest disorders may carry germline mutations in the *PHOX2B* gene. (See Section 4.22.4 for the description of this syndrome subtype.)

4.22.3. CLINICAL FEATURES

Familial cases of NB tend to occur at younger ages than sporadic cases; the average age of diagnosis in familial cases is 9 months versus 2–3 years. It is rare for NB to be diagnosed beyond age 7.

For the most part, familial NB appears to be a site-specific hereditary cancer syndrome. However, it is important to note that it is a newly recognized condition and there may be other associated features, which have not yet been recognized.

4.22.4. SYNDROME SUBTYPES

- PHOX2B *mutations*—Children who have *PHOX2B* mutations tend to have familial NB as well as other disorders related to an abnormal development of neural crest tissue. These disorders include congenital central hypoventilation syndrome and Hirschsprung's disease.

4.22.5. RESOURCES FOR FAMILIES

- Children's Neuroblastoma Cancer Foundation: http://www.cncfhope.org/post/topid/1133
- Neuroblastoma Support Group: http://www.mdjunction.com/neuroblastoma

4.23. NEUROFIBROMATOSIS, TYPE 1 (ALSO VON RECKLINGHAUSEN DISEASE)

Frequency: 1 in 3000 individuals
Inheritance: AD
Genes: *NF1* at 17q11.2
Gene test: Clinically available

4.23.1. CANCER RISKS

Malignant peripheral nerve sheath tumors (MPNSTs) occur in 3–15% of individuals with Neurofibromatosis, type 1 (NF1), making them the most frequently occurring malignancy in this syndrome. MPNSTs were previously termed neurofibroscarcomas or malignant schwannomas and develop in deep soft tissue at the nerve trunks or along nerve fibers.

The hallmark feature of NF1 is the presence of multiple café au lait spots and cutaneous and subcutaneous neurofibromas. Individuals with NF1 may have only a few of these neurofibromas or they may have hundreds of these benign tumors.

Individuals with NF1 are at risk for developing other tumors of the central nervous system, including neurofibromas (peripheral, nodular, or plexiform subtypes), astrocytomas, ependymomas, NBs, optic and nonoptic gliomas, and primitive neuroectodermal tumors (PNETs). Additional benign and malignant tumors associated with NF1 include carcinoid tumors, PCCs, GISTS, intestinal hamartomas, leukemias (especially juvenile chronic myelo-monocytic leukemia), undifferentiated sarcomas, rhabdomyosarcomas, WTs, and Lisch nodules. The carcinoid and GIST tumors occur most frequently in the small intestine (duodenum). Women with NF1 appear to have moderate increased risks of breast cancer.

4.23.2. DIAGNOSTIC CRITERIA

Individuals meet the clinical criteria for NF1 if they have at least two of the following features:

- Six or more café au lait spots (macules) over 5 mm in greatest diameter in prepubertal individuals and over 15 mm in greatest diameter in postpubertal individuals
- Two or more neurofibromas of any type or one plexiform neurofibroma
- Freckling in the axillary or inguinal regions
- Optic glioma
- Two or more Lisch nodules

- A distinctive osseous lesion such as sphenoid dysplasia or thinning of the long bones
- A first-degree relative diagnosed with NF1

Although genetic testing is available, the diagnosis of NF1 is typically based on clinical criteria. Many cases of NF1 are diagnosed by age 4. Although nearly all children with NF1 meet clinical criteria by age 8, only half of them meet the criteria by age 1. Therefore, young children with multiple café au lait spots but no other features of NF1 should still be strongly suspected as having the syndrome. Positive family history is often lacking in NF1; up to 50% of cases are *de novo*.

4.23.3. Clinical Features

NF1 is one of the most common genetic disorders. There is wide expressivity to this syndrome, with some individuals severely affected and others only mildly affected. In addition to the development of café au lait spots and neurofibromas and the heightened risk of other tumors, individuals with NF1 may also exhibit learning disabilities, skeletal abnormalities, bone disease, and vascular problems.

4.23.4. Syndrome Subtypes

None.

4.23.5. Resources for Families

- Children's Tumor Foundation: http://www.ctf.org/
- Neurofibromatosis, Inc.: http://www.nfinc.org
- Neurofibromatosis online support group: http://dailystrength.org/c/Neurofibromatosis/support-group
- Neurofibromatosis online support group: http://www.mdjunction.com/neurofibromatosis

4.24. Neurofibromatosis, Type 2

Frequency:	1 in 35,000
Inheritance:	AD
Genes:	*NF2* at 22q12.2
Gene test:	Clinically available

4.24.1. CANCER RISKS

Individuals with neurofibromatosis, type 2 (NF2) have an increased risk of developing multiple vestibular schwannomas (previously termed acoustic neuromas), spinal schwannomas, meningiomas, and neurofibromas. These tumors can be difficult to manage clinically yet rarely become malignant. About half of the individuals with NF2 develop cranial or spinal meningiomas. The average age of diagnosis is 18–24 years, although some people with NF2 are not identified until they are much older. Individuals with NF2 also have a small but increased risk of developing astrocytomas, ependymomas, and gliomas. Retinal hamartomas and cafe au lait spots are also observed in people with NF2.

4.24.2. DIAGNOSTIC CRITERIA

Two sets of diagnostic criteria have been developed for NF2. The criteria set forth by the National Institutes of Health Consensus Conference are as follows:

- Bilateral eighth nerve masses seen by MRI with gadolinium, or
- First-degree relative with NF2 plus one of the following:
    - Computed tomography (CT) or MRI evidence of a unilateral eighth nerve mass
    - A plexiform neurofibroma
    - Neurofibromas (two or more)
    - Gliomas (two or more)
    - Posterior subcapsular cataract at a young age
    - Two or more meningiomas
    - Imaging evidence of an intracranial or a spinal cord tumor

The Manchester Criteria for NF2 are as follows:

- Bilateral vestibular schwannomas, or
- A first-degree relative with NF2 and a unilateral vestibular schwannoma or any two of the following: meningioma, schwannoma, glioma, neurofibroma, posterior subcapsular lenticular opacities, or
- Unilateral vestibular schwannoma and any two of the following: meningioma, schwannoma, glioma, neurofibroma, posterior subcapsular lenticular opacities, or
- Multiple meningiomas and unilateral vestibular schwannoma or any two of the following: schwannoma, glioma, neurofibroma, cataract

An individual who develops a vestibular schwannoma under age 30 should be strongly suspected of having NF2. It is estimated that about 50% of NF2 cases are *de novo*.

In contrast to NF1, it is rare for individuals with NF2 to develop six or more café au lait spots.

4.24.3. CLINICAL FEATURES

In general, NF2 is considered an adult-onset condition, although it may be underrecognized in childhood. In many cases, the initial symptom of NF2 is hearing loss due to the vestibular schwannomas. Vestibular schwannomas, which are typically bilateral, can also cause problems with balance and tinnitus (ringing in the ears). Individuals with NF2 may also develop cataracts, facial palsy, neuropathy, and muscle weakness.

4.24.4. SYNDROME SUBTYPES

None.

4.24.5. RESOURCES FOR FAMILIES

- Children's Tumor Foundation: http://www.ctf.org/
- Neurofibromatosis, Inc.: http://www.nfinc.org
- Neurofibromatosis Support Group: http://dailystrength.org/c/Neurofibromatosis/support-group
- Neurofibromatosis Support Group: http://www.mdjunction.com/neurofibromatosis

4.25. NEVOID BASAL CELL CARCINOMA SYNDROME (ALSO GORLIN SYNDROME, BASAL CELL NEVUS SYNDROME)

Frequency: 1 in 40,000
Inheritance: AD
Genes: *PTCH* at 9q22.3
Gene test: Clinically available

4.25.1. CANCER RISKS

Individuals with nevoid basal cell carcinoma syndrome (NBCCS) have markedly increased risks for developing multiple BCCs. The associated skin cancers can occur in early childhood; however, on average, individuals with NBCCS develop their initial BCCs at around age 25. People who have fairer skin that does not tan have higher risks of developing BCCs than those with darker skin. Caucasians with NBCCS have a 90% risk of developing skin cancer while African Americans with NBCCS have about a 40% risk.

Individuals with NBCCS also have increased risks for developing PNETs (also termed medulloblastomas) and meningiomas.

Most people with NBCCS develop keratocysts of the jaw as well as other sebaceous and dermoid cysts. Over 90% of affected adults have a characteristic cluster of cells in the brain termed ectopic calcification of the falx cerebri. There is also a small increased risk of cardiac fibromas and fetal rhabomyomas. Women with NBCCS have an estimated 20% risk for developing ovarian fibromas and there may also be an increased risk of ovarian fibrosarcomas.

4.25.2. DIAGNOSTIC CRITERIA

Individuals meet diagnostic criteria for NBCCS if they have two major or one major and two minor criteria:

Major criteria:

- Two or more BCCs or one BCC under age 30 or the presence of more than 10 basal cell nevi
- Any odontogenic keratocyst (proven on histology) or polyostotic bone cyst
- Palmar or plantar pits (three or more)
- Ectopic calcification; lamella or early (before age 20) falx calcification
- Family history of NBCCS

Minor criteria:

- Congenital skeletal anomaly: bifid, fused, splayed, or missing rib; or bifid, wedged, or fused vertebrae
- Head circumference >97th percentile with frontal bossing
- Cardiac or ovarian fibroma
- Medulloblastoma (often PNET)
- Lymphomesenteric or pleural cysts
- Congenital malformation: cleft lip and/or palate, polydactyly, eye anomaly (cataract, coloboma, microphthalmia)

Over 60% of people who meet clinical criteria for NBCCS will be found to have detectable mutations or deletions in the *PTCH* gene. It is estimated that 20–40% of cases represent *de novo* mutations.

4.25.3. CLINICAL FEATURES

Many individuals with NBCCS have characteristic physical features. About 90% of individuals develop the jaw swellings (keratocysts), which can actually cause the jaw to fracture and often leads to significant dental problems. Other features can include macrocephaly, frontal bossing, coarse facial features, and facial milia (tiny keratin-filled cysts).

Many people with NBCCS have some type of skeletal anomalies, such as spina bifida occulta or rib anomalies. Epidermal cysts and palmoplantar pits are also common and their presence can be used in the diagnosis of NBCCS.

4.25.4. SYNDROME SUBTYPES
None.

4.25.5. RESOURCES FOR FAMILIES

- BCNNS Life Support Network: http://www.bccns.org
- Gorlin Syndrome Group (UK): http://www.gorlingroup.org

4.26. PARAGANGLIOMA–PHEOCHROMOCYTOMA SYNDROME, HEREDITARY (INCLUDING CARNEY–STRATAKIS SYNDROME)

Frequency:	1 in 1 million (in the Dutch population)
Inheritance:	PGL1 and PGL2: AD with paternal imprinting; PGL3 and PGL4: AD
Genes:	PGL1: *SDHD* at 11q23
	PGL2: *SDHAF2* (*SDH5*) at 11q13.1
	PGL3: *SDHC* at 1q21
	PGL4: *SDHB* at 1p36
	TMEM127 at 2q11
Gene Tests:	Clinically available

4.26.1. CANCER RISKS

For people with hereditary paraganglioma–pheochromocytoma (PGL-PCC) syndrome, the risk of developing a PGL or PCC may be about 29% by age 30 and 77% by age 50. Individuals who have inherited an *SDHD* mutation from their father have nearly a 50% likelihood of developing a PGL or PCC by age 30 and an 86% risk by age 50. Individuals who have inherited an *SDHD* mutation from their mothers rarely have increased tumor risks.

It is estimated that 10% of PGLs and PCCs are malignant at diagnosis. The malignant potential seems highest in the extra-adrenal sympathetic PGLs. People with *SDHB* mutations have the highest risk of presenting with a malignant PGL or PCC and also have increased risks of developing renal cell carcinoma.

Individuals with hereditary PGL-PCC syndrome are also at increased risk to develop GISTs. Individuals who develop both a PGL and a GIST are said to have Carney–Stratakis syndrome. Nonmedullary thyroid cancers and other endocrine tumors may also be part of PGL-PCC syndrome.

4.26.2. DIAGNOSTIC CRITERIA

There are no generally accepted criteria for hereditary PGL-PCC syndrome. PGLs and PCCs are rare tumors, which makes it appropriate to consider genetic testing even in isolated cases. However, the likelihood that an individual has hereditary PGL-PCC syndrome is higher in the following scenarios:

- An individual has developed two or more PGL or PCC tumors.
- An individual has developed one PGL or PCC tumor *and* has a relative with a PGL or PCC tumor.
- An individual has a PGL or PCC tumor, but does not meet criteria for Von Hippel–Lindau (VHL) syndrome, NF1, or MEN2.

4.26.3. CLINICAL FEATURES

PGLs are neuroendocrine tumors that occur along the paravertebral axis, which stretches from the base of the skull down to the pelvis. PGLs that occur in the adrenal gland are termed PCCs. PGLs are categorized by their location and whether or not they secrete catecholamines (e.g., epinephrine, norepinephrine, or dopamine). Secreting PGLs are also called chromaffin tumors. Most PCCs and extra-adrenal PGLs that occur in the abdomen, pelvis, or thorax are sympathetic (secreting) tumors while 95% of head and neck PGLs are parasympathetic (nonsecreting) tumors. People with hereditary PGL-PCC syndrome have higher risks of developing multifocal, bilateral, and recurrent tumors.

Secreting PGLs and PCCs can cause a variety of continual or episodic symptoms due to the surges of extra catecholamines. These symptoms include high blood pressure and pulse, headaches, profuse sweating, palpitations, pallor, anxiety, and panic attacks.

Nonsecreting head and neck PGLs have few if any warning symptoms, making them difficult to detect; their most frequent site of occurrence is in the carotid body. Researchers are developing a tumor block test; which looks for immunohistochemistry (IHC) of the *SDH* genes.

4.26.4. SYNDROME SUBTYPES

- *Carney–Stratakis syndrome*—Individuals who develop a PGL tumor and a GI tumor (GIST).

- *Paraganglioma, subtype 1*—PGL1 syndrome is caused by a germline mutation in the *SDHD* gene. Individuals with *SDHD* mutations seem to have the highest risks for developing the parasympathetic head and neck PGLs and their median age for developing a PGL or PCC tumor is 28 years. Pedigrees of families with *SDHD* mutations should be consistent with the parent-of-origin effect, that is, the familial pattern of cancer follows a dominant mode of inheritance and most individuals with PGL tumors have affected fathers rather then affected mothers. Most cases of PGL-PCC syndrome in the Dutch population are caused by three *SDHD* founder mutations termed Asp92Tyr, Leu95Pro, and Leu139Pro.

- *Paraganglioma, subtype 2*—Families with PGL2 syndrome have patterns of PGL and PCC tumors consistent with PGL-PCC syndrome. The underlying gene has recently been identified as being the *SDHAF2 (SDH5)* gene, which encodes for a mitochondrial protein.

- *Paraganglioma, subtype 3*—PGL3 syndrome is caused by an underlying mutation in the *SDHC* gene. *SDHC* gene mutations are rare and thus, there is limited information regarding cancer risks. However, it appears as though individuals with *SDHC* gene mutations develop head and neck PGLs as well as the abdominal PGLs.

- *Paraganglioma, subtype 4*—PGL4 syndrome is associated with germline mutations in the *SDHB* gene. Individuals with *SDHB* mutations have higher risks for developing PCCs or sympathetic extra-adrenal PGLs than those with other PGL-PCC gene mutations. Parasympathetic head and neck PGLs also occur in people with *SDHB* mutations. Individuals with *SDHB* mutations have increased risks for developing other forms of cancer, as well, including renal cell carcinoma and non-medullary thyroid cancers.

4.26.5. RESOURCES FOR FAMILIES

- PheoPara Alliance: http://www.pheo-para-alliance.org
- Pheochromocytoma Support Board: http://www.pheochromocytomasupportboard.yuku.com
- Pheochromocytoma Information: http://www.vhl.org/pheo/index.php
- Pheochromocytoma Support Group: http://www.pheochromocytoma.org

4.27. PEUTZ-JEGHERS SYNDROME

Frequency:	From 1 in 25,000 to 1 in 280,000
Inheritance:	AD
Genes:	*STK11* at 19p13.3
Gene test:	Clinically available

4.27.1. CANCER RISKS

PJS is characterized by the development of hamartomatous polyposis throughout the GI tract, especially in the small intestine. Individuals may also develop adenomatous polyps.

Individuals with PJS have about an 85% lifetime risk of cancer. PJS-associated cancers occur most frequently in the GI tract, namely the colon, rectum, small intestine, stomach, esophagus, and pancreas. The risk of a GI tract malignancy is about 57%; the specific risk of colorectal cancer is about 39%. Other malignancies possibly associated with PJS include kidney cancer, lung cancer, and thyroid cancer.

Women with PJS are also at increased risk for developing breast cancer, granulosa type ovarian cancer, fallopian tube cancer, uterine cancer, and a rare aggressive form of cervical cancer termed cervical adenoma malignum. In one series, the risk of breast cancer by age 40 was 8% and by age 60 was 31%. Almost all affected women develop sex cord tumors with annular tubules (SCTAT), which are benign sex cord tumors of the ovary.

Men with PJS are at increased risk for developing benign sertoli tumors of the testes. Affected men may also be at increased risks to develop breast cancer and prostate cancer.

4.27.2. DIAGNOSTIC CRITERIA

An individual may be diagnosed with PJS if the following clinical criteria are met:

- An individual has a histologically confirmed hamartomatous GI polyp with the distinctive PJS morphology *and* two of the following three findings:
  - Small bowel polyposis
  - Mucocutaneous hyperpigmentation of the buccal mucosa, lips, fingers, toes, and/or external genitalia
  - A family history of PJS demonstrating AD inheritance

PJS should be suspected in anyone who has two or more histologically confirmed hamartomatous polyps. Individuals who have an affected first-degree relative can be diagnosed with PJS solely on the presence of the characteristic pigmented spots (see below).

4.27.3. CLINICAL FEATURES

Almost all individuals with PJS develop multiple polyps in the GI tract, although the total number of polyps and associated medical problems varies greatly even among members of the same family. The major problems caused by these polyps are chronic bleeding, anemia, obstruction, and malignant potential.

One of the classic signs of PJS is the presence of dark blue to dark brown hyperpigmented macules, which develop on the lips, buccal mucosa, eyes, nostrils, and anal area. These pigmented spots are present in over 95% of people with PJS and generally appear in early childhood. However, as people age, these macules may fade and become less noticeable. (See Section 5.3.4 for additional information about PJS.)

4.27.4. SYNDROME SUBTYPES

None.

4.27.5. RESOURCES FOR FAMILIES

- Peutz Jeghers Syndrome Online Support Group: http://www.peutz-jeghers.com
- Peutz Jeghers Syndrome Support Group: http://www.mdjunction.com/peutz-jeghers-syndrome

4.28. PTEN HAMARTOMA SYNDROME (PHS) (ALSO COWDEN SYNDROME; INCLUDES BANNAYAN–RILEY–RUVALCABA SYNDROME AND PROTEUS SYNDROME)

Frequency: From 1 in 200,000 to 1 in 250,000 in the Netherlands
Inheritance: AD
Genes: *PTEN* at 10q23.3
Gene test: Clinically available

4.28.1. CANCER RISKS

Women with PHS have a 25–50% lifetime risk of breast cancer and a 6–10% risk of endometrial cancer. The risk of thyroid cancer for men and women is about 10%. Most cases of thyroid cancer are of the follicular subtype, but the papillary subtype is also seen. The risk of clear cell renal cell carcinoma also seems to be increased in people with PHS. Men with PHS may be at increased risk to develop breast cancer. Additional malignancies that may be part of the PHS phenotype include uterine, colon, and kidney cancers. People with PHS are at increased risk to develop lipomas, fibromas, and GI hamartomas, all of which are benign tumors that may require resection depending upon their location and symptomatology.

4.28.2. DIAGNOSTIC CRITERIA

An individual meets clinical criteria for PHS if he or she meets any one of the following criteria:

- Pathognomonic mucocutaneous lesions alone if there are:
    - Six or more facial papules, at least three of which are trichilem-momas, or
    - Cutaneous facial papules and oral mucosal papillomatosis, or
    - Oral mucosal papillomatosis and acral keratoses, or
    - Six or more palmoplantar keratoses
- Two or more major criteria (listed below)
- One major and at least three minor criteria (listed below)
- At least four minor criteria (listed below)

Pathognomonic criteria:

- Adult Lhermitte–Duclos disease (LDD), defined as the presence of a cerebellar dysplastic gangliocytoma
- Mucocutaneous lesions: trichilemmomas (facial), acral keratoses, papillomatous lesions, mucosal lesions

Major criteria:

- Breast cancer
- Thyroid cancer (nonmedullary), especially follicular thyroid epithe-lial cancer
- Macrocephaly (occipital frontal circumference $\geq$97th percentile)
- Endometrial carcinoma

Minor criteria:

- Other thyroid lesions (e.g., adenoma, multinodular goiter)
- Mental retardation (IQ $\leq$ 75)
- Hamartomatous intestinal polyps
- Fibrocystic disease of the breast
- Lipomas

- Fibromas
- Genitourinary tumors (especially renal cell carcinoma)
- Genitourinary malformation
- Uterine fibroids

Given the rarity of the syndrome and the general frequency of some of the minor criteria currently listed (especially uterine fibroids and fibrocystic breast disease), genetic testing may be the most definitive way to make a diagnosis of PHS. It is estimated that 80% of individuals who meet clinical criteria for PHS will have a detectable mutation in the *PTEN* gene. Individuals with macrocephaly and some form of autism also appear to have a higher likelihood of having a *PTEN* mutation and should be offered genetic testing.

4.28.3. CLINICAL FEATURES

PHS is thought to be rare, but is almost certainly underreported. The hallmark features of PHS are the mucocutaneous lesions, particularly on the face, which include trichilemmomas, acral keratoses, papillomatous papules, and mucosal lesions. Individuals with PHS typically have large-sized heads. The macrocephaly (usually dolichocephaly) is typically greater than two standard deviations above the normal head size. Other features of PHS include fibrocystic breast disease, thyroid disease, lipomas, fibromas, and oral mucosal papillomatosis (furrowed or cobblestoned tongue or gums). A subset of individuals with Cockayne syndrome (CS) have *PTEN* mutations. CS displays developmental delay, autism, mental retardation, or adult-onset LDD. LDD is caused by a cerebellar gangliocytoma, which can lead to an altered gait (ataxia), increased intracranial pressure, and seizures.

4.28.4. SYNDROME SUBTYPES

- *Bannayan–Riley–Ruvalcaba (BRR) syndrome*—BRR is characterized by macrocephaly, lipomas, hemangiomata, hamartomas, and develop-mental delay. Children with BRR are usually identified during infancy or early childhood. It is estimated that 60% of children with BRR will have a detectable mutation or deletion in the *PTEN* gene.
- *Proteus syndrome*—Proteus syndrome is characterized by congenital malformations, hamartomatous polyposis, epidermal and connective tissue nevi, and hyperostoses. Between 20–50% of children with proteus or proteus-like syndrome have *PTEN* mutations.

4.28.5. RESOURCES FOR FAMILIES

- PTEN World: www.ptenworld.com
- Cowden Syndrome: A Guide for Patient and Their Families: http://www.uihealthcare.org/2column.aspx?id=22923
- Bannayan-Ruvalcaba-Riley syndrome: http://www.uihealthcare.org/2column.aspx?id=22904

4.29. RENAL CELL CARCINOMA, HEREDITARY PAPILLARY

Frequency: Rare
Inheritance: AD
Genes: *MET* at 7q31
Gene test: Clinically available

4.29.1. CANCER RISKS

Individuals with hereditary papillary renal cell carcinoma (HPRCC) syndrome have lifetime risks of kidney cancer that approach 100%. The kidney cancers that occur in HPRCC are type I papillary renal cell carcinomas. Benign papillary renal adenomas have also been reported.

Other possible associated features of HPRCC include carcinomas of the stomach, rectum, lung, pancreas, and bile duct.

4.29.2. DIAGNOSTIC CRITERIA

There are no formally agreed-upon clinical criteria for HPRCC, but candidates for genetic analysis of the *MET* proto-oncogene include:

- An individual with bilateral and multifocal type I papillary renal cell carcinoma even in the absence of additional family history.
- An individual with a single or multifocal papillary renal cell carcinoma, type I plus a first- or second-degree relative diagnosed with renal cell carcinoma, type I.

4.29.3. CLINICAL FEATURES

Individuals with HPRCC can develop the distinctive papillary renal cell carcinomas from ages 19 to 80, but typically occur between ages 35 and 55. It may turn out that the HPRCC-associated carcinomas arise primarily from the papillary renal adenomas, which are also an established feature of the syndrome.

4.29.4. SYNDROME SUBTYPES

None.

4.29.5. RESOURCES FOR FAMILIES

- Information about Papillary Renal Cell Carcinoma: http://www. atlasgeneticsoncology.org/Tumors/kidney5003.html
- Information about HPRCC: http://www.cancer.net/patient/cancer +types/hereditary+papillary+renal+cell+carcinoma
- Kidney Cancer Association: www.KidneyCancer.org

4.30. RETINOBLASTOMA, HEREDITARY

Frequency: From 1 in 13,500 to 1 in 20,000 total cases of retinoblastoma (RB; about 40% of cases are hereditary)
Inheritance: AD
Genes: *RB1* at 13q14
Gene test: Clinically available

4.30.1. CANCER RISKS

At least 90% of children with familial RB will develop either unilateral or bilateral tumors in the developing retina. Affected children who develop pinealoblastoma (a tumor in the pineal gland behind the eye) are said to have trilateral RB.

Individuals with hereditary RB have about a 26% likelihood of developing a second primary cancer and the risk may be more than 50% in those who received radiation therapy. Osteosarcomas are the most frequent second cancer. Other sarcomas that occur in hereditary RB include chondrosarcomas, fibrosarcomas, rhabdomyosarcomas, and leiomyosarcomas. Additional forms of cancer seen in hereditary RB include leukemia, lymphoma, melanoma, brain tumors, sebaceous carcinomas of the eyelid, and malignant phyllodes tumors. Individuals with hereditary RB who smoke cigarettes appear to have increased risks of lung and bladder cancer.

Associated benign tumors include retinomas, other benign retinal tumors, and lipomas.

4.30.2. DIAGNOSTIC CRITERIA

An individual meets clinical criteria for hereditary RB if at least one of the following criteria is met:

- Bilateral RB
- Unilateral RB plus a positive family history
- RB (unilateral or bilateral) plus a second primary cancer

All children who are diagnosed with RB should be offered genetic testing.

It is estimated that 90% of individuals with hereditary RB will be found to have a detectable mutation or deletion in the *RB1* gene. Genetic testing involves the analysis of the *RB1* alleles in blood and tumor specimens.

It is estimated that 60% of RB cases are unilateral and nonhereditary, 15% of cases are unilateral and hereditary, and 25% of cases are bilateral and hereditary. It is not uncommon for children with RB to have negative family histories, because up to one-third of cases are due to *de novo* mutations.

The estimated risks of RB for children, given the following conditions:

- If parent has unilateral RB and no family history: 2–6%
- If parent has bilateral RB regardless of family history: 40%
- If sibling has RB tumor and positive family history: 40%

The estimated risks of RB for siblings, given the following conditions:

- If sibling has unilateral RB and no family history: 3%
- If sibling has bilateral RB and no family history: 2–10%
- If sibling has RB tumor and positive family history: 40%

4.30.3. CLINICAL FEATURES

RB is a malignant tumor of the developing retina. The average age of diagnosis is 24 months for unilateral cases of RB and 15 months for bilateral cases. It is rare for a child to be diagnosed with RB after the age of 5. Children may first present with a "cat's eye reflex," which is a white spot (leukoria) or with eye problems, such as strabismus.

Dr. Knudsen used the two forms of RB (familial and sporadic) to demonstrate the important two-hit model of carcinogenesis. (See Section 3.2.2 for a description of this model.)

4.30.4. SYNDROME SUBTYPES

- *13q deletion syndrome*—About 5–7% of children with hereditary RB will have 13q deletion syndrome. In addition to developing RB tumors, affected children may also have developmental delay, birth defects, and distinctive facial features.

- *Low penetrant RB*—A small percentage of hereditary RB families have a milder phenotype, with the associated risks of RB being about 25% rather than the more typical 90%. Affected children are also more likely to develop unilateral than bilateral RBs.

4.30.5. RESOURCES FOR FAMILIES

- Canadian Retinoblastoma Society: http://www.rbsociety.ca
- Retinoblastoma International: http://www.retinoblastoma.net
- The United Kingdom Childhood Eye Cancer Trust: http://www.chect.org.uk

4.31. ROTHMUND–THOMSON SYNDROME

Frequency: Rare
Inheritance: Autosomal recessive
Genes: *RECQL4* at 8q24.3
Gene test: Clinically available

4.31.1. CANCER RISKS

Individuals with Rothmund–Thomson syndrome (RTS) have an estimated 32% risk of developing osteosarcoma. In one series of RTS patients, the median age of developing osteosarcoma was 11.5 years (range 4–41 years).

There is also a 5% risk of developing some type of skin cancer, such as squamous cell carcinoma, BCC, spindle cell carcinoma, and Bowen disease.

Benign skin lesions are also associated features of RTS, including actinic keratoses, warty dyskeratosis, and poikiloderma.

Additional malignancies include tongue cancer and acute myelogenous leukemia. Cases of aplastic anemia have also been reported. Affected children may also develop aplastic anemia, progressive leukopenia, or myelodysplasia.

4.31.2. DIAGNOSTIC CRITERIA

The diagnosis of RTS is based on clinical findings, particularly the presence of the characteristic sun-sensitive rash. This rash appears as redness (erythema), swelling, and blistering on the face and typically spreads to the buttocks and extremities. The typical age for the rash to appear is between 3 and 6 months of age (range is from birth to 24 months).

Children are said to have "probable RTS" if their rashes are atypical, but they have at least two of the following features:

- Poikiloderma (telangiectasias, reticulated pigmentation, punctate dermal atrophy)
- Sparse hair, eyelashes, eyebrows
- Small stature
- Skeletal and dental abnormalities
- Cataracts
- Osteosarcoma (or other associated cancer)

About two-thirds of children with features of RTS will be found to have a detectable mutation in the *RECQL4* gene.

4.31.3. CLINICAL FEATURES

Only a small number of individuals have been identified with this rare condition. In addition to the characteristic rash, children with RTS may also exhibit small stature, skeletal abnormalities, dental problems, cataracts, and/or sparse hair on their scalps, eyebrows, and eyelashes. There is also a higher incidence of infertility among affected individuals.

4.31.4. SYNDROME SUBTYPES

None.

4.31.5. RESOURCES FOR FAMILIES

- Rothmund-Thomson Syndrome (RTS) Place: http://www.rtsplace.org
- Rothmund-Thomson Syndrome on-line support group: http://www.mdjunction.com/rothmund-thomson-syndrome

4.32. TUBEROUS SCLEROSIS COMPLEX (TSC)

Frequency:	1 in 5800 live births
Inheritance:	AD
Genes:	*TSC1* at 9q34
	TSC2 at 16p13.3
Gene test:	Clinically available

4.32.1. CANCER RISKS

TSC is characterized by the presence of multiple, rare benign and malignant lesions. Individuals with TSC have a 6–14% risk of childhood brain tumors, most of which are subependymal giant cell astrocytomas. There is also a 2–5% risk of clear cell, papillary, or chromophobe renal cell carcinomas. Childhood cases of renal cell carcinoma have been reported, although the average age of onset is 28 years. Individuals with TSC may also develop malignant angiomyolipomas though cases are rare.

Malignancies that may be associated with TSC include WT, Hurthle cell thyroid carcinoma, chordomas, or pancreatic islet cell tumors. Over half of the children with TSC are born with cardiac rhabdomyomas, although these benign tumors usually regress after birth.

TSC is associated with multiple benign lesions involving the skin, brain, kidneys, heart, lungs, and endocrine system. These lesions include:

- *Skin*—shagreen patch (skin plaques), acrochordons, facial angiofibromas, ungual fibromas (papules)
- *Brain*—Childhood brain tumors, including cortical and subcortical tubers (glial hamartomas), subependymal glial nodules
- *Eye*—retinal hamartomas or acromic patches
- *Kidney*—renal lipomas, angiomyolipomas, ococytomas, multiple cysts
- *Pancreas*—adenomas
- *Heart*—cardiac rhabdomyomas
- *Lungs*—lymphangiomyomatosis (LAM) of the lung
- *Endocrine system*—PGL, adrenal angiomyolipomas, adenomas of parathyroid and adrenal gland

4.32.2. DIAGNOSTIC CRITERIA

The diagnostic criteria for TSC are as follows:
Major features:

- Facial angiofibromas or forehead plaque
- Nontraumatic ungula or periungual fibromas
- Hypomelanotic macules (three or more)
- Shagreen patch
- Multiple retinal nodular hamartomas
- Cortical tuber
- Subependymal nodule
- Subependymal giant cell astrocytoma
- Cardiac rhabdomyoma, single or multiple
- LAM
- Renal angiomyolipoma

Minor features:

- Multiple randomly distributed pits in dental enamel
- Hamartomatous rectal polyps
- Bone cysts
- Cerebral white matter radial migration lines
- Gingival fibromas
- Nonrenal hamartoma
- Retinal achromic patch

- "Confetti" skin lesions
- Multiple renal cysts

Definite TSC: Two major features or one major feature plus two minor features

Probable TSC: One major feature plus one minor feature

Possible TSC: One major feature or two or more minor features

About 80% of individuals who meet clinical criteria for TSC are found to have mutations in the *TS* gene. More than 60% of TSC cases are due to *de novo* mutations. It is worth noting that up to one-quarter of TSC cases represent cases of somatic mosaicism, which is associated with a milder phenotype.

4.32.3. CLINICAL FEATURES

Almost all children with TSC develop some type of benign lesions involving their kidneys, brains, and skin. Children may also develop permanent teeth that have multiple enamel pits. Cognitive and behavioral problems are common among children with TSC. At least 80% of children have seizures and about 50% will have severe learning disabilities, hyperactivity, and/or autism.

4.32.4. SYNDROME SUBTYPES

- *Tuberous sclerosis (TS)/polycystic kidney disease (PKD) contiguous gene syndrome*—A small subset of children with TSC will also be found to have infantile severe polycystic kidney disease. These children have a contiguous gene syndrome involving the *TSC2* and *PKD1* genes, which lie next to each other on chromosome 16. To date, all cases of TS/PKD contiguous gene syndrome have been caused by *de novo* deletions.

4.32.5. RESOURCES FOR FAMILIES

- Tuberous Sclerosis Alliance: http://www.tsalliance.org
- Tuberous Sclerosis Association (UK): http://www.tuberous-sclerosis.org
- Tuberous Sclerosis Canada: http://www.tscanada.ca

4.33. Von Hippel Lindau Syndrome

Frequency: 1 in 36,000
Inheritance: AD
Genes: *VHL* at 3p25
Gene test: Clinically available

4.33.1. Cancer Risks

Individuals with VHL are at increased risk for developing clear cell renal cell carcinomas. The incidence of renal cell carcinoma in VHL is between 25% and 40% and the mean age of onset is about 40 years (range: 16–69 years). Individuals with VHL also have about a 7–25% risk of developing islet cell tumors of the pancreas; these pancreatic tumors occur in a subset of VHL families, suggesting that they may only occur with certain mutations. Carcinoid tumors have also been reported in families with VHL.

Individuals with VHL are also at risk for developing tumors involving their eyes and ears. About 70% of individuals with VHL develop retinal angiomas, which are benign tumors that can compromise vision. The average age of onset for retinal angiomas is 21–28 years, but childhood cases can also occur. Endolymphatic sac tumors (ELSTs), which are papillary adenocarcinomas of the inner ear, occur in about 10–15% of individuals with VHL and can cause significant hearing loss as well as vertigo and tinnitus.

PCCs are rare adrenal gland tumors that occur in 3–17% of individuals with VHL. PCCs are typically benign tumors that secrete catecholamines, triggering high blood pressure, heart palpitations, and increased risks of stroke. Malignant PCCs can also occur. PGLs, which are extra-adrenal gland tumors, have also been reported in people with VHL.

Men with VHL may develop epididymal cystadenomas and women with VHL may develop cystadenomas of the broad ligaments (of the uterus).

Hemangioblastomas are pathognomonic characteristics of VHL. Individuals with VHL may develop one or more hemangioblastomas in the cerebellum or spine with about 80% occurring in the cerebellum. Although hemangioblastomas are benign tumors, they can cause significant morbidity given their location.

One of the characteristic features of VHL is the development of cysts and benign tumors (adenomas or angiomas) in the kidney, liver, pancreas, spleen, and (rarely) the adrenal gland.

4.33.2. Diagnostic Criteria

The clinical criteria of VHL are as follows:

- An individual, with no family history of VHL, who presents with two or more characteristic lesions of VHL, which are defined as two hemangioblastomas of the retina or brain or a single hemangioblastoma in association with one of the following: a kidney or pancreatic cyst; renal cell carcinoma; adrenal or extra-adrenal PCC, ELST, papillary cystadenoma of the epididymis or broad ligament, or neuroendocrine tumors of the pancreas.

- An individual, with a positive family history of VHL, who has at least one of the following characteristic lesions of VHL: retinal angioma, spinal or cerebellar hemangioblastoma, PCC, multiple pancreatic cysts, epididymal or broad ligament cystadenomas, multiple renal cysts, or renal cell carcinomas before age 60.

Nearly all people who meet clinical criteria for VHL are found to have a mutation or deletion in the *VHL* gene. About 20% of cases are *de novo* and cases of somatic mosaicism have also been reported. VHL was originally described by a physician in the Black Forest region of Germany and there is a German founder mutation involving codon 169 (tyr to his).

It is estimated that 10–15% of people with ELSTs will be found to have a mutation in the VHL gene.

4.33.3. Clinical Features

VHL is often diagnosed in early adulthood, although childhood symptoms (usually retinal angiomas) can occur. VHL has a wide expressivity with some people severely affected and others with only mild symptoms of the disorder. However, almost all individuals with VHL will manifest at least one of the characteristic lesions or cysts by age 65. The leading causes of death in VHL are from either the hemangioblastomas or kidney cancer.

4.33.4. Syndrome Subtypes

VHL is sometimes divided into two main subtypes:

- *VHL, type 1*—Individuals with VHL, type 1 rarely develop PCCs, but they do develop the other manifestations of VHL. VHL, type 1 is caused by truncating mutations or missense mutations that do not disrupt the folding of the VHL protein.
- *VHL, type 2*—Individuals with VHL, type 2 are at high risk for developing PCCs as well as the other features of VHL. VHL, type 2 can be further divided into the following three subgroups:
    - *VHL, type 2A*—Individuals with VHL, type 2A are at high risk for developing PCCs, but have lower risks of renal cell carcinomas.

- *VHL, type 2B*—Individuals with VHL, type 2B are at high risk for developing PCCs and are at high risk for developing renal cell carcinomas.
- *VHL, type 2C*—By definition, individuals with VHL, type 2C develop PCCs, but do not develop renal cell carcinomas.

4.33.5. RESOURCES FOR FAMILIES

- VHL Family Alliance: http://www.vhl.org
- VHL National and International Support Groups: www.vhl.org/support/intlsprt.php

4.34. WERNER SYNDROME (ALSO TERMED PROGERIA OF THE ADULT)

Frequency: From 1 in 50,000 to 1 in 1,000,000 in the general population
               From 1 in 20,000 to 1 in 40,000 in Japan
Inheritance: Autosomal recessive
Genes: *WRN* at 8p12-p11.2
Gene test: Available on a research basis only

4.34.1. CANCER RISKS

Associated cancers include soft tissue sarcomas, osteosarcomas, melanomas, nonmedullary thyroid cancer, and hematologic malignancies. The thyroid cancers can be follicular, papillary, or anaplastic subtypes. Many of the associated melanomas are a subtype termed acral lentiginous melanomas, which typically occur on the soles of the feet or in the nasal mucosa.

Additional malignancies that may be associated with Werner syndrome (WS) include meningiomas and gastric, breast, liver (hepatocellular), and bile duct cancers.

4.34.2. DIAGNOSTIC CRITERIA

The clinical criteria of WS are as follows:
  Cardinal signs of WS (onset over age 10):

- Bilateral ocular cataracts
- Characteristic skin (including tight skin, atrophic skin, pigmentary alterations, ulceration, hyperkeratosis, and regional subcutaneous atrophy)
- Characteristic facies (e.g., pinched nasal bridge that gives the person a "bird-like" appearance)

- Short stature
- Premature graying and/or thinning of scalp hair
- Parental consanguinity or affected sibling

Additional signs of WS:

- Type 2 diabetes mellitus
- Hypogonadism
- Osteoporosis
- Radiographic evidence of osteosclerosis of distal phalanges of fingers or toes
- Soft-tissue calcification
- Evidence of premature atherosclerosis (e.g., history of myocardial infarction)
- Neoplasms (including soft tissue sarcomas, osteosarcomas, and melanomas)
- Abnormal voice (high-pitched, squeaky or hoarse)
- Flat feet

Definite diagnosis: All cardinal signs plus any two additional signs

Probable diagnosis: First three cardinal signs plus any two other signs

Possible diagnosis: Cataracts or dermatologic findings plus any four other signs

About 90% of individuals who have a definite diagnosis of WS by clinical criteria are found to have mutations in the *WRN* gene. One *WRN* founder mutation termed IVS 25-1G > C accounts for 60% of cases in Japan.

Individuals with probable or possible diagnoses of WS have lower likelihoods of positive genetic test results, although genetic testing may be useful in sorting out the diagnosis.

4.34.3. Clinical Features

Following a normal childhood, individuals with WS develop multiple "old age" complaints in their twenties or thirties. The median age of diagnosis is 38 and the average lifespan in WS is age 54. The main causes of death are myocardial infarctions and cancer. Malignancies tend to develop between the ages of 25 and 64 years.

Other features associated with WS include ocular cataracts, premature graying hair and/or balding, decreased muscle mass, osteoporosis of the long bones, arteriosclerosis, scleroderma, skin ulcers, endocrine failure, type 2 diabetes, and reduced fertility. Interestingly, children who manifest any of these symptoms before age 10 are unlikely to have WS. The earliest sign of WS (often noted retrospectively) may be the lack of growth during puberty.

4.34.4. SYNDROME SUBTYPES

None.

4.34.5. RESOURCES FOR FAMILIES

- International Registry of Werner Syndrome: http://www.wernersyn drome.org/registry/registry.html
- The Werner Syndrome Support Group: http://www.MDJunction. com/werner-syndrome

4.35. WILMS TUMOR, FAMILIAL (INCLUDES DENYS-DRASH SYNDROME, FRASIER SYNDROME, WAGR SYNDROME)

Frequency:	1 in 10,000 annual cases of WT
	Fewer than 5% of cases are familial
Inheritance:	AD
Genes:	WT1 at 11p13
	WT2 (BWS) at 11p15.5
	WT3 localized to 16q
	FWT1 localized to 17q12-q21
	FWT2 localized to 19q
	WT5 localized to 7p11.2-p15
Gene test:	WT1 testing is clinically available

4.35.1. CANCER RISKS

WT arises from an embryonal stem cell in the kidney and is sometimes referred to as a nephroblastoma. In familial WT, 5–10% of the kidney tumors are bilateral.

Second primary tumors are rare in familial WT. If they occur, it is likely caused by the chemotherapy and radiation treatments more than the underlying genotype.

In terms of benign lesions, children with familial WT may have nephrogenic rests (benign foci of embryond kidney cells), which are thought to be precursors for WT.

4.35.2. DIAGNOSTIC CRITERIA

Bilateral cases of WT are assumed to represent familial cases. Unilateral cases of WT are diagnosed as familial if there is either:

- A positive family history of the disorder. About 1–2% of affected children have a family history of WT.
- The presence of features associated with Drash syndrome or WAGR (Wilms tumor, aniridia, genitourinary anomalies, and mental retardation) syndrome (see subtypes). About 2–3% of children with WT have one of these two syndromes.

Less than 5% of isolated WT cases are found to have a *WT1* mutation. The likelihood of a positive *WT1* result may be as high as 30% if the child has bilateral or multifocal disease and the child was diagnosed at a younger age (age 1 vs. age 4). Most germline *WT1* mutations represent *de novo* cases.

The *WT2* gene comprises a small region of the *BWS* gene, which causes BWS. Not surprisingly, children with BWS are at increased risk to develop WT.

Non-syndromic cases of WT are often due to a genetic imprinting error involving chromosomal region 11p15. (See Section for more information about this mechanism.)

4.35.3. CLINICAL FEATURES

WT is the most common solid tumor in childhood. About 5–10% of cases are bilateral or multifocal tumors. The average age of diagnosis for unilateral WT cases is 42–47 months and the average age of diagnosis for bilateral cases is 30–33 months.

4.35.4. SYNDROME SUBTYPES

- *Denys-Drash syndrome (DDS)*—DDS is characterized by the undermasculinization of external genitalia in a chromosomally female (46, XX) infant. Affected children have ambiguous to normal-appearing female genitalia and diffuse mesangial sclerosis, which can cause early-onset renal failure. Urinary tract malformations are also common. Children with DDS have greater than 90% risks of developing WT.
- *Frasier syndrome (FS)*—FS is characterized by the undermasculinization of external genitalia in a chromosomally male (46, XY) infant. Affected children have ambiguous to normal-appearing female genitalia and focal segmental glomerulosclerosis. Cases of WT and gonadoblastoma have been reported in children with FS.
- *WAGR syndrome*—The following features are associated with WAGR syndrome: WT, aniridia (absence of the iris), genitourinary abnormalities, and mental retardation. WAGR syndrome, an example of a contiguous gene syndrome, is caused by a large 11p deletion (that includes the 11p13 region). Children with 11p13 deletions have an estimated 40–50% risk of developing WT. The risk of bilateral disease is higher in WAGR syndrome than in familial WT, possibly because of the high number of nephrogenic rests, which are present in affected children.

4.35.5. Resources for Families

- National Wilms Tumor Study: http://www.nwtsg.org
- Wilms Tumour dot com: http://www.wilmstumour.com

4.36. Xeroderma Pigmentosum (Includes XP/CS Complex, XP Variant)

Frequency:	1 in 1,000,000 (United States)
	1 in 22,000–40,000 (Japan)
Inheritance:	Autosomal recessive
Genes:	*XPA* at 9q22.3
	XPB (ERCC3) at 2q21
	XPC at 3p25.1
	XPD (ERCC2) at 19q13.2
	XPE (DDB2) at 11p12-p11
	XPF (ERCC4) at 16p13.3-p13.13
	XPG (ERCC5) at 13q33
	XP-V (POLH) at 6p21.1-p12
Gene test:	*XPA* and *XPC* testing are clinically available

4.36.1. Cancer Risks

Individuals with xeroderma pigmentosum (XP) have astonishingly high rates of skin cancer, which include BCCs, squamous cell carcinomas, and melanomas. Affected individuals are estimated to have a 1000-fold increased risk for developing a cutaneous malignancy and the initial skin cancer diagnosis often occurs under age 10. Individuals with XP typically develop multiple skin cancers over their lifetime.

Malignancies of the eye and mouth are also common in XP. These neoplasms include ocular melanoma, squamous cell carcinoma of the eye, ephithelioma of the eyelid, squamous cell carcinoma of the tongue, and other cancers of the oral cavity.

Affected individuals may also have 10- to 20-fold increased risks for developing internal malignancies. In addition, lung cancer rates appear to be increased in people with XP, especially if they smoke cigarettes.

Leukemia, brain tumors (especially gliomas), and cancers of the uterus, breast, stomach, kidney and testes may also be associated features of XP.

The benign tumors associated with XP include conjunctival papilloma, actinic keratosis, keratoacanthoma, angioma, fibroma, telangietasia, and epithelioma of the eyelid.

4.36.2. Diagnostic Criteria

The clinical diagnosis of XP is based on the following skin and eye characteristics:

- *Skin manifestations*—include xerosis (dry skin), poikiloderma (reddish or brown mottled pigmentation), marked freckling prior to age 2, and the development of severe sunburns, blisters, or rashes despite minimal sun exposure. These characteristic skin changes are present in about 50% of individuals with XP by 18 months and about 95% of individuals by age 15. In some people with XP, the primary skin manifestation is the onset of multiple skin cancers during childhood.

- *Eye manifestations*—include cataracts, photophobia, keratitis, loss of eye lashes, and atrophy of the eye lids. The ocular problems occur in the portion of the eye that is exposed to ultraviolet light (i.e., the conjunctiva and cornea) rather than the retina, which is protected from ultraviolet light.

About one-third of individuals with XP also have acquired microcephaly or another abnormality of the central nervous system.

The *XP* genes are involved in nucleotide excision repair, which is the primary mechanism for repairing genetic damage caused by exposure to ultraviolet radiation. About 50% of XP cases are found to have two abnormal copies of either the *XPA* or *XPC* gene.

4.36.3. CLINICAL FEATURES

The diagnosis of XP is often made by age 18 based on the characteristic skin and eye findings. Symptoms—such as severe freckling, blistering, and irregular pigmentation—indicate an abnormal sensitivity to ultraviolet radiation. Individuals with XP have chronic dermatologic problems and need to be vigilant about avoiding sun exposure. Vision problems and cognitive impairments are also common. About 30% of individuals with XP have mild to severe neurological problems, including diminished deep tendon reflexes, progressive hearing loss, mental retardation, microcephaly, and spasticity.

4.36.4. SYNDROME SUBTYPES

- *Cerebro-oculo-facial-skeletal syndrome (COFS)*—COFS is characterized by progressive neurological impairments, microcephaly, intracranial calcifications, ocular anomalies (microcornea, optic atrophy, cataracts), joint contractures, and growth failure. Individuals with COFS may also have high sensitivities to UV radiation, and, therefore, they may be at increased risk for developing skin, eye, and oral cancers. Some individuals with COFS have germline mutations in the *ERCC2* and *ERCC5* genes.

- *XP/CS complex*—Children with XP/CS complex have features of both XP and Cockayne syndrome (CS). This condition is also referred to as "XP with neurological disease." Affected children have the high risks of skin cancer associated with XP as well as the features of CS that include dwarfism, microcephaly, progressive neurological abnormalities (including spasticity and ataxia), mental retardation, retinal degeneration hypogonadism, and a premature aged appearance. Affected individuals do not seem to have the increased risk of internal organ cancer that is typically associated with XP, nor do they have the skeletal dysplasia seen in CS. Individuals with XP/CS complex have mutations or deletions involving the *XPB (ERCC3)*, *XPD (ERCC2)*, or *XPG (ERCC5)* genes.

- *XP/Trichothiodystrophy (TDD) syndrome*—XP/TDD syndrome is characterized by mental retardation, sulfur-deficient brittle hair, and ichthyosis. Individuals with XP/TDD may also have high sensitivities to UV radiation, and, therefore, they may be at high risk for developing skin, eye, and oral cancers. Some individuals with XP/TDD syndrome have germline mutations in the *ERCC2* and *ERCC3* genes.

- *XP Variant*—Children with the XP Variant subtype are still at increased risk for developing skin cancers and eye problems, but they tend to develop fewer cancers and the onset of disease typically occurs at older ages (e.g., the third decade of life rather than childhood). Neurological abnormalities are rare in children with XP Variant. Children with XP Variant have a defect in the *XPV (POLH)* gene. This condition was once termed pigmented xerodermoid.

4.36.5. RESOURCES FOR FAMILIES

- Xeroderma Pigmentosum Society: http://www.xps.org
- XP Family Support Group: http://www.xpfamilysupportgroup.org
- Xeroderma Pigmentosum Support Group (UK): http://joomla.xpsupportgroup.org.uk

4.37. FURTHER READING

Aarnio, M, Sankila, R, Pukkala, E, et al. 1999. Cancer risk in mutation carriers of DNA-mismatch-repair genes. Int J Cancer 81:214–218.

Agarwal, R, and Robson, M. 2009. Inherited predisposition to gastrointestinal stromal tumor. Hematol Oncol Clin North Am 23:1–13.

Alter, BP. 2003. Cancer in Fanconi anemia, 1927–2001. Cancer 97:425–440.

Alter, BP, Rosenberg, PS, and Brody, LC. 2007. Clinical and molecular features associated with biallelic mutations in FANCD1/BRCA2. J Med Genet 44:1–9.

Amos, CI, Frazier, ML, and McGarrity, TJ. 2007. Peutz-Jeghers syndrome. Gene Reviews. http://www.genetests.org.

Aretz, S, Koch, A, Uhlhaas, S, et al. 2006. Should children at risk for familial adenomatous polyposis be screened for hepatoblastoma and children with apparently sporadic hepatoblastoma be screened for APC germline mutations? Pediatr Blood Cancer 47:811–818.

Aretz, A, Stienen, D, Uhlhaus, S, et al. 2007. High proportion of large genomic deletions and geneotype phenotype update in 80 unrelated families with juvenile polyposis syndrome. J Med Genet 44:702–709.

Asthagiri, AR, Parry, DM, Butman, JA, et al. 2009. Neurofibromatosis type 2. Lancet 373:1974–1986.

Attard, TM, Giglio, P, Koppula, S, et al. 2007. Brain tumors in individuals with familial adenomatous polyposis: a cancer registry experience and pooled case report analysis. Cancer 109:761–766.

Ball, SE, McGuckin, CP, Jenkins, G, et al. 1996. Diamond-Blackfan anaemia in the U.K.: analysis of 80 cases from a 20-year birth cohort. Br J Haematol 94:645–653.

Baser, ME, Kuramoto, L, Joe, H, et al. 2004. Genotype-phenotype correlation for nervous system tumors in neurofibromatosis 2: a population-based study. Am J Hum Genet 75:231–239.

Beech, DJ. 2004. Genetics of Multiple Endocrine Neoplasia. In Ellis, CN, Jr. (ed), Inherited Cancer Syndromes: Current Clinical Management. Springer-Verlag, New York.

Biasco, G, Velo, D, Angriman, I, et al. 2009. Gastrointestinal stromal tumors: report of an audit and review of the literature. Eur J Cancer Prev 18:106–116.

Birch, JM, Hartley, AL, Tricker, KJ, et al. 1994. Prevalence and diversity of constitutional mutations in the p53 gene among 21 Li-Fraumeni families. Cancer Res 54:1298–1304.

Bleesing, JJH, Johnson, J, and Zhang, K. 2007. Autoimmune lymphoproliferative syndrome. Gene Reviews. http://www.genetests.org.

Boikos, SA, and Stratakis, CA. 2007. Carney complex: the first 20 years. Curr Opin Oncol 19:24–29.

Burt, RW, and Jasperson, KW. 2008. APC-associated polyposis conditions. Gene Reviews. http://www.genetests.org.

Chow, E, and Macrae, F. 2005. A review of juvenile polyposis syndrome. J Gastroenterol Hepatol 20:1634–1640.

Cleaver, JE. 2005. Cancer in xeroderma pigmentosum and related disorders of DNA repair. Nat Rev Cancer 5:564–573.

Coleman, JA, and Russo, P. 2009. Hereditary and familial kidney cancer. Curr Opin Urol 19:478–485.

Croitoru, ME, Cleary, ZSP, Di Nicola, N, et al. 2005. Association between biallelic and monoallelic germline MYH gene mutations and colorectal cancer risk. JNCI 96:1631–1634.

Curatolo, P, Bombardieri, R, and Jozwiak, S. 2008. Tuberous sclerosis. Lancet 372:657–668.

Czene, K, and Hemminki, K. 2003. Familial papillary renal cell tumors and subsequent cancers: a nationwide epidemiological study from Sweden. J Urol 169:1271–1275.

Daly, MB, Axilbund, JE, Bryant, E, et al. 2006. Genetic/familial high-risk assessment: breast and ovarian cancer. J Natl Compr Canc Netw 4:156–176.

Dome, JS, and Huff, V. 2006. Wilms tumor overview. Gene Reviews. http://www.genetests.org.

Ellis, CN, Jr. 2004. Polyposis syndromes. In Ellis, CN, Jr. (ed), Inherited Cancer Syndromes: Current Clinical Management. Springer-Verlag, New York.

Eng, C. 2004. Cowden syndrome. In Eeles, RA, Easton, DF, Ponder, BAJ, and Eng, C (eds), Genetic Predisposition to Cancer, 2nd edition. Arnold Publishers, London, UK, 155–166.

Ertem, D, Acar, Y, Kotiloglu, E, et al. 2001. Blue rubber bleb nevus syndrome. Pediatrics 107:418–421.

Evans, DG. 2006. Neurofibromatosis 2. Gene Reviews. http://www.genetests.org.

Falchetti, A, Marini, F, and Brandi, ML. 2005. Multiple endocrine neoplasia type 1. Gene Reviews. http://www.genetests.org.

Ferner, RE, Huson, SM, Thomas, N, et al. 2007. Guidelines for the diagnosis and management of individuals with neurofibromatosis 1. J Med Genet 44:81–88.

Fishman, SJ, Smithers, CJ, Folkman, J, et al. 2005. Blue rubber bleb nevus syndrome. Surgical eradication of gastrointestinal bleeding. Ann Surg 241:253–528.

Friedman, JM. 2007. Neurofibromatosis 1. Gene Reviews. http://www.genetests.org.

Gazda, H, Grawbowska, A, Merida-Long, LB, et al. 2006. Ribosomal protein S24 gene is mutated in Diamond-Blackfan anemia. Am J Hum Genet 79:1110–1118.

Giardiello, RM, and Trimbath, JD. 2006. Peutz-Jeghers syndrome and management recommendations. Clin Gastroenterol Hepatal 4:408–415.

Glasock, JM, and Carty, S. 2002. Multiple endocrine neoplasia type I: fresh perspective on clinical features and penetrance. Surg Oncol 11:143–150.

Goldstein, AM, Struewing, JP, Fraser, MC, et al. 2004. Prospective risk of cancer in CDKN2A germline mutation carriers. J Med Genet 41:421–424.

Gonzalez, KD, Noltner, KA, Buzin, CH, et al. 2009. Beyond Li Fraumeni syndrome: clinical characteristics of families with p53 germline mutations. J Clin Oncol 27:1250–1256.

Gorlin, RJ. 2004. Gorlin syndrome. Genet Med 6:530–539.

Goto, M, Miller, RW, Ishikawa, Y, et al. 1996. Excess of rare cancers in Werner syndrome (adult progeria). Cancer Epidemiol Biomarkers Prev 5:239–246.

Greer, KJ, Kirkpatrick, SJ, Weksberg, R, et al. 2008. Beckwith-Wiedemann syndrome in adults: clinical observations from one family and recommendations for care. Am J Med Genet A 146A:1707–1712.

Haidle, JL, and Howe, JR. 2008. Juvenile polyposis syndrome. Gene Reviews. http://www.genetests.org.

Hansson, J. 2008. Familial melanoma. Surg Clin North Am 88:897–916.

Hearle, NC, Schumacher, V, Menko, FH, et al. 2006. Frequency and spectrum of cancers in the Peutz-Jeghers syndrome. Clin Cancer Res 2:3209–3215.

Hobart, JA, and Eng, C. 2009. PTEN hamartoma tumor syndrome: an overview. Genet Med 11:687–694.

Holman, JD, and Dyer, JA. 2007. Genodermatoses with malignant potential. Curr Opin Pediatr 19:446–454.

Jimenez, C, Cote, G, Arnold, A, et al. 2006. Review: should patients with apparently sporadic pheochromocytomas or paragangliomas be screened for hereditary syndromes? J Clin Endocrinol Metab 91:2851–2858.

Karurah, P, MacMillan, A, Byd, N, et al. 2007. Founder and recurrent CDH1 mutations in families with hereditary diffuse gastric cancer. JAMA 297:2360–2372.

Kaurah, P, and Huntsman, DG. 2006. Hereditary diffuse gastric cancer. Gene Reviews. http://www.genetests.org.

Kleinerman, RA, Tucker, MA, Tarone, RE, et al. 2005. Risk of new cancers after radio-therapy in long-term survivors of retinoblastoma: an extended follow-up. J Clin Oncol 23:2272–2279.

Kohlmann, W, and Gruber, SB. 2006. Hereditary non-polyposis colon cancer. Gene Reviews. http://www.genetests.org.

Kouvaraki, MA, Shaprio, SE, Perrier, ND, et al. 2005. RET proto-oncogene: a review and uptake of genotype–phenotype correlations in hereditary medullary thyroid cancer and associated endocrine tumors. Thyroid 15:531–544.

Kraemer, KH. 2008. Xeroderma pigmentosum. Gene Reviews. http://www.genetests.org.

Leistritz, DF, Hanson, N, Martin, GM, et al. 2007. Werner syndrome. Gene Reviews. http://www.genetests.org.

Li, FP, and Fraumeni, JF, Jr. 1969. Soft-tissue sarcomas, breast cancer, and other neo-plasms: a familial syndrome? Ann Intern Med 71:747–752.

Lichon, V, and Khachemoune, A. 2007. Xeroderma pigmentosum: beyond skin cancer. J Drugs Dermatol 6:281–288.

Lindor, NM, Jalal, SM, Kumar, S, et al. 2007. Multiple primary tumors associated with chromosome 9p deletion. Am J Med Genet 143:95–97.

Lindor, NM, McMaster, ML, Lindor, CJ, et al. 2008. Concise handbook of familial cancer susceptibility syndromes—second edition. J Natl Cancer Inst Monogr 38:1–93.

Linehan, WM, Pinto, PA, Bratslavsky, G, et al. 2009. Hereditary kidney cancer: unique opportunity for disease-based therapy. Cancer 115:2252–2261.

Lipton, JM, and Ellis, SR. 2009. Diamond-Blackfan anemia: diagnosis, treatment, and molecular pathogenesis. Hematol Oncol Clin North Am 23:261–282.

Lo Muzio, L. 2008. Nevoid basal cell carcinoma syndrome (Gorlin syndrome). Orphanet J Rare Dis 3:32. http://www.ojrd.com/content/3/1/32.

Lohmann, DR, and Gallie, BL. 2007. Retinoblastoma. Gene Reviews. http://www.genetests.org.

Lonser, RR, Glenn, GM, Walther, M, et al. 2003. Von Hippel-Lindau disease. Lancet 361:2059–3067.

Lubbe, SJ, DiBernardo, MC, Chandler, IP, et al. 2009. Clinical implications of the colorectal cancer risk associated with MUTYH mutation. J Clin Oncol 27:3975–3980.

Lynch, HT, Lynch, PM, Lanspa, SJ, et al. 2009. Review of the Lynch syndrome: history, molecular genetic, screening, differential diagnosis, and medicolegal ramifica-tions. Clin Genet 71:1–18.

Marshall, M, and Solomon, S. 2007. Hereditary breast-ovarian cancer: clinical findings and medical management. Plast Surg Nurs 27:124–127.

Masciari, S, Larsson, N, and Senz, J. 2007. Germline E–cadherin mutations in familial lobular breast cancer. J Med Genet 44:726–731.

Mavrou, A, Tsangaris, GT, Roma, E, et al. 2008. The ATM gene and ataxia telangiec-tasia. Anticancer Res 28:401–405.

McWhinney, SR, Pasini, B, and Stratakis, CA. 2007. International Carney Triad and Carney-Stratakis consortium. Familial gastrointestinal stromal tumors and germ-line mutations. NEJM 357:1054–1056.

Muftuoglu, M, Oshima, J, von Kobbe, C, et al. 2008. The clinical characteristics of Werner syndrome: molecular and biochemical diagnosis. 124:369–377.

Nielsen, M, Franken, PF, Reinards, THCM, et al. 2005. Multiplicity in polyp count and extracolonic manifestations in 40 Dutch patients with MYH associated polyposis coli (MAP). J Med Genet 42:e54.

Nielsen, M, Joerink-van de Beld, MC, Jones, N, et al. 2009. Analysis of MUTYH genotypes and colorectal phenotypes in patients with MUTYH-associated polyposis. Gastroenterology 136:471–476.

Nieuwenhuis, MH, and Vasen, HF. 2007. Correlations between mutation site in APC and phenotype of familial adenomatous polyposis (FAP): a review of the literature. Crit Rev Oncol Hematol 67:153–161.

Northrup, H, and Au, KS. 2005. Tuberous sclerosis complex. Gene Reviews. http://www.genetests.org.

Online Mendelian Inheritance in Man, OMIM (TM). McKusick-Nathans Institute of Genetic Medicine, Johns Hopkins University (Baltimore, MD). http://omim.org.

Pasini, B, McWhinney, SR, Bei, T, et al. 2008. Clinical and molecular genetics of patients with the Carney-Stratakis syndrome and germline mutations of the genes coding for the succinate dehydrogenase subunits SDHB, SDHC, and SDHD. Eur J Hum Genet 16:79–88.

Petrucelli, N, Daly, MB, Bars Culver, JO, et al. 2007. Breast cancer. Gene Reviews. http://www.genetests.org.

Piecha, G, Chudek, J, and Wiecek, A. 2008. Multiple endocrine neoplasia type 1. Eur J Intern Med 19:99–103.

Pithukpakorn, M, and Toro, JR. 2007. Hereditary leiomyomatosis and renal cell cancer. Gene Reviews. http://www.genetests.org.

Raue, F, and Frank-Raue, K. 2007. Multiple endocrine neoplasia type 2: 2007 update. Horm Res 68(Suppl. 5):101–104.

Renwick, A, Thompson, D, Seal, S, et al. 2006. ATM mutations that cause A-T are breast cancer susceptibility alleles. Nat Genet 38:873–875.

Roach, ES, Gomez, MR, and Northrup, H. 1998. Tuberous sclerosis complex consensus conference: revised clinical diagnostic criteria. J Child Neurol 13:624–628.

Sanz, M, and German, J. 2006. Bloom's syndrome. Gene Reviews. http://www.genetests.com.

Schimke, RN, Collins, DL, and Stolle, CA. 2007. Von Hippel-Lindau syndrome. Gene Reviews. http://www.genetests.org.

Schmidt, L, Nickerson, ML, Angelan, D, et al. 2004. Early onset hereditary papillary renal carcinoma germline missense mutations in the tyrosine kinase domain of the MET proto-oncogene. J Urol 172:1256–1261.

Schneider, K, and Garber, J. 2010. Li-Fraumeni syndrome. Gene Reviews. http://www.genetests.org.

Scott, RH, Stiller, CA, Walker, L, et al. 2006. Syndrome and constitutional chromosomal abnormalities associated with Wilms tumour. J Med Genet 43:705–715.

Scott, RH, Walker, L, Olsen, OE, et al. 2006. Surveillance for Wilms' tumor in at risk children: pragmatic recommendations for best practice. Arch Dis Child 91:995–999.

Shuman, C, Smith, AC, and Weksberg, R. 2005. Beckwith-Wiedemann syndrome. http://www.genetests.org.

Stein, JL, and Eng, C. 2006. PTEN hamartoma tumor syndrome (PHTS). Gene Reviews. http://www.genetests.org.

Stewart, L, Glenn, GM, Stratton, P, et al. 2009. Association of germline mutations in the fumarate hydratase gene and uterine fibroids in women with hereditary leiomyomatosis and renal cell cancer. Arch Dermatol 144:1584–1592.

Stratakis, C. 2008. Carney complex. Gene Reviews. http://www.genetests.org.

Taylor, SF, Cook, AE, and Leatherbarrow, B. 2006. Review of patients with basal cell nevus syndrome. Ophthal Plast Reconstr Surg 22:259–265.

Timmers, HJ, Gimenez-Roquepio, AP, Mannelli, M, et al. 2009. Clinical aspects of SDHx-related pheochromocytoma an paraganglioma. Endocr Relat Cancer 16:391–400.

Toro, JR. 2008. Birt Hogg Dube syndrome. http://www.genetests.org.

Toro, JR, Wei, MH, Glenn, GM, et al. 2008. BHD mutations, clinical and molecular genetic investigations of Birt-Hogg-Dube syndrome: a new series of 50 families and a review of published reports. J Med Genet 45:321–331.

Toshiyasu, T. 2008. Fanconi anemia. Gene Reviews. http://www.genetests.org.

Umar, A, Boland, CR, Terdiman, JP, et al. 2004. Revised Bethesda guidelines for hereditary nonpolyposis colorectal cancer (Lynch syndrome) and microsatellite instability. JNCI 96:261–268.

Wang, LL, and Plon, SE. 2006. Rothmund-Thomson syndrome. Gene Reviews. http://www.genetests.org.

Wang, LL, Levy, ML, Lewis, RA, et al. 2001. Clinical manifestations in a cohort of 41 Rothmund-Thomson syndrome patients. Am J Med Genet 102:11–17.

Wiesner, GL, and Snow-Bailey, K. 2005. Multiple endocrine neoplasia type 2. Gene Reviews. http://www.genetests.org.

Wilkes, D, McDermott, DA, and Basson, CT. 2005. Clinical phenotypes and molecular genetic mechanisms of Carney complex. Lancet Oncol 6:501–508.

Williams, VC, Lucas, J, Babcock, MA, et al. 2009. Neurofibromatosis type 1 revisited. Pediatrics 123:124–133.

Wong, P, Verselis, SJ, Garber, JE, et al. 2006. Prevalence of early onset colorectal cancer in 397 patients with classic Li-Fraumeni syndrome. Gastroenterology 130:73–79.

Worth, A, Thrasher, AJ, and Gaspar, HB. 2006. Autoimmune lymphoproliferative syndrome: molecular basis of disease and clinical phenotype. Br J Haematol 133:124–140.

Zbar, B, Alvrd, WG, Glenn, G, et al. 2002. Risk of renal and colonic neoplasms and spontaneous pneumothorax in the Birt-Hogg-Dube syndrome. Cancer Epidemiol Biomarkers Prev 11:393–400.

5

ALL ABOUT BREAST CANCER

> We are working hard toward the day when our daughters and nieces will never
> have to hear the words "you have breast cancer."
>
> *(Love and Lindsey, p. 527)*

5.1. OVERVIEW OF BREAST CANCER

This section begins with a description of normal breast anatomy followed
by an overview of risk factors and tumor types.

5.1.1. BASIC ANATOMY OF THE BREAST

The basic anatomy of the normal breast is illustrated in Figure 5.1. The major
components of the breast are presented in the succeeding sections.

5.1.1.1. Breast Tissue

The breast tissue sits on top of the chest muscle extending from the collarbone down to the lower ribs and across the chest from the breastbone to
underneath the armpits. In women, the breast tissue is composed of about
15–20 lobes, which contain the many milk-producing lobules and the systems
of narrow tubules termed ducts. Breast tissue also contains networks of
arteries, veins, nerves, and lymphatics.

Counseling About Cancer, Third Edition. Katherine A. Schneider.
© 2012 Wiley-Blackwell. Published 2012 by John Wiley & Sons, Inc.

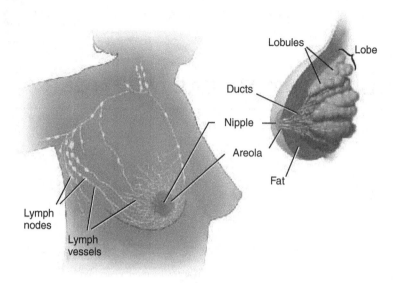

FIGURE 5.1. Normal anatomy of the breast. Source: National Cancer Institute at the National Institute of Health, What you need to know about breast cancer (October 15, 2009, p. 2). http://www.cancer.gov/cancertopics/wyntk/breast/page2.

5.1.1.2. Connective and Fibrous Tissue

The breast tissue is held together on a sturdy grid of fibrous and connective tissue. These supporting tissues are called stroma. The layers of stroma and fat protect the lobules and ducts.

5.1.1.3. Ducts

The ducts are thin hollow tubules that transport milk to the nipples in a lactating woman. Resembling spokes on a wheel, the ducts branch into thousands of terminal buds that contain the lobules. In females, the breast ductal system first develops during puberty and it remains dynamic in response to fluctuations in hormone levels during the monthly menstrual cycles and pregnancy.

5.1.1.4. Fat

Protective layers of fat and breast tissue surround the milk ducts and lobules. In an average-sized woman, about one-third of the breast is composed of fat. As women age, the amount of breast tissue decreases and the amount of breast fat increases.

5.1.1.5. Lobules

The lobules reside in the cul-de-sacs of the breasts, which are named terminal ductal lobular units. Each lobule contains clusters of tiny milk-producing glands. The production of breast milk is triggered by hormonal signals that occur during and after pregnancy. Multiple hormones, especially estrogen and progesterone, are important for the production of milk.

5.1.1.6. Lymph Vessels

The lymphatic system runs through the breast tissue into the lymph nodes, which trap bacteria and other potentially harmful substances (including cancer cells). The lymph nodes that are in closest proximity to the breast are located in the axilla (under the armpit), behind the breastbone, and above the collarbone.

5.1.1.7. Nipple and Areola

The nipple has sebaceous glands that secrete milk in a woman who is lactating. The areola is the darker area of the breast that surrounds the nipple. The areola contains a small amount of muscle cells as well as glands that look like small raised bumps termed Montgomery's glands.

5.1.1.8. Skin

The outer layer of the breast is composed of a layer of dermal cells.

5.1.2. RISK FACTORS FOR BREAST CANCER

Breast cancer is a multifactorial disease that can be caused by a variety of factors. The following features presented in the succeeding sections are proven or suspected risk factors for breast cancer.

5.1.2.1. Age

Two-thirds of breast cancer cases occur in women over age 50. As women get older, their risk of breast cancer increases. (See Table 5.1.) At age 20, the average risk of breast cancer is one in 1837, while at age 70, the risk is one in eight. Various theories abound for why the risk of breast cancer increases with age, but likely theories include a lifetime of carcinogenic exposures, a less efficient immune system, and the increased number of DNA errors that occur as we age.

TABLE 5.1. THE ABSOLUTE RISK OF BREAST CANCER FOR WOMEN IN THE UNITED STATES BY AGE

If Current Age Is:	Absolute Risk of Developing Breast Cancer in the Next 10 Years Is:
20	1 in 1837 (0.05%)
30	1 in 234 (0.4%)
40	1 in 70 (1.4%)
50	1 in 28 (2.5%)
60	1 in 28 (3.9%)
70	1 in 26 (3.9%)

Source: American Cancer Society (2007).

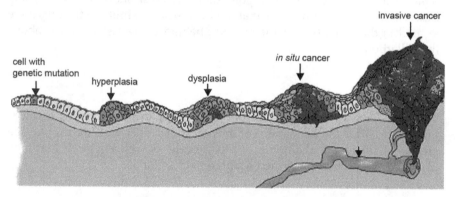

FIGURE 5.2. A model illustrating progression from normal breast cells to invasive cancer. Source: National Institutes of Health (NIH). Cell Biology and Cancer. NIH Curriculum Supplement Series. Teacher's Guide: Understanding Cancer. Available at: http://science-education.nih.gov/supplements/nih1/cancer/guide/understanding1.htm.

5.1.2.2. Alcohol Use

Alcohol use, even in moderate amounts, increases the body's level of estrogen. Thus, it is not surprising that drinking two or more alcoholic beverages a day has been shown to increase a woman's risk of breast cancer. The greater the number of alcoholic drinks consumed, the higher the risk of breast cancer. Binge drinking defined as episodic excessive drinking is also associated with heightened breast cancer risks.

5.1.2.3. Benign Breast Conditions

The progression from a normal cell to a fully malignant one is not as clearly delineated in breast cancer as it is in colon cancer. However, Figure 5.2 illustrates one possible chain of events, in which cells progress from an increased number of normal cells (hyperplasia) to an increased number of abnormal cells (atypical hyperplasia) to a frank malignancy (invasive carcinoma).

TABLE 5.2. ATYPICAL BREAST CELLS AND THE RELATIVE RISKS OF INVASIVE BREAST CANCER

No increased risk
- Nonproliferative fibrocystic change
- Fibroadenoma
- Solitary papilloma

Slightly increased risk (1.5–2 times)
- Proliferative fibrocystic change
- Usual ductal hyperplasia
- Sclerosing adenosis (florid)
- Radial scar
- Complex fibroadenoma (approximately 3 times risk)

Moderately increased risk (4–5 times)
- Atypical ductal hyperplasia (no family history)
- Atypical lobular hyperplasia

High risk (8–10 times)
- DCIS, low grade
- LCIS
- Atypical ductal hyperplasia (positive family history)

Very high risk (>8–10 times)
- DCIS, high grade

Source: Berry, GJ, Dorfman, RF, Gratzinger, D. et al. 2005. From Rouse, RV (ed.), Surgical Pathology Criteria. Stanford University School of Medicine. http://surgpathcriteria.stanford.edu.

Table 5.2 lists the risks of invasive cancer for certain benign or abnormal breast conditions. One of these breast conditions is atypical hyperplasia. The presence of atypical hyperplasia in one breast seems to increase the risk of cancer for both breasts. Whether the malignant tumor arises from these atypical cells or they are simply a harbinger of malignant potential is unclear. Atypical hyperplasia occurring in the milk ducts is associated with higher risks of cancer than atypical hyperplasia that occurs in the lobules. Atypical ductal hyperplasia is associated with a 15% lifetime risk of breast cancer; this cancer risk may be even higher if there is a positive family history of breast cancer. Another risk factor for breast cancer is postmenopausal breast density. Young women almost always have dense breasts, but breast density in older women seems to be associated with a small increased risk of breast cancer. Fibrocystic breast disease, fibroadenomas, and solitary papillomas do not appear to increase the risk of breast cancer.

5.1.2.4. Ethnicity

Women of Caucasian ancestry have higher risks of breast cancer than women of Hispanic, Asian, or African American descent. However, nonwhite women have a greater likelihood of dying from breast cancer than white women. The risk of breast cancer is also increased for women of Ashkenazi Jewish descent, which is partially but not completely explained by the higher incidence of *BRCA1* and *BRCA2* mutations in this population.

5.1.2.5. Family History

Breast cancer does seem to cluster in some families, even in the absence of an identifiable dominant gene mutation. Having one or more affected first- or second-degree relatives with breast cancer increases one's lifetime risk of breast cancer by two- or threefold degrees of magnitude. Women who have relatives diagnosed with premenopausal breast cancer are at higher risk to develop breast cancer than women whose relatives were diagnosed at older ages. However, it remains true that the majority of women who develop breast cancer do not have a family history of the disease.

5.1.2.6. Gender

Breast cancer is the most common cancer occurring in women and it is the second leading cause of cancer deaths among women. Over 99% of all breast cancers occur in women rather than in men. This is not surprising given that, compared to men, women have a greater amount of breast tissue, a higher number of active breast cells, and experience many more hormonal fluctuations and surges.

5.1.2.7. Genetic Predisposition

The risks of breast cancer are increased in women who have inherited mutations in the *BRCA1*, *BRCA2*, *TP53*, *PTEN*, *STK11*, or *CDH1* genes. Dominant genetic risk factors account for only 5–10% of breast cancer cases. However, they confer by far the greatest magnitude of risk compared to other risk factors. There are also several lower penetrance genes that, when mutated, confer low to moderate increased risks of breast cancer. Examples of low penetrance genes include *ATM*, *CHEK2*, and *PALB2*.

5.1.2.8. Geographic Region

The breast cancer incidence rates vary in different regions of the United States and elsewhere in the world. (See Chapter 1 for further discussion of cancer incidence rates.)

5.1.2.9. High Gail Model Score

The Gail model estimates the percentage of a woman's lifetime risk of breast cancer based on the following factors: age at menarche, age at first live birth, number of previous biopsies, presence of atypical hyperplasia, and number of affected first-degree relatives. This model is extremely useful for determining the likelihood of sporadic breast cancer and is routinely used in clinical settings. A major limitation of this model is that it does not consider second-degree relatives, virtually excluding any paternal history of breast cancer. For this reason, cancer genetic counselors rely more heavily on risk models that predict the likelihood of a *BRCA1* or *BRCA2* mutation (also see Section 5.3.1.2).

5.1.2.10. Hormones

A number of hormones affect breast cell activity, including estrogen, progesterone, prolactin, and oxytocin. Women who have a greater number of menstrual cycles over their lifetime are at higher risk to develop breast cancer than those with a lower number of cycles. This means that there are increased risks of breast cancer in women who have undergone early menarche (age <12) and/or late menopause (age >55). Breast cancer risks are also increased in women who have never been pregnant, never breast-fed, had their first full-term pregnancy at age >30, and used birth control pills or hormone replacement therapy for a prolonged time.

5.1.2.11. Obesity and Sedentary Lifestyle

There is some evidence that being overweight and/or sedentary raises the risk of breast cancer. Obesity can affect the levels of circulating hormones and women who are obese after menopause appear to have increased risks of breast cancer. High-fat diets may also seems the risk of breast cancer. The lack of regular exercise also seems to increase the risk of breast cancer and there is some evidence that a lack of physical activity during puberty may impact future breast cancer risk.

5.1.2.12. Personal History of Breast Cancer

Women who have been diagnosed with a breast carcinoma (either invasive or *in situ*) are at increased risk for developing a second breast primary. The risk of another breast cancer is about 15% if the initial tumor was in a milk duct and about 20% if it was in one of the breast lobules.

5.1.2.13. Radiation Exposure

Excessive radiation to the chest region, especially during childhood or adolescence, increases the risk of breast cancer. The link between radiation exposure and breast cancer comes from several sources, including adolescent girls with scoliosis who received serial X-rays, girls with Hodgkin disease who were treated with radiation therapy, and female survivors of the Hiroshima or Nagasaki atomic bombings, all of whom were shown to have increased rates of breast cancer. The greater the dosage of radiation, the higher the subsequent risk of breast cancer. Also, the age of the radiation exposure is important, with prepubescent girls having the highest lifetime risks of breast cancer.

5.1.3. BENIGN BREAST LESIONS

Some breast lesions are considered harmless while others increase the risk of cancer. The most common types of benign breast lesions are described below.

5.1.3.1. Cyst

Breast cysts are fluid-filled sacs that can cause the breast to feel lumpy or tender. Simple cysts are not associated with increased risks of breast cancer, but their presence may make it harder to evaluate the surrounding breast tissue for malignant cells. It may be necessary to aspirate a lesion in order to confirm that it is a fluid-filled cyst rather than a solid mass. Complex cysts may contain a cluster of abnormal or malignant cells.

5.1.3.2. Fibroadenoma

Fibroadenomas are benign growths that are not associated with higher risks of breast cancer. Fibroadenomas are described as smooth round lumps that can move easily within the breast tissue (as opposed to malignant tumors, which are typically fixed). Some women develop a single breast fibroadenoma while others develop multiple fibroadenomas over their lifetime. Fibroadenaomas are common in young women in their teens or in their twenties, but can occur at other ages as well. In menopausal women, for example, the use of hormone replacement therapy (HRT) can trigger the growth of fibroadenomas. The average fibroadenoma grows to a certain size (often the size of a marble) and then typically remains dormant for its life span, which can range from several months to several years. Sometimes it is necessary to biopsy the fibroadenoma to confirm that it is not a slow-growing malignancy.

Rare types of fibroadenomas include hamartomas, papillomas, and giant fibroadenomas. Hamartomas and papillomas are not linked to higher cancer risks but are seen in women with PTEN Hamartoma syndrome (PHS). Giant fibroadenomas can grow to the size of a lemon but are usually benign. About 1% of giant fibroadenomas contain a rare malignant tumor termed cystosarcoma phylloides.

5.1.3.3. Microcalcifications

Microcalcifications are tiny specks of calcium that can show up on a mammogram. While microcalcifications occur in normal breast tissue, certain patterns of these tiny specks are associated with breast neoplasms. The detection of multiple, widely scattered or large-sized microcalcifications is not worrisome, but the detection of a few tightly clustered tiny-sized specks may be a warning sign that an invasive or *in situ* tumor is present. About 20% of microcalcifications are associated with a malignant tumor.

5.1.4. Intraductal Breast Cancers

Intraductal breast cancers are early-stage malignant tumors that have not begun to spread beyond their site of origin. The two major types of intraductal or Stage 0 breast cancer are ductal carcinoma *in situ* (DCIS) and lobular carcinoma *in situ* (LCIS).

5.1.4.1. DCIS

DCIS represents about 2.5% of breast cancer cases. In DCIS, the malignant cells are present in the lining of a milk duct, but have not penetrated further into the breast. Unlike LCIS, which has a low rate of invasiveness, some cases of DCIS will transform into invasive cancer if not removed. The three main subtypes of DCIS are: micropapillary, cribiform, and comedo. The comedo type is a high-grade tumor that is associated with the highest risk of invasive cancer. About 20–25% of women with low-grade DCIS will go on to develop invasive cancer; the percentage is higher with high-grade DCIS.

5.1.4.2. LCIS

LCIS represents about 2.5% of breast cancer cases. In LCIS, the malignant cells have formed in the lining of a lobule but have not spread further into the breast. The presence of LCIS in a breast increases the risk of cancer in both breasts. Since LCIS has a low risk of transforming into an invasive tumor, it is unclear whether invasive lobular carcinomas usually arise from LCIS or whether LCIS is a more generalized risk factor. Women with LCIS have a risk of invasive breast cancer of about 1% per year with a maximum lifetime risk of about 15%.

5.1.5. Invasive Breast Cancers

Invasive breast cancers are tumors that have metastatic potential. This includes Stage I–Stage IV breast cancers. The vast majority of invasive breast cancers have arisen from the glandular tissues of the breast. There are over

30 histologically distinct types of breast cancer. The most common forms of invasive breast cancer are listed below.

5.1.5.1. Infiltrating Ductal Carcinoma

About 65% of all breast cancers originate in the epithelial cells (lining) of a milk duct. Infiltrating ductal cancer is a tumor that spreads through the duct wall into the surrounding breast tissue. Women with ductal carcinoma have an estimated 15% risk of contralateral cancer. Some breast neoplasms are combinations of infiltrating ductal carcinomas and other tumor types, such as lobular, mucinous, or papillary carcinomas.

5.1.5.2. Infiltrating Lobular Carcinoma

About 10–15% of breast cancers are lobular carcinomas. Women who develop breast cancer after taking HRT are more likely to develop lobular carcinomas than other types. Lobular carcinomas can grow larger than ductal carcinomas but can be more difficult to detect. Women with lobular cancer may notice a thickening of breast tissue rather than a palpable lump. Women with lobular carcinomas have a 20% risk of contralateral cancer.

5.1.5.3. Tubular Carcinoma

About 6–8% of all breast cancers are tubular carcinomas. Tubular breast cancers appear as cylindrical shapes under the microscope. These tumors tend to be low-grade, well-differentiated tumors and are less aggressive than some of the other types of breast cancer.

5.1.5.4. Medullary Carcinoma

About 6% of breast cancers are of the medullary subtype. Medullary breast cancer resembles the color of the brain medulla. This type of breast cancer occurs more frequently among younger (premenopausal) women.

5.1.5.5. Mucinous Carcinoma

About 3% of all breast cancers are mucinous (also called colloid) carcinomas. Mucinous tumors make a glue-like mucus, hence the name. These tumors tend to be low grade, well differentiated, and less aggressive than some of the other ductal subtypes.

5.1.5.6. Paget Disease of the Breast

Paget disease of the breast represents 3% of breast cancer cases. The initial signs of Paget disease are an eczema-like itchiness, redness, and flaking of the nipple that does not get better over time. Other symptoms are hypersensitivity, pain, crusting, ulceration, and weeping. It is not clear whether the cancer starts in the breast sinus and travels up to the nipple or whether it originates in the nipple itself. Paget disease is typically unilateral (skin rashes on both breasts are less likely to be Paget disease). About half of the women with Paget disease do not have a detectable mass. Some women who have Paget disease will be found to have another *in situ* or invasive tumor. Paget disease by itself is typically low grade and slow growing.

5.1.5.7. Inflammatory Breast Cancer

Inflammatory breast cancer represents about 1% of breast cancers. The earliest signs of inflammatory breast cancer may be a redness and warmth of the skin of the breast; many women with inflammatory disease do not develop a detectable mass or lump in their breasts. Inflammatory breast cancer tends to be a high-grade, aggressive cancer.

5.1.5.8. Papillary Carcinoma

About 1% or less of breast cancers are papillary carcinomas. These tumors contain cells that form tiny finger-like projections (called fronds). Papillary breast tumors often develop underneath the nipple and areola.

5.1.5.9. Sarcoma

Sarcomas of the breast are rare, representing only 0.1% of breast cancer cases. Breast sarcomas are tumors that have arisen from the connective tissue grid (fibrosarcoma) or fat (liposarcoma) of the breast. Breast sarcomas are associated with Li–Fraumeni syndrome (LFS).

5.1.5.10. Cystosarcoma Phylloides (Malignant)

Fewer than 1% of breast tumors are cystosarcoma phylloides and only 5% of cystosarcoma phylloides are malignant. The originating cell is thought to be one of the supporting stromal cells. This low-grade tumor is often encased in a giant fibroadenoma. Cases of malignant cystosarcoma phylloides have been reported in women who have LFS.

5.1.5.11. Other Types of Breast Cancer

There are other types of cancer that occur infrequently within the breast. These malignancies include sebaceous carcinomas, lymphomas, sweat gland carcinomas, and angiosarcomas, which are rare cancers of the blood vessels of the breast or underarm.

5.2. BREAST CANCER MANAGEMENT: SCREENING, DIAGNOSIS, AND TREATMENT

5.2.1. SCREENING AND PREVENTION GUIDELINES

The American Cancer Society (ACS) guidelines for breast cancer in the general population are listed in Table 5.3. Women who have one or more close relatives with breast cancer are generally recommended to begin breast cancer monitoring 7–10 years earlier than the youngest case of breast cancer in the family.

The United States Preventive Services Task Force, a panel of independent experts, issued the following recommendations about breast cancer screening in 2009:

- Women who are age 50–74 should have mammograms every 2 years
- Women who are age 40–49 should not have routine mammograms
- Women who are age 75 or older do not need mammograms
- Women should no longer be told to perform breast self-examinations (BSEs)
- There is no additional benefit to clinical breast examinations by physicians nor is there proven benefit to digital mammography or magnetic resonance imaging (MRI) over film mammography.

Although the policies (and insurance coverage) of breast cancer screening in the United States remain unchanged, it is worth noting that the Task Force guidelines are based on current scientific research and are similar to the screening policies in many European countries.

TABLE 5.3. ACS BREAST CANCER SCREENING GUIDELINES

For women at average risk:
- Annual mammography beginning at age 40.
- Clinical breast exams should be part of a woman's periodic health examination, about every 3 years for women in their twenties and thirties and annually for women age 40 and older
- Women should report any breast change promptly to their health-care provider. Beginning in their twenties, women should be told about the benefits and limitations of breast self-examination (BSE). It is acceptable for women to choose not to do BSE or to do it occasionally.
- Older women should continue annual mammography, regardless of age, as long as the woman does not have serious chronic health problems. For women with serious health problems or short life expectancy, evaluate ongoing early detection testing in terms of benefits and limitations.

Source: American Cancer Society (2011).

TABLE 5.4. WARNING SIGNS OF BREAST CANCER

A lump or thickening in or near the breast or in the underarm that persists through the menstrual cycle

A mass or lump, which may feel as small as a pea

A change in the size, shape, or contour of the breast

A bloodstained or clear fluid discharge from the nipple

A change in the feel or appearance of the skin on the breast or nipple (dimpled, puckered, scaly, or inflamed)

Redness of the skin on the breast or nipple

An area that is distinctly different from any other area on either breast

A marble-like hardened area under the skin

Source: WebMD (2010).

While imaging technologies have gotten better at picking up early-stage breast lesions, the first signs of breast cancer are often detected by the women themselves. The warning signs for breast cancer are listed in Table 5.4. The most common sign of breast cancer is an abnormal lump. However, it is important to remember that the majority of breast lumps turn out to be benign growths or cysts.

Women are more likely to notice an abnormal breast lump while washing in the shower or rolling over in bed than during a self-breast examination. Although monthly self-breast exams are still included in the ACS guidelines, there is increasing evidence that it is a greater source of anxiety for women than a useful screening technique.

In Dr. Susan Love's Breast Book, fourth edition (2005), the following strategies are suggested to women who want to reduce their risks of breast cancer:

- Take a multivitamin and make sure it includes adequate folic acid
- Exercise for at least 30 minutes a day, 5 days a week
- Maintain a normal weight, especially if you are postmenopausal
- Have your children before age 35 if you have a choice
- Breast-feed your children
- Avoid unnecessary X-rays
- Drink alcohol in moderation and make sure you take folic acid when you do drink
- Avoid taking hormones (HRT, fertility drugs) unless necessary
- Evaluate any breast symptoms or changes that develop
- Have a mammogram when appropriate
- Consider raloxifene if you need to take a drug to prevent bone loss postmenopausally

Keep in mind that it is not clear how effective these strategies are in reducing the risk of breast cancer in women with inherited susceptibilities.

5.2.2. STRATEGIES FOR DIAGNOSING BREAST CANCER

The diagnostic tests described in this section are the main ones that are used to identify and stage breast cancer.

5.2.2.1. Clinical Breast Examination

The clinical breast exam involves a careful, methodical palpation of each breast and under each armpit. These exams are performed by a physician, nurse practitioner, or physician's assistant. The clinician will look at the size and shape of the breasts and will check for rashes, dimpling, or enlarged lymph nodes. Cancerous lumps tend to feel different than benign ones; lumps that are oddly shaped, hard, and firmly attached are more likely to be malignant tumors. Lumps that are round, smooth, soft, and moveable are more likely to be fibroadenomas (see Section 5.1.3.2).

5.2.2.2. Mammogram

A mammogram is an X-ray of the breast tissue. Mammography is useful at detecting tumors that are not yet palpable and will not be detected via clinical exam. Mammograms are either classified as screening or diagnostic procedures. A screening mammogram looks for microcalcifications and any other possible signs of a lesion in a woman who has no symptoms of breast cancer. A diagnostic mammogram will hone in and evaluate a particular area of the breast that is of concern. Mammograms are less informative in women with dense breasts due to cysts, benign growths, or young age.

5.2.2.3. Breast MRI

An MRI study provides an enhanced view of the breast. MRI technology uses a magnet linked to a computer that detects the uptake of a dye (usually gadolinium), which is injected into the woman. A breast MRI looks for an unusual number or cluster of blood vessels, which could be indicative of a tumor that has created its own food supply through angiogenesis. Breast MRIs appear to be a good screening modality to use in women with dense tissue. However, slow-growing tumors with few blood vessels may be missed by this technology. Therefore, breast MRI exams are typically used as an adjunct to rather than a replacement of mammography. The main limitation of breast MRI is that it is a relatively new technology and thus, it may detect unusual findings that require additional—and sometimes quite unnecessary—follow-up tests.

5.2.2.4. Ultrasound

Ultrasonography is used as a follow-up test to an abnormal clinical breast exam, mammogram, or breast MRI. Ultrasound exams use sound waves that bounce off the breast tissue and are used to create a computerized image. An ultrasound can confirm the presence of a possible mass and can assess whether it is more likely to be a harmless cyst or a solid lesion that requires biopsy. Follow-up or serial ultrasound scans may be helpful in determining if the shape and size of a lesion have changed; fibroadenomas and cysts tend to fluctuate in size in response to the woman's menstrual cycle while malignant tumors do not.

5.2.2.5. Positron Emission Tomography Scan

Positron emission tomography (PET) scanning looks at how fast glucose is being absorbed by certain tissues. Women are given radioactive glucose molecules and then undergo the scanning procedure, which is similar to a computed tomography (CT) scan. The PET scanner is linked to a computer, which produces digital images of the area. In general, breast tumors use more glucose than normal tissue so the identification of high absorption of glucose suggests the presence of a neoplasm. PET technology is also useful in determining the extent of local spread in people with invasive disease.

5.2.2.6. Biopsy

The identification of a solid mass often triggers the need for a biopsy. A biopsy can evaluate the cells of the mass to look for evidence of malignancy or malignant potential. Typically, the area of the breast is locally anesthetized and a needle and syringe are used to remove fluid and/or cells. Any fluid and cells obtained from a biopsy will be sent to the pathology department for careful evaluation. There are two main types of surgical biopsy: an incisional biopsy, which takes a small sample from the mass for analysis, and an excisional biopsy, which removes the entire mass. A biopsy that identifies the presence of a malignant tumor typically leads to additional biopsies of the neighboring lymph nodes to determine the extent of spread. The spread of cancer cells to the lymph nodes happens in a fairly predictable fashion, so rather than sampling multiple lymph nodes, which increases the risk of lymphedema (i.e., a lymphatic obstruction that causes fluid retention and swelling), the surgeon will often sample one or two main nodes (termed sentinel nodes) that lie nearest to the tumor. If the sentinel node biopsy is negative for cancer cells, then no further sampling of the lymph nodes is performed. If the sentinel node is positive for cancer cells, then a more complete study of the other lymph nodes will be conducted.

5.2.2.7. Tumor Grading

Tumor grading is the process of determining the specific characteristics of a tumor. (Refer to Section 2.2.2 for more information on tumor grading). The specific characteristics of the tumor will help guide the clinician in recommending therapies that have the greatest chance of success. More and more, cancer treatments are targeted to tumors with certain biological, histological, or genetic properties. In breast neoplasms, it is important to determine whether the tumor has receptors for estrogen and/or progesterone. The presence of these receptors means that the tumor needs these hormones in order to grow. Therefore the cancer treatment can include antihormones to "starve" the tumor. Breast tumor analysis also looks for the presence of human epidermal growth factor receptor-2 (Her2/neu). Tumors that are estrogen receptor positive tend to be less aggressive and tumors that contain amplified copies of the Her2/neu oncogene tend to be more aggressive. So-called triple-negative breast tumors are ones that do not contain estrogen receptors, progesterone receptors, or the Her2/neu growth factor. Tumors that are triple negative may be more difficult to treat and are also associated with germline *BRCA1* or *BRCA2* mutations. Her2/neu positive tumors may be associated with LFS.

5.2.2.8. Cancer Staging

Breast cancers are staged from Stage 0 to Stage IV and predictably, survival rates decrease with each advancing stage. (See Section 2.2.3 for more information about cancer staging.) The clinical staging system used for breast cancer is listed in Table 5.5.

5.2.2.9. Additional Studies

Once a breast neoplasm has been identified, it is important to determine the extent of spread to other organs. In the case of breast cancer, the most common sites of metastases are the bones, liver, lungs, and brain. Patients will undergo a series of blood tests that may include an evaluation of liver function, bone enzymes, and the presence of the carcinoembryonic antigen (CEA) tumor marker. Additional radiology procedures may include X-rays, CT scans, or MRIs of the spine, hips, abdomen, and head.

5.2.3. STRATEGIES FOR TREATING BREAST CANCER

Similar to other solid tumors, the local treatment of breast cancer consists of surgery and radiation therapy, while systemic treatment of breast cancer involves chemotherapy, hormonal therapy, and biological therapy. A general description of these therapies is provided below.

TABLE 5.5. THE TNM CANCER STAGING CLASSIFICATIONS FOR BREAST
CANCER

Stage 0	Tis N0 M0
Stage 1A	T1 N0 M0
Stage 1B	T0 N1mi (micrometastases) M0 or T1 N1mi M0
Stage IIA	T0 N1 M0 or T1 N1 M0 or T2 N0 M0
Stage IIB	T2 N1 M0 or T3 N0 M0
Stage IIIA	T0 N2 M0 or T1 N2 M0 or T2 N2 M0 or T3 N1 M0 or T3 N2 M0
Stage IIIB	T4 N0 M0 or T4 N1 M0 or T4 N2 M0
Stage IIIC	Any T N3 M0
Stage IV	Any T Any N M1

T (Primary Tumor): T0 = No evidence of primary tumor; Tis = Carcinoma in situ; T1 = Tumor
≤20 mm; T2 = Tumor >20 mm but ≤50 mm; T3 = Tumor >50 mm; T4 = Tumor of any size with
direct extension to chest wall and/or skin. N (Regional Lymph Nodes): N0 = No regional
lymph node metastases; N1 = Metastases to movable ipsilateral level I, II axillary lymph
node(s); N2 = Metastases in ipsilateral level I, II axillary lymph nodes fixed or matted or in
clinically detected ipsilateral internal mammary nodes in the absence of clinically evident axillary lymph node metastases; N3 = Metastases in ipsilateral infraclavicular (level III axillary)
lymph node(s) with or without level I, II axillary lymph node involvement or in clinically
detected ipsilateral internal mammary lymph node(s) with clinically evident level I, II axillary
lymph node metastases, or metastases in ipsilateral supraclavicular lymph nodes(s) with or
without axillary or internal mammary lymph node involvement; M (Distant Metastases):
M0 = No clinical or radiological evidence of distant metastases; M1 = Distant detectable
metastases.

Source: American Joint Committee on Cancer (2010), pp. 421–442.

5.2.3.1. Surgery

The major treatment decision for newly diagnosed breast cancer patients is
whether to have a mastectomy, which removes most of the breast tissue, or
a lumpectomy (also termed partial mastectomy), which removes the tumor
and a surrounding margin of normal tissue. Survival rates appear similar
for both surgical procedures, although it is not clear whether this is the case
for women with inherited breast cancer. Mastectomy may be recommended
if there are:

- concerns about cancer spread (the tumor is large or aggressive)
- two or more primary tumors in different areas of the breast
- diffuse microcalcifications throughout the breast
- persistent positive margins following lumpectomy
- concerns about the effectiveness or safety of radiation therapy due
  to pregnancy, the presence of an autoimmune disease, a prior history
  of radiation therapy (e.g., survivors of Hodgkin disease), or an
  increased risk of radiation-induced second tumors

Most women who have mastectomies undergo the modified radical mastectomy procedure. In this procedure, the surgeon removes the majority of breast tissue and the nipple and areola but does not take all of the lymph nodes under the arms. It is important for women to realize that it is not possible to remove all breast tissue since breast cells are interwoven into the chest wall. Most women who have mastectomies choose to have breast reconstruction. Breast reconstruction can include the use of saline or silicone implants or can use a patch of skin and muscle from the woman's back or abdomen to form the breast, which is termed the latissimus flap or TRAM-flap procedure respectively. Some women undergoing prophylactic mastectomy choose to retain their own nipples and areolae for a better cosmetic outcome.

5.2.3.2. Radiation

Radiation therapy generally targets the remaining breast tissue, the neighboring lymph nodes, and the chest wall. Radiation can be given by external beams or with surgically implanted radiation seeds. Protocols vary, but a typical regimen is to have radiation treatments for 5 days a week for a period of 6 weeks. The dosage of radiation and the overall length of treatment can be decreased or increased depending on the tumor response and the occurrence of serious side effects. Women may undergo neoadjuvant radiation as a first-line treatment in an effort to shrink the tumor to increase the chances that it can be surgically resected. Women who undergo lumpectomies will need to undergo postadjuvant radiation treatments. Women who have mastectomies may also require postadjuvant radiation treatments to the chest wall if the tumor is especially large or if there are multiple positive lymph nodes. Radiation can also be done to shrink the tumor for palliative purposes in order to relieve pressure on nerves or bones.

5.2.3.3. Chemotherapy

Chemotherapy is recommended if there is any evidence that the cancer has spread beyond the initial site or if the tumor is aggressive or large (greater than 3 cm). Chemotherapy regimens may include the following agents: cyclophosphamide, methotrexate, 5-fluorouracil, doxorubicin, and anthracycline. The sequence and combination of chemotherapeutic agents varies depending on the tumor characteristics and the stage of disease. The dosages and the overall length of treatment can be decreased or increased depending on the tumor response and the occurrence of serious side effects. A typical regimen is to have chemotherapy once every 3 weeks for 6–12 cycles. Neoadjuvant chemotherapy may be given in hopes of shrinking the tumor to increase the surgical options. Chemotherapy agents can also be used for palliative purposes.

5.2.3.4. Hormonal Therapy

Hormonal therapy may be used as a first line of treatment in women with advanced disease or may be used to reduce the risk of recurrence for women who are in remission. This type of therapy involves reducing the number of hormones that could potentially feed any remaining cancer cells. Women with hormone-positive tumors are typically prescribed an antihormonal drug, such as tamoxifen or raloxifene, for 5 years posttreatment. Tamoxifen, for example, binds the estrogen receptors, thus interfering with their ability to function and reduces the risk of recurrence by about 50%. Aromatase inhibitors are another type of hormonal therapy that shows great promise. Aromatase inhibitors halt the production of estrogen produced by organs other than the ovaries. These include the adrenal glands, fat, breast, brain, and muscles. Arimidex and Femara temporarily block the production of estrogen from these sources; Aromasin permanently inactivates its production. For premenopausal women, shutting down the ovaries (ovarian ablation) may be recommended. Ovarian ablation can be accomplished temporarily by the use of monthly injections or permanently by undergoing a surgical oophorectomy.

5.2.3.5. Biological Therapy

Biological agents include cancer vaccines, monoantibody-based agents, and inhibitors of tumor angiogenesis. Many of these therapies are still investigational, including PARP inhibitors, which show great promise in treating BRCA-related breast and ovarian tumors. One example of a biological agent currently used to treat breast cancer is trastuzumab, which is a monoclonal antibody that binds to (and nullifies) the Her2/neu growth factor. Patients who have positive tumors are typically given a neoadjuvant or postadjuvant course of trastuzumab.

5.2.4. TREATMENT OPTIONS BY STAGE OF DIAGNOSIS

This section provides an overview of the standard treatment options for individuals with breast cancer based on their clinical stage at diagnosis.

5.2.4.1. Stage 0

Women with LCIS do not usually require any treatment beyond the removal of the abnormal cells. In contrast, women with DCIS generally undergo lumpectomy followed by radiation therapy. The underarm lymph nodes are not generally biopsied unless the tumor is especially large or high grade. Tamoxifen will be given if the tumor is estrogen receptor positive. In a small number of DCIS cases, women may undergo a mastectomy rather than lumpectomy. Women with Stage 0 breast cancer have a 98–100% survival rate.

5.2.4.2. Stage I

Women with Stage I breast cancer typically undergo lumpectomy followed by radiation therapy. However, mastectomy may be recommended if the tumor is especially large or aggressive or if radiation is contraindicated. Tamoxifen will generally be given if the tumor is estrogen receptor positive. A sentinel node biopsy may be done. Women with Stage I breast cancer have an 85–97% survival rate.

5.2.4.3. Stage II

Women with Stage II breast cancer typically undergo lumpectomy and radiation therapy followed by tamoxifen if the tumor is estrogen receptor positive. Mastectomy may also be recommended. Lymph nodes will be sampled to determine involvement. Women are generally given adjuvant chemotherapy and/or hormonal therapy. Women with Stage II breast cancer have a 70–90% survival rate.

5.2.4.4. Stage III

Women with Stage IIIA breast cancer typically undergo lumpectomy and radiation therapy or mastectomy. Women with Stage IIIB or Stage IIIC breast cancer typically undergo neoadjuvant chemotherapy and/or radiation with hopes of shrinking the tumor to an operable level. Lymph node dissection will also be done. Other options for women with Stage III breast cancer include hormonal therapy and biological therapy. Women with Stage III breast cancer have a 40–70% survival rate.

5.2.4.5. Stage IV

Women with Stage IV breast cancer will undergo hormonal therapy, chemotherapy, and/or biological therapy such as Herceptin. For women with Stage IV breast cancer, the main concern may be the sites of metastases rather than the tumor itself. For this reason the focus is on systemic therapies rather than local therapy (surgery or radiation). However, radiation therapy is sometimes used for pain management. Women with Stage IV breast cancer have a 5–20% survival rate.

5.2.4.6. Recurrent Breast Cancer

The treatment of recurrent breast cancer depends on the location and the extent of the recurrence. For a local recurrence, more extensive breast surgery may be performed. If distant metastases have occurred, then treatment will include chemotherapy, hormonal therapy, or biological therapy.

TABLE 5.6. HEREDITARY CANCER SYNDROMES THAT HAVE INCREASED RISKS OF BREAST CANCER

Breast cancer is a major feature in:
- Hereditary Breast–Ovarian Cancer syndrome
- Hereditary Diffuse Gastric Cancer syndrome
- Li–Fraumeni syndrome
- Peutz–Jeghers syndrome
- PTEN Hamartoma syndrome

Breast cancer is a minor feature in:
- Autoimmune Lymphoproliferative syndrome
- Ataxia Telangiectasia
- Bloom syndrome
- Melanoma, cutaneous malignant
- Werner syndrome
- Xeroderma Pigmentosum

Sources: Lindor et al. (2008); Petrucelli et al. (2011).

5.3. BREAST CANCER SYNDROMES

Of the people with personal or family histories of breast cancer, many are interested in discussing the option of *BRCA1* and *BRCA2* testing. However, it is important to keep in mind that breast cancer is also an associated feature of other hereditary cancer syndromes.

The major hereditary breast cancer syndromes are: Hereditary Breast–Ovarian Cancer syndrome (HBOCS), Hereditary Diffuse Gastric Cancer (HDGC) syndrome, LFS, Peutz–Jeghers syndrome (PJS), and PHS. In these five syndromes, the risk of breast cancer is substantially increased. Additional hereditary cancer syndromes that confer heightened breast cancer risk are listed in Table 5.6.

This section focuses on the five major breast cancer syndromes in terms of tumor characteristics, family history assessment, and management recommendations.

5.3.1. HEREDITARY BREAST–OVARIAN CANCER SYNDROME

HBOCS accounts for 60–75% of inherited cases of breast cancer. It is estimated that 5% of all breast cancer patients have a germline *BRCA1* or *BRCA2* mutation. Women with HBOCS have a 50–85% lifetime risk of breast cancer risk. Men who have a *BRCA1* mutation have an estimated 3% risk of breast cancer and men with a *BRCA2* mutation have an estimated 6% risk of breast cancer. (See Section 4.7 for detailed information about HBOCS.)

5.3.1.1. HBOCS Tumor Types

- *Breast cancer*—Invasive lobular and ductal carcinomas of various histologies have been reported in people with *BRCA1* and *BRCA2* mutations. The malignancies originate from the epithelial layer of cells in the breast. DCIS is also a feature of HBOCS. Compared to sporadic breast cancers, *BRCA1*-related breast tumors are more likely to have a medullary histopathology and a "basal phenotype" (i.e., the tumor expresses basal keratin by immunohistochemistry) and to be high grade, lymph node positive, estrogen receptor negative, progesterone receptor negative, and negative for the Her2/neu growth factor. *BRCA2*-related breast tumors tend to resemble sporadic breast cancers and do not appear to have a specific histopathology subtype. Compared to *BRCA1*-related tumors, *BRCA2*-related tumors are less likely to be triple negative (negative for estrogen receptors, progesterone receptors, and Her2/neu growth factor) or to have a basal phenotype.

- *Ovarian cancer*—Over 90% of the ovarian tumors occurring in women with *BRCA* mutations are serous adenocarcinomas. Compared to mucinous ovarian tumors, serous adenocarcinomas are more likely to be bilateral and of a higher grade. However, the survival rate of women with *BRCA*-related ovarian cancer seems to be better than for women with sporadic ovarian carcinomas.

- *Other cancers*—Other malignancies associated with HBOCS include:
  - Fallopian tube cancer
  - Primary peritoneal cancer
  - Prostate cancer
  - Pancreatic cancer
  - Melanoma, cutaneous, and ocular (primarily *BRCA2* carriers)

5.3.1.2. HBOCS Family History Assessment

The likelihood of a *BRCA* gene mutation is higher among individuals who have developed breast cancer under age 40, have Ashkenazi Jewish heritage, have developed contralateral breast cancer, and/or have personal or family histories of ovarian, pancreatic, or male breast cancer. It is estimated that two-thirds of families with three or more cases of breast or ovarian cancer will be found to have *BRCA* mutations.

Several empirical risk models have been developed to help assess the likelihood of a *BRCA1* or *BRCA2* mutation. These models may be useful in determining the value in genetic testing, although clinicians are cautioned that each model has its weaknesses. The most widely used model in clinical practice is BRCAPRO (Bayes Mendel Group, Johns

TABLE 5.7. MANAGEMENT GUIDELINES FOR INDIVIDUALS WITH HBOCS

For Women with HBOCS:
- Recommend clinical breast exam semi-annually starting at age 25 years.
- Recommend mammography annually starting at age 25 years or 5–10 years earlier than the earliest known breast cancer diagnosis in the family (whichever is earliest).
- Recommend breast magnetic resonance imaging (MRI) annually starting at age 25 years or 5–10 years earlier than the earliest known breast cancer diagnosis in the family (whichever is earliest).
- Recommend prophylactic salpingo-oophorectomy between ages 35 and 40 years or upon completion of child bearing.
- For women who have not undergone oophorectomy, discuss the options of pelvic exam, trans-vaginal ultrasound, and CA-125 test semi-annually starting at age 25–35 years.
- Discuss the option of performing monthly breast self-examinastion (BSE) starting in early adulthood.[a]
- Discuss the option of undergoing prophylactic mastectomy as a strategy for reducing breast cancer risk.
- Discuss the chemoprevention options, which can reduce the risk of breast or ovarian cancer.
- Discuss any clinical studies designed for women with BRCA mutations.

For Men with HBOCS:
- Recommend annual digital rectal exam and prostate-specific antigen (PSA) testing starting at age 40.
- Recommend clinical breast exam annually or semi-annually.
- Consider recommending the use of mammography if gynecomastia or other breast cancer risk factors are present.
- Discuss option of monthly BSEs starting in early adulthood.[a]

Source: Petrucelli et al. (2007) and National Comprehensive Cancer Network Clinical Practice Guidelines in Oncology. Genetic/familial high risk assessment: breast and ovarian. V.I.2009, www.nccn.org.

[a]Given recent evidence that BSE's are not effective screening tools, clinicians may wish to de-emphasize this recommendation.

Hopkins Medical Institutions: http://astor.som.jhmi.edu/BayesMendel/ brcapro.html.Baltimore, Maryland). The BRCAPRO model determines the probability of BRCA1 and BRCA2 mutations based on the following factors: the patient's age, the patient's personal history of breast and ovarian cancer, the history of breast and ovarian cancer among first- and second-degree relatives, and the presence of Ashkenazi Jewish heritage.

5.3.1.3. HBOCS Management Recommendations

The management recommendations for women with BRCA mutations are listed in Table 5.7. Screening with mammography and breast MRI begins at age 25 unless the family history dictates an earlier onset. Clinical breast exams should also be performed every 6 months beginning at age 25. Although BSE is included in these recommendations, recent studies suggest that there may be little value to performing monthly BSEs.

The best way for female BRCA carriers to reduce their risks of breast cancer is to surgically remove most of the breast tissue. This procedure, termed prophylactic mastectomy, reduces the risk of breast cancer by 90–95%. There may be less of a benefit for women who are of older ages. Premenopausal women who surgically remove their ovaries also cut their risk of breast cancer by about 50%. Chemoprevention is another useful strategy for reducing breast cancer risks. The use of the antihormonal agent, Tamoxifen, appears to reduce the risk of breast cancer by about 50% for women in the general population and for women with BRCA2 mutations; however, it may be less effective in women with BRCA1 mutations.

Monitoring for ovarian cancer consists of assessing the level of CA-125 tumor markers in the blood and performing transvaginal ultrasound exams. However, these strategies are decidedly poor at detecting early-stage ovarian cancer. For this reason, it is recommended that female BRCA carriers undergo prophylactic oophorectomy, which is the surgical removal of the ovaries, between the ages of 35 and 45. Prophylactic oophorectomy reduces the risk of ovarian cancer by 70–95%; premenopausal women reap the greatest benefits from surgery. The fallopian tubes should also be removed during this surgery since fallopian tube cancer is an established feature of HBOCS. The use of oral contraceptives for at least 6 months also reduces the risk of ovarian cancer by 50% in the general population and in female BRCA carriers.

Men with BRCA mutations should have clinical breast exams and can consider baseline mammography. Male BRCA carriers can consider having annual mammograms if gynecomastia or glandular breast density is present. They should also be screened for prostate cancer with annual prostate exams and prostate-specific antigen (PSA) blood tests beginning at age 40.

Individuals with BRCA2 mutations also have small increased risks for developing cutaneous or ocular melanoma. Although the HBOCS screening guidelines do not include careful skin or eye exams, clinicians can consider whether this might be beneficial.

Primary peritoneal cancer and pancreatic cancer are also features of HBOCS; however, there are no established guidelines for the early detection or prevention of either of these malignancies in people with HBOCS.

5.3.2. HEREDITARY DIFFUSE GASTRIC CANCER SYNDROME

Women with CDH1 mutations have an estimated 39% risk of developing breast cancer. However, the amount of breast cancer attributable to CDH1 is thought to be extremely low. Men with CDH1 mutations do not seem to have an increased risk of breast cancer.

About 5–10% of all gastric cancers are due to an inherited susceptibility. The percentage of cases attributable to *CDH1* mutations is not known. The lifetime risk of developing diffuse gastric cancer is about 67% in men with a *CDH1* mutation and about 83% in women with a *CDH1* mutation. (See Section 4.12.1 for additional information about HDGC.)

5.3.2.1. HDGC Tumor Types

- *Breast cancer*—HDGC-related breast cancers are almost always invasive lobular carcinomas. However, cases of invasive ductal carcinomas have also been reported in women with HDGC.

- *Stomach cancer*—People with HDGC are at high risk for developing diffuse gastric cancer, also termed signet ring adenocarcinoma of the stomach. Diffuse gastric cancer accounts for about 35% of all stomach cancer diagnoses. The other major type of stomach cancer, termed intestinal-type gastric cancer, is not associated with *CDH1* mutations. Diffuse gastric cancer causes a thickening of the stomach wall (called "linitis plastica") rather than a discrete tumor. Diffuse gastric cancer is less likely than the intestinal-type gastric cancer to occur in the distal stomach and less likely to be associated with *Helicobacter pylori* infection. Intramucosal (*in situ*) signet ring cell adenocarcinomas of the stomach may also be an associated feature of HDGC.

- *Other cancers*—Individuals with HDGC may also be at increased risk for developing signet ring colon cancer and islet cell pancreatic cancer.

5.3.2.2. HDGC Family History Assessment

The identification of a patient with HDGC hinges on the presence of diffuse gastric cancer. Since two-thirds of gastric cancers are *not* the diffuse subtype, obtaining medical records documentation is important. HDGC-related gastric cancer typically occurs under age 40, so the age of onset is an important variable.

Approximately one-third of families meeting clinical criteria for HDGC will be found to have a *CDH1* mutation. Individuals with diffuse gastric cancer have a higher likelihood of having a *CDH1* mutation if they have relatives with diffuse gastric cancer, lobular breast cancer, signet ring colon cancer, and possibly relatives born with cleft lip and/or palate.

5.3.2.3. HDGC Management Recommendations

The management recommendations for individuals with HDGC are listed in Table 5.8. The value of these surveillance strategies remains unproven.

TABLE 5.8. MANAGEMENT GUIDELINES FOR INDIVIDUALS WITH HDGC
SYNDROME

For women with HDGC:
- Monthly breast self-exam beginning at age 18 years.[a]
- Clinical breast exam every 6–12 months beginning at age 18 years.
- Mammogram every 12 months beginning at age 35 or 5–10 years prior to the earliest diagnosis in the family.
- Consider supplemental breast MRI exam or breast ultrasound exam every 12 months beginning at age 35.

For men and women with HDGC:
- Endoscopy examination of the stomach with multiple random biopsies of the gastric wall every 6–12 months beginning at age 16.
- Consider the option of chromoendoscopy instead of the regular endoscopy exam every 6–12 months beginning at age 16.
- Consider the option of prophylactic gastrectomy, 5 years prior to the earliest case in the family.
- In HDGC families with colon cancer, undergo colonoscopy exam every 12–18 months, beginning 5–10 years prior to the earliest case in the family.

Sources: Kaurah and Huntsman (2006); Lindor et al. (2008, p. 44).

[a]Given recent evidence that BSEs are not effective screening tools, clinicians may wish to de-emphasize this recommendation.

Surveillance endoscopy may be inadequate for people at high risk for developing diffuse gastric cancer. The earliest signs of diffuse gastric cancer are subtle changes of the stomach wall that may be missed by this procedure. Conducting multiple random biopsies is helpful, but this technique may also miss early-stage cancer. For this reason, some clinicians recommend that individuals with HDGC undergo specialized endoscopic procedures termed chromoendoscopy. Chromoendoscopy utilizes a special red dye and penta-gastrin stimulation during the procedure, which may make it a more effective strategy for detecting early signs of diffuse gastric cancer.

Given the high mortality associated with gastric cancer and the inadequate screening techniques, at-risk individuals may wish to consider prophylactic gastrectomy. Gastrectomy, which is the surgical removal of the stomach, dramatically reduces the risk of gastric cancer, but it is associated with a number of long-term sequelae.

Women with HDGC should begin having annual mammograms at age 35 and they may wish to consider having breast MRI exams as well.

5.3.3. LI-FRAUMENI SYNDROME

Individuals with LFS have high risks of developing breast cancer, sarcomas, brain tumors, and adrenal cortical carcinomas (ACCs). In addition to these

LFS-related core cancers, individuals are at increased risk for developing a variety of other malignancies during childhood and adulthood.

LFS accounts for less than 1% of total breast cancer cases. However, women with very early onset breast cancer (diagnosed under age 30) have a higher probability of having a *TP53* mutation.

Women with LFS have an estimated 90% risk of breast cancer, often in their twenties or thirties. Men with LFS appear to have only slightly increased risks of breast cancer. The overall risk of malignancy in LFS is 90% or more for women and 65–70% for men. The risk of developing a second primary cancer is about 50%. (See Section 4.16 for additional information about LFS).

5.3.3.1. LFS Tumor Types

- *Breast cancer*—Women with LFS have markedly increased rates for developing invasive ductal and lobular breast carcinomas as well as DCIS. LFS-related breast tumors seem more likely to be Her2-neu positive. Other LFS-related breast malignancies include rare tumor types such as breast sarcomas and malignant cystophylloides tumors.

- *ACC*—ACCs are rare tumors of the adrenal gland. In LFS, the cases of ACC typically occur under age 50 (and often occur in childhood).

- *Brain tumor*—Several types of benign and malignant brain tumors have been reported in LFS families. LFS-related brain tumors include choroid plexus carcinoma, ependymoma, astrocytoma, and glioblastoma. Other tumors of the central nervous system, such as neuroblastomas and primitive neuroectodermal tumors, may also occur in people with LFS. In LFS, the brain tumors often develop in childhood and typically occur under age 50.

- *Sarcoma*—A variety of malignant tumors of bone, muscle, and connective tissue have been reported in people with LFS. Malignant sarcomas include osteosarcomas, fibrosarcomas, and rhabdomyosarcomas. The one exception is Ewing sarcoma, which does not appear to be a feature of LFS. Individuals with LFS may also be at increased risk for developing benign or precancerous tumors of bone, muscle, and connective tissue.

- *Other cancers*—Dr. Frederick P. Li once remarked that "all organs are potentially at risk" in LFS. Malignancies known or suspected to be at increased risk in LFS include:
  - Colorectal cancer
  - Leukemia and lymphoma
  - Lung cancer
  - Melanoma
  - Thyroid cancer

5.3.3.2. LFS Family History Assessment

In one series of breast cancer patients diagnosed under age 30, 4% of the patients had germline *TP53* mutations. The breast cancer patients under age 30 who also have a relative with one of the other LFS-related core malignancies (brain tumor, sarcoma, or ACC) had a 16% likelihood of a *TP53* mutation (Gonzalez et al., 2009). The likelihood of identifying a *TP53* mutation in a breast cancer patient diagnosed over age 45 is exceedingly low unless there is additional personal or family history suggestive of LFS.

Of individuals who meet criteria for classic LFS, 75% will be found to have a detectable *TP53* mutation and an additional 4% will be found to have a large rearrangement. About 10–20% of individuals who meet criteria for LFS-like syndrome will be found to have a *TP53* mutation. The likelihood of finding a *TP53* mutation is higher in people who have personal and family histories that include the core malignancies (breast cancer, sarcoma, brain tumor, and ACC), rare tumor types, unusually young ages of onset, childhood cancers, adult onset malignancies under age 45, and multiple primaries.

The highest rate of *TP53* mutations has been seen in series of patients with childhood choroid plexus carcinoma or ACC; 50% or more of these individuals are positive for *TP53* mutations.

5.3.3.3. LFS Management Recommendations

The management recommendations for individuals with LFS are listed in Table 5.9.

Women with LFS have extremely high risks of breast cancer—and it is one of the few LFS-related malignancies for which effective monitoring is available. It is recommended that women undergo annual breast MRI exams beginning by age 20. Annual mammograms are also recommended; however, this recommendation is somewhat controversial because of the concerns about cumulative radiation exposure. Individuals with LFS do appear to have increased risks for developing radiation-induced malignancies, although the degree of risk from a single mammogram is thought to be small.

Women with LFS should also consider the option of prophylactic mastectomies as the best strategy for reducing their breast cancer risks.

In terms of the risks of other solid tumors, clinical researchers are exploring the options of annual imaging studies, including PET scan, abdominal ultrasound, and brain MRI.

Individuals with LFS who experience any symptoms or warning signs of cancer are urged to seek prompt medical attention and undergo the appropriate follow-up tests to rule out a malignant tumor.

The risk of childhood malignancies is high in LFS. Clinical researchers are currently exploring the usefulness of more extensive monitoring protocols for infants and children who are known or suspected of having LFS.

TABLE 5.9. MANAGEMENT GUIDELINES FOR INDIVIDUALS WITH LI-FRAUMENI SYNDROME

For women with LFS:
- Recommend clinical breast exam semi-annually starting at age 20–25 years.
- Recommend mammography screening annually starting at age 20–25 years or 5–10 years earlier than the earliest known breast cancer diagnosis in the family (whichever is earliest).
- Recommend breast MRI screening annually starting at age 20–25 years or 5–10 years earlier than the earliest known breast cancer diagnosis in the family (whichever is earliest).
- Discuss the option of undergoing prophylactic mastectomy as a strategy to reduce breast cancer risk.
- Discuss the option of performing monthly BSE starting in early adulthood.[a]

For men and women with LFS:
- Recommend comprehensive physical exam, annually, which should include careful skin and neurologic exams.
- Recommend colonoscopy exams every 2–5 years starting at age 20–25 years
- Consider recommending additional cancer screening tests between birth to age 24 months to look for tumors in the abdomen and brain.
- Consider recommending additional cancer screening tests, which target malignancies occurring in the patient's family.
- Provide patient education regarding the signs and symptoms of cancer.
- Maintain a low threshold for ordering follow-up tests to rule out malignancy.
- Discuss options to participate in novel imaging technologies or clinical research studies.

Source: Schneider K and Garber J: 2010. Li-Fraumeni syndrome. Gene Reviews. Pagon RA, Bird TD, Dolan. CR et al. eds. Seattle WA: Univ Wash, Seattle, 1993. www.genereviews.org; National Comprehensive Cancer Network Clinical Practice Guidelines in Oncology. Genetic/familial high risk assessment: breast and ovarian. V.I.2009, www.nccn.org.

[a]Given recent evidence that BSE's are not effective screening tools, clinicians may wish to de-emphasize this recommendation.

5.3.4. PEUTZ–JEGHERS SYNDROME

PJS is associated with gastrointestinal (GI) polyposis and the distinctive skin and mucosal lesions (macules). Individuals with PJS are at increased risk for developing specific GI and reproductive malignancies.

Breast cancer is also a feature of PJS. The risk of breast cancer for women with PJS may be as high as 30%. Male breast cancer has also been reported in PJS. (See Section 4.27 for additional information about PJS.)

5.3.4.1. PJS Tumor Types

- *GI tumors*—One of the hallmark features of PJS is the presence of hamartomatous polyps throughout the GI tract. The histopathology of the hamartomas reveals mucosa containing smooth muscle bundles that have a characteristic branching tree appearance. PJS-associated polyps are most common in the small intestine, but also occur frequently in the colon, rectum, pancreas, and stomach. The number of polyps can range from several to hundreds and the onset of polyps often occurs in childhood or early adolescence. Cases of polyps have also been reported in very young children. Hamartomas have a low likelihood of transforming into malignant tumors; however, these lesions can cause significant morbidity, including chronic bleeding and obstructions. Precancerous adenomatous polyps also occur in people with PJS. Colorectal cancer is the most frequently occurring cancer in PJS. People with PJS also have increased risks for developing other GI cancers, including cancer of the small intestine, pancreas, stomach, and esophagus.

- *Breast cancer*—Most PJS-associated breast cancers are ductal carcinomas, which is similar to the general population. Invasive lobular carcinomas can also occur. The breast neoplasms in PJS do not seem to display a specific histology.

- *Female reproductive cancers*—Women with PJS have increased risks for developing ovarian adenocarcinomas, often of the mucinous granulosa subtype. Almost all women with PJS develop benign ovarian sex cord tumors with annular tubules (SCTAT). The PJS-associated SCTAT tumors tend to be bilateral, multifocal small tumors that seldom become malignant. In contrast, sporadically occurring SCTAT tumors are more likely to be large, unilateral tumors that have a 20% risk of malignant transformation. Women with PJS are also at increased risk for developing a rare aggressive form of cervical cancer termed adenoma malignum of the cervix. Cases of fallopian tube and endometrial cancer have also been reported in women with PJS.

- *Male reproductive cancers*—Men with PJS have small increased risks for developing estrogen-secreting Sertoli cell tumors of the testes, which can lead to gynecomastia.

5.3.4.2. PJS Family History Assessment

The clinical diagnosis of PJS rests on the presence of GI hamartomatous polyps in the GI tract (especially the small intestine) and the characteristic macules on the lips, fingers, penis, or anus. Almost all families who meet clinical criteria for PJS will be found to have a mutation in the *STK11* gene.

PJS should also be considered in women who have personal histories of adenoma malignum cervical cancer or SCTAT tumors of the ovary.

5.3.4.3. PJS Management Recommendations

The screening recommendations for individuals with PJS are listed in Table 5.10.

The breast cancers associated with PJS can develop in premenopausal women, which is the rationale for the recommendation that breast imaging studies begin at age 25. In addition, adult women with PJS should be screened for other reproductive cancers and can also consider the option of complete hysterectomy. Men with PJS should be screened for testicular tumors. Breast screening is not necessary for men with PJS unless they have gynecomastia.

The main recommendations for people with PJS involve screening for the benign hamartomas and the premalignant adenomas in the GI tract. These polyps can occur in childhood and screening should begin between the ages of 8 and 10. The GI screening can begin earlier if the child has any symptoms or if younger cases of polyps have occurred in the family.

Since the PJS-associated neoplasms can occur throughout the digestive tract, it presents significant challenges from the screening perspective. The real challenge is the identification of the polyps, especially in the stomach and small intestine. Newer technologies such as video capsule or double balloon and endoscope should be considered. All identified polyps should be removed. Even though the hamartomas rarely pose a risk of malignancy,

TABLE 5.10. MANAGEMENT GUIDELINES FOR INDIVIDUALS WITH PJS

For women with PJS:
- Clinical breast exam every year beginning at age 20.
- Mammogram every 2–3 years beginning at ages 20–25.
- Pelvic exam, pelvic ultrasound, and Pap test every year beginning at age 20.
- Consider hysterectomy and salpingo-oophorectomy upon completion of child bearing.

For men with PJS:
- Testicular exam every year beginning at age 10.

Men and women:
- Upper endoscopy every 2 years beginning at ages 8–10.
- Small bowel follow-through (barium study) every 2 years beginning at ages 8–10.
- Consider video capsule endoscopy or double-balloon endoscopy instead of the barium study every 2 years beginning at ages 8–10.
- Colonoscopy exam every 2–3 years beginning at age 25.
- Endoscopic ultrasound (if available) or abdominal ultrasound with special attention to the pancreas every 1–2 years beginning at age 30.

Sources: Amos et al. (2007); Lindor et al. (2008, p. 70).

these polyps can cause significant morbidity. Pancreatic screening can be done, but there is limited information regarding its efficacy.

5.3.5. PTEN Hamartoma Syndrome

PHS is thought to account for less than 1% of total breast cancer cases; however, it is almost certainly underreported. The major features of PHS include macrocephaly, mucocutaneous lesions, hamartomas, thyroid cancer, and breast cancer. (See Section 4.28 for detailed information on PHS and also on Bannayan–Riley–Ruvalcaba syndrome, which is not included in this section).

Women with PHS have a 25–50% lifetime risk of breast cancer. Cases of male breast cancer have also been reported.

5.3.5.1. PHS Tumor Types

- *Breast*—Most PHS-associated breast cancers are ductal carcinomas (either invasive or *in situ*), although lobular carcinomas have also been reported. There is an increased risk of both bilateral and multi-focal breast cancer. PHS is characterized by exuberant growth, which is exemplified by the extent and variety of benign breast tumors associated with this syndrome. This can include breast papillomas, hamartomas, fibroadenomas, fibrocystic breast disease, ductal hyperplasia, and LCIS. Two-thirds of women with PHS have some type of benign yet atypical breast cells.

- *Colon/rectum*—Individuals with PHS may develop GI hamartomas, especially in the colon and rectum. The hamartomas in PHS appear different from the ones that occur in PJS and are less likely to cause problems, such as bleeding, obstruction, or malignant transformation. In fact, people with PHS appear to have only slightly increased risks of colorectal cancer.

- *Skin*—Characteristic facial lesions are a pathognomonic feature of PHS. These benign skin lesions include:
  - Acral keratoses
  - Papillomatous papules
  - Trichilemmomas

- *Thyroid*—Individuals with PHS have increased risks for developing thyroid cancer. Most cases are epithelial carcinomas of the follicular subtype. Papillary thyroid carcinomas are also seen in PHS. Benign thyroid lesions include adenomas and multinodular goiters.

- *Uterus*—Women with PHS are at increased risk for developing uterine adenocarcinomas. Benign uterine tumors, including fibroids and hamartomas, are frequent in women with PHS.

- *Other*—Other benign and malignant neoplasms associated with PHS include:
  - Cerebellar dysplastic gangliocytoma (Lhermitte–Duclos)
  - Renal cell carcinoma

5.3.5.2. PHS Family History Assessment

Individuals with breast, thyroid, uterine or renal cell carcinoma are more likely to have *PTEN* mutations if they have personal histories of macrocephaly (with frontal bossing), facial papules, signs of exuberant growth (e.g., multiple hamartomas, lipomas, or papillomas), and/or autism. Some of the features of PHS, such as lipomas and fibrocystic breast disease, are common in the general population; therefore, it is useful to focus on the less common features when assessing the potential value of *PTEN* genetic testing.

About 80% of individuals who meet clinical criteria for PHS will be found to have a mutation in the *PTEN* gene. The majority of individuals with

TABLE 5.11. MANAGEMENT GUIDELINES FOR INDIVIDUALS WITH PTEN-HAMARTOMA SYNDROME

For women with PHS:
- Recommend clinical breast exam annually or semiannually starting at age 25 years.
- Recommend mammography annually starting at age 30–35 years or 5–10 years earlier than the earliest known breast cancer diagnosis in the family (whichever is earliest).
- Recommend breast MRI exams annually starting at age 30–35 years or 5–10 years earlier than the earliest known breast cancer diagnosis in the family (whichever is earliest).
- Discuss the options for endometrial cancer screening.
- Discuss the option of performing monthly BSE starting in early adulthood.[a]
- Discuss options of undergoing prophylactic mastectomy and/or hysterectomy as strategies for reducing cancer risks.

For men and women with PHS:
- Recommend comprehensive physical exam annually starting at age 18 years, with particular attention to breast and thyroid exam.
- Recommend thyroid ultrasound annually starting at age 18 years
- Consider recommending careful skin examination annually.
- Consider recommending colonoscopy every 5–10 years starting at age 50 years or earlier if any symptoms arise or there is a family history of colorectal cancer.

Source: Stein J and Eng C (2006) Cowden syndrome. Gene Reviews. Pagon RA, Bird TD, Dolan. CR et al. eds. Seattle: University of Washington, Seattle, 1993. www.genereviews.org; and National Comprehensive Cancer Network Clinical Practice Guidelines in Oncology. Genetic/familial high risk assessment: breast and ovarian. V.I.2009, http://www.nccn.org.

[a]Given recent evidence that BSE's are not effective screening tools, clinicians may wish to de-emphasize this recommendation.

PHS will have some features of the disorder by the third decade of life. This can be helpful in determining the probability of a *de novo* versus inherited *PTEN* mutation.

5.3.5.3. PHS Management Recommendations

The screening recommendations for individuals with PHS are listed in Table 5.11. In PHS, the highest risks of malignancy are in the breast, thyroid, and uterus.

Breast cancer can occur in premenopausal women with PHS, which is why imaging studies begin at age 25–30 and include breast MRI. The extent of benign breast disease may make it difficult to identify malignant or premalignant lesions. Perpetual biopsies can be anxiety-provoking for patients and the resulting scar tissue may make it even more difficult to screen for breast cancer in the future. For prevention, women with PHS can consider taking an antihormonal agent such as tamoxifen and can also consider the option of prophylactic bilateral mastectomies. It is important to realize that no studies have assessed the efficacy of breast MRI, tamoxifen, or prophylactic mastectomy in women with PHS.

In terms of the uterine cancer risks, pelvic exams and endometrial biopsies are recommended. The option of hysterectomy may also be discussed.

Thyroid cancers can occur in early adulthood so screening should start at age 18. Screening typically consists of a clinical palpation of the thyroid and an ultrasound exam.

5.4. FURTHER READING

American Cancer Society. 2007. Breast Cancer Facts and Figures, 2007–2008. American Cancer Society, Atlanta, GA, 1–36.

American Cancer Society. 2011. Breast Cancer: Early Detection. http://www.cancer.org/Cancer/BreastCancer/MoreInformation/BreastCancerEarlyDetection/breast-cancer-early-detection.

American Joint Committee on Cancer. 2010. Cancer Staging Handbook, 7th edition. Springer, New York.

Amos, CI, Frazier, ML, and McGarrity, TJ. 2007. Peutz-Jeghers syndrome. Gene Reviews (online). Pagon, RA, Bird, TD, and Dolan, CR (eds). University of Washington, Seattle, 1993. http://www.genetests.org.

Berliner, JL, and Fay, AM. 2007. Risk assessment and genetic counseling for hereditary breast and ovarian cancer: recommendations of the National Society of Genetic Counselors. J Genet Couns 16:241–260.

Dollinger, M, Rosenbaum, EH, Tempero, M, et al. 2002. Breast. In Everyone's Guide to Cancer Therapy, 4th edition. Andrews McMeel Pub, Kansas City, MO.

Frank, TS, Manley, SA, Olopade, OI, et al. 1998. Sequence analysis of BRCA1 and BRA2: correlation of mutations with family history and ovarian cancer risk. J Clin Oncol 16:2417–2425.

Gonzalez, KD, Noltner, KA, Buzin, CH, et al. 2009. Beyond Li-Fraumeni syndrome: clinical characteristics of families with p53 germline mutations. J Clin Oncol 27:1250–1256.

Haites, N, and Gregory, H. 2002. Overview of the clinical genetics of breast cancer. In Morrison, PJ, Hodgson, SV, and Haites, NE (eds), Familial Breast and Ovarian Cancer: Genetics, Screening, and Management. Cambridge University Press, Cambridge, UK.

Kaurah, P, and Huntsman, DG. 2006. Hereditary diffuse gastric cancer. Gene Reviews. (online). Pagon, RA, Bird, TD, and Dolan, CR (eds). 1993. University of Washington, Seattle, 1993. http://www.genetests.org.

Lindor, NM, McMaster, ML, Linder, CJ, et al. 2008. Concise Handbook of Familial Cancer Susceptibility Syndromes. J Natl Cancer Inst Monogr 38:1–93.

Link, J, Cullinane, C, Kakkis, J, et al. 2007. The Breast Cancer Survival Manual, 4th edition. Holt Paperbacks, New York.

Love, S, and Lindsey, K. 2005. Dr. Susan Love's Breast Book, 4th edition. Da Capo Press, Cambridge, MA.

Petrucelli, N, Daly, MB, and Feldman, GL. 2011. BRCA1 and BRCA2 Hereditary Breast and Ovarian Cancer. Gene Reviews (online). Pagon, RA, Bird, TD, and Dolan, CR, et al. (eds). University of Washington, Seattle, 1993. http://www.genetests.org.

Web MD. 2010. Breast Cancer Guide. Web MD, LLC. http://www.webmd.com/breast-cancer/guide/default.htm.

ALL ABOUT COLORECTAL CANCER

In 2000 [Katie Couric] famously televised her own colonoscopy on the *Today* show as a way to demystify a procedure that many people were too embarrassed to discuss. "I've heard every colonoscopy joke there is," she says. "People might feel like, 'Shut up already. Here she is, talking about colons again.' But I think the benefits far outweigh the negatives."

(Evans, R, Ladies Home Journal, March 2010, p. 88)

6.1. OVERVIEW OF COLORECTAL CANCER

This section begins with a description of the normal anatomy of the colon and rectum followed by an overview of risk factors and tumor types.

6.1.1. BASIC ANATOMY OF THE COLON AND RECTUM

The colon and rectum are part of the lower gastrointestinal (GI) tract, which is also referred to as the large intestine. The large intestine consists of the appendix, cecum, colon, rectum, and anal canal. In adults, the large intestine is about 5 feet (1.5 meters) in length. The normal anatomy of the colon and rectum are shown in Figure 6.1.

The main components of the colon and rectum are described below.

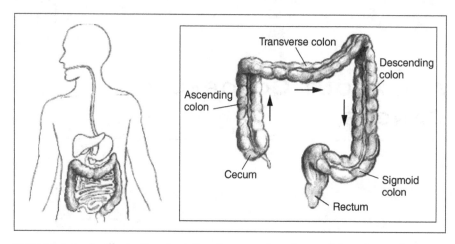

FIGURE 6.1. An illustration depicting the normal anatomy of the colon and rectum.
Source: http://www.wellsphere.com/digestive-health-article/anatomic-problems.

6.1.1.1. Colon

The colon is a long tubular structure that begins at the small intestine (and cecum) and ends at the rectum. The main functions of the colon are to form and temporarily store stool (feces) and to propel the stool toward the anal canal for expulsion from the body. Within the colon, numerous enzymes and bacteria reabsorb any excess water and remaining nutrients from the stool. It is estimated that 400 types of bacteria normally reside in the colon (and other parts of the large intestine). The colon is subdivided into the following sections:

- *The ascending colon (right-sided colon)*—This is the first segment of the colon. It begins at the juncture of the small intestine and ends at the transverse colon. In adults, it is about 25 cm in length.

- *The transverse colon (middle colon)*—This is the second segment of the colon. The transverse colon lies completely within the peritoneum and stretches horizontally between the ascending colon and the descending colon. In adults, it is about 45 cm in length.

- *The descending colon (left-sided colon)*—This is the third segment of the colon. It begins at the transverse colon and ends at the sigmoid colon. It is also retroperitoneal (i.e., the peritoneum covers its anterior side). In adults, it is about 15 cm in length.

- *The sigmoid colon (left-sided colon)*—This is the fourth segment of the colon that lies between the descending colon and the rectum. It is considered to be part of the "left-sided" colon together with the descending colon. In adults, it is about 40 cm in length.

6.1.1.2. Rectum

The rectum is a tubular organ that connects the sigmoid colon to the anal canal. In adults, the rectum is about 12 cm long. The lower third of the rectum is not covered by the peritoneal lining and is sometimes called the "rectal ampulla." The function of the rectum is the same as listed above for the colon, with the only difference being that the stool has very few nutrients or excess water by this point. After having had every ounce of nutritional value wrung from it, the stool is then pushed toward the anal canal for elimination from the body. In adults, the rectum is 12 inches in length.

6.1.1.3. Colorectal Walls

The walls of the tubular-shaped colon and rectum are composed of the following four layers of tissue (see Fig. 6.2):

- *Mucosa*—The mucosa is the innermost layer of the colorectal wall. The mucosal layer is composed primarily of epithelial cells that form the inner lining of the colorectum. Normal epithelial cells have a short life span, renewing themselves approximately every 6 days. The continual growth of the epithelial cells as well as their direct contact with the contaminants present in the fecal matter make these cells vulnerable to carcinogenic transformation. The colorectal mucosa also contains other types of cells, including:
  - Glandular cells (crypts), which secrete hormones to absorb the final drops of water and nutrients from the fecal matter and help with the propulsion of stool.
  - Goblet cells, which produce mucus to help keep bacteria out of the bloodstream.
  - Collagen cells (lamina propria), which form a protective mesh of tissue around the crypts and other cells of the mucosa.
  - Lymphocytes and other cells of the immune system, which may help protect the other cells from infection and may play another as-yet undetermined role within the colon and rectum.
- *Submucosa*—The second layer of the colorectal wall holds the network of arteries, veins, and nerves that run throughout the colon and rectum.
- *Muscularis externa*—The third layer of the colorectal wall is composed of the muscles that propel the stool through the colon and rectum.
- *Serosa*—The fourth and outermost section of the colorectal wall is the serosa, which maintains the positioning of the colon and rectum within the lower abdomen. This layer of tissue may also be termed the adventitia.

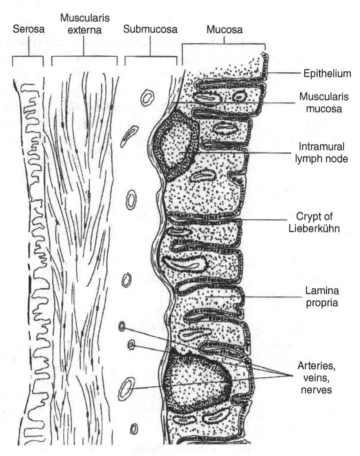

FIGURE 6.2. A microscopic view of the four main layers of cells that make up the colorectal walls. The mucosa, which is the innermost layer, is the initial site of most CRCs. Source: Adrouny (2002), 9, fig 1.1 by Alan Estridge. Reproduced by permission of University Press of Mississippi.

6.1.1.4. Blood Vessels

The blood vessels that nourish the colon and rectum form an apron-shaped pattern around the large intestine. These blood vessels are part of the mesentery system of arteries and veins. The blood vessels that provide nutrients to the ascending colon and transverse colon originate from the superior mesenteric artery. The blood vessels that provide nutrients to the descending colon, sigmoid colon, and rectum originate from the inferior mesenteric artery.

6.1.1.5. Lymphatics

The lymphatic system collects any fluid that leaks out from blood vessels and accumulates between cells so that it can be filtered through the lymph nodes, and then returned to the circulatory system. The main purposes of the lymph nodes are to trap debris and to monitor the need for any immune responses. There are three main clusters of lymph nodes near the colon and rectum:

- The paracolic nodes, which are located near the outside surface of the colon.
- The intermediate nodes, which are located along the major blood vessels supplying the colon.
- The central nodes, which are located near the aorta and lungs.

6.1.2. RISK FACTORS FOR COLORECTAL CANCER

Colorectal cancer (CRC) is a multifactorial disease that can be caused by a variety of factors. The features described in this section are proven or suspected risk factors for CRC.

6.1.2.1. Age

The risk of colon cancer increases with age. More than 90% of CRC cases occur in people over age 50. In the United States, the average age of CRC in the general population is 62. Less than 1% of cases of CRC occur below age 20.

6.1.2.2. Alcohol Use

The use of alcohol increases the risk of CRC. In one study, people who drank more than seven alcoholic drinks a week increased their risk of CRC by about 60% compared with people who drank less alcohol per week. Individuals who have more than three alcoholic drinks a day seem to have the highest risks of colon cancer. It does not seem to matter whether the consumed alcoholic drinks are wine, beer, or hard liquor.

6.1.2.3. Diabetes

Individuals with type II diabetes are at increased risk to develop CRC. The risk of CRC may be 20–40% higher in people who are insulin dependent compared with those who metabolize sugar normally. Diabetics who develop CRC also appear to have a poorer prognosis.

6.1.2.4. Dietary Factors

Carcinogens that are present in digested food can disturb the glandular cells in the lining of the colon wall. Cancers may occur more frequently in the colon and rectum than in the small intestine because fecal matter (containing possible carcinogens) is stored in the colorectum for a longer amount of time, thus increasing the likelihood of damaging the epithelial lining of the colon wall. Diets that contain high quantities of red meats, processed meats, and fat (which are more difficult for the body to digest) increase the risk of CRC while diets rich in fruits, vegetables, and fiber decrease the risk of CRC. Individuals who have low levels of vitamin D, potassium, and calcium may also have increased risks of CRC.

6.1.2.5. Ethnicity

African Americans have one of the highest incidences of CRC, although the reason for this is not clear. Individuals of Ashkenazi Jewish heritage also have increased risks of CRC, primarily due to the excessive prevalence of the I1307K mutation in the *APC* gene. The presence of the I1307K mutation confers a small to moderate increased risk of CRC.

6.1.2.6. Family History

Individuals who have a close relative diagnosed with precancerous polyps (adenomas) or CRC have increased risks of developing CRC. (See Table 6.1.) The risk of CRC to age 79 ranges from 4% if the individual has no affected relatives to 16% if two or more relatives have been diagnosed with CRC.

6.1.2.7. Gender

Men appear to have a higher incidence of developing precancerous and cancerous tumors in the colon compared with women, especially at older ages (69 years or older). In addition, the incidence of rectal cancer is much higher in men than in women. Men have an estimated 4:1 ratio of being diagnosed with rectal cancer compared with women.

TABLE 6.1. Estimated Risk of Colorectal Cancer (CRC) Based on Family History

First-Degree Relative (FDR)	Relative Risk	Absolute Risk (to 79) (%)
None with CRC	1	4
1 FDR: adenoma	2.0 (95% CI, 1.6–2.6)	8
1 FDR: CRC	2.3 (95% CI, 2.0–2.5)	9
1 FDR: CRC <45 years	3.9 (95% CI, 2.4–6.2)	15
2 FDRs: CRC	4.3 (95% CI, 3.0–6.1)	16

Source: National Cancer Institute, Genetics of Colorectal Cancer (PDQ), p.3. http://www.cancertopics/pdg/genetics/colorectal/HealthProfessional _12.

CI, confidence interval.

6.1.2.8. Genetic Predisposition

The risk of CRC is greatly increased in people who have inherited mutations in the *MSH2, MLH1, MSH6, APC, MYH, PMS2, TACSTD1, SMAD4, BMPR1A,* and *STK11* genes. These genetic risk factors account for only 5–10% of CRC cases. However, they confer the greatest magnitude of risk compared to other factors. Aberrant methylation of a mismatch repair gene also accounts for some cases of nonhereditary CRC. For example, mutations in the *BRAF* gene (especially the V600E mutation) are present in about 8% of sporadic CRCs. *BRAF* mutations are frequently associated with methylated *MLH1* genes. There are also several lower penetrance genes, which, when mutated, confer low to moderate increased risks of CRC. The best known example of a low penetrance gene is the I1307K mutation in the *APC* gene, which confers a low to moderate increased risk of CRC.

6.1.2.9. Inflammatory Bowel Disease

Individuals who have inflammatory bowel disease (IBD)—for example, ulcerative colitis or Crohn's disease—are at increased risk for developing invasive CRC. The average age of CRC in people with IBD is age 48. IBD causes recurrent inflammations and ulcerations in the mucosa cells of the wall of the colon or rectum, which can ultimately lead to the formation of a tumor. The exact risk of CRC associated with IBD depends on the severity of the condition (the number of flare-ups), the extent of the colon and rectum that is affected, and the length of time that the person has had the condition. Ulcerative colitis tends to aggravate the epithelial cells in the mucosal lining, while Crohn's disease can cause inflammation and ulcers throughout all the layers of the colorectal walls. Individuals who have irritable bowel syndrome do not appear to have increased risks of CRC.

6.1.2.10. Microsatellite Instability-High Tumor

Individuals with colorectal tumors that display high levels of microsatellite instability (MSI) are more likely to have Lynch syndrome, which is caused by a germline mutation in a mismatch repair gene. A panel of five or more markers is used to determine the MSI status. Possible MSI results are as follows:

- *MSI stable*—no instability in any of the markers
- *MSI low*—instability in <30% of the markers
- *MSI high*—instability in >30% of the markers

MSI has been called the "fingerprint" of Lynch syndrome. About 90% of Lynch syndrome-associated colorectal tumors are MSI high while only 15%

of sporadic tumors are MSI high. The main cause of sporadic MSI is somatic methylation of the *MLH1* gene.

6.1.2.11. Obesity

Individuals who are morbidly overweight are at increased risk for developing colon cancer. This is especially true for obese individuals who have a body mass index (BMI) of 25 or greater. A high BMI score appears to be more of a risk factor for colon cancer than for rectal cancer. Overeating and a sedentary lifestyle may also be risk factors for CRC.

6.1.2.12. Personal History of CRC or Adenomas

A prior personal history of CRC increases the risk of developing a second colorectal primary. The development of a colorectal adenoma also increases the risk of CRC, especially if the person has developed a large-sized adenoma (greater than 1 cm) or has developed multiple adenomas.

6.1.2.13. Radiation Exposure

Individuals who receive radiation therapy in the lower abdomen or pelvic region are at increased risk for developing CRC.

6.1.2.14. Tobacco Use

The use of tobacco also appears to increase the risk of developing colorectal adenomas and cancer. In one study, the risk of dying from colon cancer was 34% higher in male smokers and 43% higher in female smokers compared with nonsmokers. The risk of dying from colon cancer was associated with the number of daily cigarettes smoked and the number of years that a person had smoked. Pipe smokers were also found to have an increased risk of CRC.

6.1.3. Benign Colorectal Lesions

About 95% of CRCs arise from polyps (mostly adenomas). These polyps come in two basic shapes—pedunculated or sessile. Pedunculated polyps have a rounded, mushroom-like appearance and a slender stalk, which is attached to the mucosal lining. Sessile polyps are finger-like protuberances that sit directly on the mucosal lining. Some sessile polyps lie flat against the colorectal wall, which make them more difficult to detect (and remove). Tubular adenomas are pedunculated polyps and villous adenomas are sessile polyps. (See Fig. 6.3.) By age 50, it is estimated that one in four people will have a colorectal polyp; however, only a few of these

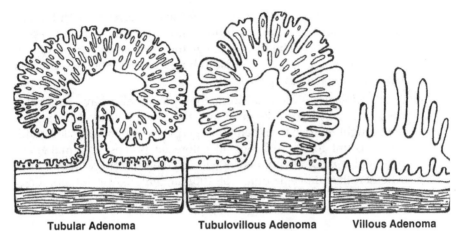

Tubular Adenoma   **Tubulovillous Adenoma**   **Villous Adenoma**

FIGURE 6.3. An illustration depicting the three major types of adenomas. Source: Adrouny (2002), 18, fig 2.2 by Alan Estridge. Reproduced by permission of University Press of Mississippi.

polyps will be precancerous. A polyp is more likely to transform into a malignant tumor if it is glandular, large in size, and/or has occurred in the ascending colon. An adenoma that is less then 1 cm has less than a 1% risk of malignancy, while a 2-cm adenoma has a 15% or greater likelihood of containing malignant cells. The major types of polyps are described below.

6.1.3.1. Adenomas

Adenomas arise from the glandular cells that lie in the innermost mucosal lining of the colon. About 70% of all polyps are characterized as adenomas. Adenomatous polyps are considered precancerous lesions because of their high potential for neoplastic transformation. In general, it takes 5 years for an adenoma to transform into a malignant tumor. Adenomatous polyposis is defined as the presence of at least 100 adenomas in the colon and rectum. There are several types of adenomas, including:

- *Tubular adenomas*—Tubular adenomas are pedunculated polyps. Tubular adenomas are the most common type of tumor that occurs in the colon. About 90% of sporadic tubular adenomas occur in the rectum or sigmoid colon. Tubular adenomas confer about a 2% risk of malignancy.
- *Villous adenomas*—Villous adenomas are sessile polyps. This type of polyp occurs much less frequently than tubular adenomas, but when present, it confers a 35% risk of malignancy. Villous adenomas are also termed papillary adenomas.

- *Tubulovillous adenomas*—These polyps have features of both tubular and villous adenomas. Some tubulovillous adenomas have a sessile or flat appearance. The risk of malignancy associated with a tubulovillous adenoma is about 20%. Tubulovillous adenomas are also termed villoglandular polyps.

- *Sessile adenomas*—These adenomatous polyps also have some features of hyperplastic polyps. In fact, these rare precancerous polyps are thought to arise from benign hyperplastic polyps. Sessile adenomas account for 0.1–0.5% of all colorectal polyps. The malignant potential of these adenomas depends on their histology type, that is, whether they have features of tubular, villous, or tubulovillous polyps.

6.1.3.2. Hamartomas

A hamartoma is a pedunculated polyp composed of normal cells that has formed an atypical (and disorganized) mass. Hamartomas have a low likelihood of becoming malignant or causing morbidity. A juvenile polyp is a type of hamartoma that has distinctive characteristics and often (though not always) occurs in childhood. Juvenile polyposis is defined as the development of five or more juvenile polyps. Peutz–Jegher polyps also have distinctive characteristics.

6.1.3.3. Hyperplastic Polyps

Hyperplastic polyps are benign lesions that represent an increased number of normal (and orderly) colorectal cells. Hyperplastic polyps do not typically increase the risk of CRC. However, these polyps are generally removed during a colonoscopy and sent to pathology to confirm the absence of atypical or malignant cells. A rare type of precancerous adenoma, termed a sessile serrated adenoma, can arise from a hyperplastic polyp. Some people develop multiple hyperplastic polyps over their lifetime, which raises the suspicion that they may have some increased risk of colorectal cancer.

6.1.3.4. Inflammatory Polyps

Most inflammatory polyps are actually irritations of the mucosal lining caused by chronic inflammations. This type of "pseudopolyp" often occurs in people with IBD. Another type of inflammatory polyp is the benign lymphoid polyp. Lymphoid polyps contain normal lymphatic tissue and have a low potential for malignancy. This rare type of polyp occurs more frequently in the rectum than in the colon and develops more often in children than in adults.

6.1.3.5. Leiomyomas

Leiomyomas are rare, benign tumors that arise from the smooth muscle cells of the colon or rectum. In some cases, these low-grade tumors have been misclassified as gastrointestinal stromal tumors (GISTs), which are much more likely to be malignant.

6.1.4. INTRAMUCOSAL CRC

6.1.4.1. Adenocarcinoma *In Situ*

In situ adenocarcinomas are composed of fully malignant cells, but they are either localized to one specific region of the mucosa or they are fully contained within a polyp.

6.1.4.2. Intramucosal Adenocarcinoma

Adenocarcinomas that are intramucosal are malignant tumors that have begun to spread beyond the initial lesion, but are still confined to the mucosal lining.

6.1.5. INVASIVE CRC

Invasive tumors are ones that have partially or completely penetrated through the colorectal wall. Almost 50% of CRCs occur in the lower third part of the colon (descending and sigmoid colon) and rectum. At diagnosis, about 50% of individuals with CRC show some evidence of metastatic disease. The most common sites of metastases in CRC are the neighboring organs, the peritoneum, the liver, and the lungs.

6.1.5.1. Adenocarcinoma

The vast majority of colorectal malignant tumors are adenocarcinomas, which have originated from glandular cells in the mucosa. Invasive adenocarcinomas are fully malignant tumors that are positioned to spread to local lymph nodes and neighboring organs. There are a variety of different adenocarcinoma histological subtypes. Three specific types of colorectal adenocarcinomas are described below:

- *Mucinous (colloid) carcinoma*—Mucinous carcinomas produce globules of mucus that form pools or colloid (empty-appearing) spaces. The presence of mucus seems to help the cancer cells to spread faster, which may explain why this tumor subtype is considered aggressive with a high rate of metastasis. It is estimated that about 10–15% of all adenocarcinomas are the mucinous subtype.

- *Signet ring cell carcinoma*—Signet ring cell carcinomas produce globules of mucus, similar to mucinous carcinomas, but the mucus stays trapped within the cytoplasm of the cells. This causes the nuclei to be pushed to one side, giving the cells a "ring-like" appearance under the microscope. Signet ring carcinomas are difficult to treat and tend to be even more aggressive than mucinous tumors. Only 1–2% of adenocarcinomas are the signet ring cell carcinoma subtype.

- *Squamous cell (epidermoid) carcinoma*—Squamous cell carcinomas originate from epidermoid cells in the mucosal lining. These cells are similar to cutaneous epidermoid cells, although in terms of treatment, colorectal squamous cell carcinomas are treated similarly to colorectal adenocarcinomas.

6.1.5.2. Gastrointestinal Stromal Tumors (GIST)

GISTs arise from specific cells in the autonomic nervous system termed interstitial cells of Cajal (ICCs). ICCs are nicknamed the "pacemakers" of the digestive tract. Their function is to send signals to the muscles to stimulate the digestion and movement of food and waste products through the body. GIST tumors are more typically found in the stomach or small bowel than in the colon or rectum. These rare tumors can be either malignant or benign.

6.1.5.3. Leiomyosarcoma

Leiomyosarcomas are soft tissue sarcomas that originate from the smooth muscle cells of the colon wall. Soft tissue sarcomas of the colon tend to be aggressive tumors with a high rate of metastasis. Leiomyosarcomas represent less than 2% of CRCs and the average age at diagnosis is 60 years.

6.1.5.4. Lymphoma

Lymphomas originate from a lymphocyte cell located in the wall of the colon or rectum. A number of non-Hodgkin lymphomas can occur in the colon or rectum, including follicular cell, mantle cell, large B cell, anaplastic large cell, Burkitt lymphoma, and mucosa-associated lymphoma tissue (MALT). Lymphomas are more likely to occur in the rectum than in the colon. Lymphomas represent 1% or less of colorectal malignancies.

6.1.5.5. Melanoma

Primary melanoma of the colon or rectum represents only 1–2% of colorectal malignancies. More typically, the melanoma cells found in the colon or rectum have metastasized from elsewhere in the body.

6.1.5.6. Neuroendocrine Tumors

About 4% of CRCs are large-cell or small-cell neuroendocrine carcinomas (NECs). NECs originate from one of the hormone-producing cells within the nervous system that runs throughout the colon wall. These tumors tend to be quite aggressive. In contrast, carcinoid tumors, which can also occur in the colon or rectum, tend to be slow-growing neuroendocrine tumors that have a low rate of metastasis.

6.2. CRC MANAGEMENT: SCREENING, DIAGNOSIS, AND TREATMENT

6.2.1. SCREENING AND PREVENTION GUIDELINES

The American Cancer Society guidelines for colon cancer screening in the general population are listed in Table 6.2. The standard recommendation is for each individual to have a baseline flexible sigmoidoscopy or colonoscopy at age 50. Both procedures involve inserting a scope into the rectum and colon to look for unusual growths, obstructions, or inflammations. If any polyps are detected, they are generally snared and removed in a procedure termed polypectomy. Thus, the colonoscopy and polypectomy procedures not only detect CRC, but can also prevent it. Unfortunately, a number of people delay or refuse to be scoped, because of their dislike of the necessary cleaning out preparation or fear of the procedure itself.

A sigmoidoscopy allows the gastroenterologist to examine the lower one-third segment of the colon while a colonoscopy examines the full length of the colon. Since the majority of sporadic CRCs occur in the lower part of the colon or rectum, the sigmoidoscopy procedure may be adequate for most people. However, if the individual has any additional risk factors for colon cancer, then the more comprehensive colonoscopy procedure is recommended.

Individuals with ulcerative colitis need to have annual colonoscopies beginning 15–25 years after being diagnosed if the disease is confined to the left colon and 8–10 years after diagnosis if there is an episode of pancolitis (in which the disease involves the entire colon). Individuals with Crohn's disease that involves the colon should also have more frequent colonoscopy procedures, depending upon the duration and extent of the disease.

Warning signs of CRC include general abdominal discomfort (frequent gas, pain, bloating, fullness, or cramps) and marked changes in bowel habits, especially an increase in frequency. (See Table 6.3.) Symptoms are more likely to occur if the tumor lies in the lower part of the colon or in the rectum. More advanced stages of CRC can cause significant internal bleeding, weight loss, and anemia. If the tumor has actually perforated the bowel, then it can cause excruciating pain similar to appendicitis or a gall bladder attack.

TABLE 6.2. AMERICAN CANCER SOCIETY GUIDELINES FOR COLON CANCER
SCREENING IN THE GENERAL POPULATION

Beginning at age 50, both men and women at *average risk* for developing CRC
should use one of the screening tests below. The tests that are designed to find
both early cancer and polyps are preferred.

Tests that find polyps and cancer:
- flexible sigmoidoscopy every 5 years[a]
- colonoscopy every 10 years
- double contrast barium enema every 5 years[a]
- CT colonography (virtual colonoscopy) every 5 years[a]

Tests that mainly find cancer:
- fecal occult blood test (FOBT) every year[a,b]
- fecal immunochemical test (FIT) every year[a,b]
- stool DNA test (sDNA), interval uncertain[a]

Source: American Cancer Society: http://www.cancer.org/docroot/PED/content/ped_2_3X_
ACS_Cancer_Detection_Guidelines_36.asp.

[a]Colonoscopy should be done if test results are positive.

[b]For FOBT or FIT used as a screening test, the take-home multiple sample method should be
used. An FOBT or FIT done during a digital rectal exam in the doctor's office is not adequate
for screening.

The American Cancer Society suggests the following strategies to reduce
the risks of developing CRC:

- Choose foods and beverages in amounts that help achieve and main-
  tain a healthy weight.
- Eat five or more servings of a variety of vegetables and fruits each day.
- Choose whole grains rather than processed (refined) grains.
- Limit your intake of processed and red meats.
- Avoid excessive alcohol intake; no more than one drink per day for
  women and no more than two drinks a day for men.
- Maintain an active lifestyle; engage in some type of physical activity
  for at least 30 minutes on five or more days of the week.
- Contact your physician if you have any possible symptoms of colon
  cancer .
- If you are age 50 or older, schedule a colon cancer screening test.

Other possible strategies for reducing one's risk of CRC are to limit the intake
of dietary fat, which can irritate the bowel mucosa, and to increase the intake
of dietary fiber because fiber binds to bile and keeps it from irritating the
bowel mucosa.

TABLE 6.3. WARNING SIGNS OF CRC

A change in bowel habits
Blood in stool
Diarrhea or constipation
Stool is narrower than usual
General abdominal discomfort
Unexplained weight loss
Constant tiredness
Anemia or jaundice
Vomiting or nausea

Source: Dixon (2007b): About.com: Colon Cancer http://coloncancer.about.com/od/coloncancerbasics/a/colcansymptoms.htm.

Taking supplemental calcium, folic acid, aspirin, or other nonsteroidal anti-inflammatory drugs (NSAIDs) may also reduce the risks of colorectal polyps and cancer.

Keep in mind that it is not clear how effective these strategies are in reducing the risk of CRC in people with inherited susceptibilities.

6.2.2. STRATEGIES FOR DIAGNOSING CRC

The diagnostic tests described in this section are the main ones that are used to identify and stage CRC.

6.2.2.1. Colonoscopy and Sigmoidoscopy

The colonoscopy and flexible sigmoidoscopy procedures are the main procedures used to diagnose CRC. These procedures are typically performed by a gastroenterologist. Prior to the procedure, the individual is instructed to take laxatives to clear stool out of the colon. The procedure involves inserting a long thin tube into the rectum and colon. In a flexible sigmoidoscopy, the tube is inserted into the lower one-third section of the colon. In a colonoscopy, the tube is inserted through the full length of the colon. Air is generally put into the colon to expand the colon walls and allow the surfaces to be seen more clearly. Water or a special dye may also be used to enhance the viewing of the mucosal lining. Individuals are almost always fully sedated for the colonoscopy procedure but may not be sedated for a sigmoidoscopy. Any suspicious lesions detected during the scope will be removed with a snare unless the lesion is too large for simple extraction or there are simply too many polyps. The most common side effects of a colonoscopy or sigmoidoscopy are gas pains and minor rectal bleeding. More serious complications, such as infection or perforating the colon or rectum, are rare occurrences.

6.2.2.2. Computed Tomography Colonography

Computed tomography (CT) colonography, also termed a virtual colonoscopy, is an imaging technique that creates a three-dimensional view of the colon. Preparation for this procedure involves taking laxatives similar to the colonoscopy or sigmoidoscopy. If any suspicious growths are detected by CT colonography, then the individual will need to undergo a traditional colonoscopy to reassess and remove the lesions. While CT colonography is much less invasive than a colonoscopy, there are concerns that it is not as effective at detecting flat (sessile) polyps. For this reason, virtual colonoscopies are not recommended for people who have increased risks of CRC.

6.2.2.3. Clinical Examination

A comprehensive clinical exam usually includes a digital rectal exam. The digital rectal exam is performed by a clinician who puts a lubricated gloved finger into the rectum to look for abnormalities of the rectum, prostate, or female reproductive organs. The clinician may also press on the abdomen to check for other signs of CRC such as tenderness, pain, drum-like sounds, liver enlargement, or abdominal distention.

6.2.2.4. Fecal Occult Blood Test

The fecal occult blood test (FOBT) (also termed the stool guaiac test) is a noninvasive screening test for CRC. For this analysis, an individual collects several stool samples (typically three) in a specialized specimen kit and ships it to a laboratory. The lab will then assess the stool for microscopic amounts of blood. Other laboratory analyses may also be performed, including the fecal immunochemical test (FIT) and the stool DNA (sDNA) test.

6.2.2.5. Double Contrast Barium Enema

The double contrast barium enema is a type of X-ray that can help determine the need for a colonoscopy or sigmoidoscopy. To prepare for the double contrast barium enema, the individual takes laxatives to clean out the bowel. For the procedure, the clinician inserts barium sulfate into the individual's rectum and then takes several X-rays of the colorectum from different angles. The barium sulfate creates a chalky white outline of the colon walls that can help with the detection of polyps. Air may also be used to inflate the colon and enhance the images. If any polyps are detected on these X-rays, then a follow-up colonoscopy or flexible sigmoidoscopy will be performed.

6.2.2.6. Blood Tests

Individuals who are diagnosed with CRC often have blood tests to assess the level of a tumor marker termed carcinoembryonic antigen (CEA). This is an antigen that is produced by most colorectal tumors, but not by normal cells. Thus, the levels of CEA can be used to monitor the tumor's growth or regression. Additional blood tests may include a complete blood count (CBC), a liver function test, and the CA-19 tumor marker test.

6.2.2.7. Biopsy

Colorectal lesions are typically biopsied (or removed) during the colonoscopy or sigmoidoscopy procedure. A fine-needle biopsy or core biopsy may also be performed. These biopsy procedures are usually performed in conjunction with a CT scan or ultrasound. The colorectal specimen will then be sent to the pathology department for careful review. If the tumor is malignant, then it is also important to biopsy neighboring lymph nodes. In general, 7–14 lymph nodes are sampled.

6.2.2.8. Grading the Tumor

To grade the colorectal tumor, the pathologist will consider its size, configuration, and histopathology. (See Section 2.2.2 for more information about cancer staging.) About 20% of colorectal tumors are classified as poorly differentiated (advanced) neoplasms. Additional tests can be performed on the tumor including MSI, immunohistochemistry (IHC), and a chromosome study.

6.2.2.9. Staging the Cancer

The Dukes system of colon cancer classification (Stages A through D) has been replaced by the TNM system that is used for all solid tumors. (See Section 2.2.3 for more information about cancer staging.) The clinical staging system used for CRC is listed in Table 6.4.

6.2.2.10. Additional Studies

Individuals diagnosed with CRC will typically undergo imaging studies to look for sites of metastases. CRC can metastasize to any organ, but the most common sites of distant metastasis are the liver and lungs. It is also common for the cancer to spread to other segments of the colon or rectum, the small intestine, and the peritoneum. Imaging studies to look for signs of metastatic disease will typically include a chest X-ray to focus on the lungs and an abdominal CT scan or MRI to focus on the liver.

TABLE 6.4. TNM Clinical Staging System for CRC

Stage 0	Tis N0 M0
Stage 1	T1 or T2 N0 M0
Stage IIA	T3 N0 M0
Stage IIB	T4a N0 M0
Stage IIC	T4b N0 M0
Stage IIIA	T1-T2 N1/N1c M0 or T1 N2a M0
Stage IIIB	T3-T4a N1/N1c M0 or T2-T3 N2a M0 or T1-T2 N2b M0
Stage IIIC	T4a N2a M0 or T3-T4a N2b M0 or T4b N1-N2 M0
Stage IVA	Any T Any N M1a
Stage IVB	Any T Any N M1b

T (Primary Tumor): Tis = Carcinoma in situ: intraepithelial or invasion of lamina propria; T1 = Tumor invades submucosa; T2 = Tumor invades muscularis propria; T3 = Tumor invades through the muscularis propria into the pericolorectal tissues; T4a = Tumor penetrates to the surface of the visceral peritoneum; T4b = Tumor directly invades or is adherent to other organs or structures. N (Regional Lymph Nodes): N0 = No regional lymph node metastasis; N1 = Metastasis in 1–3 regional lymph nodes; N1a = Metastasis in 1 regional lymph node; N1b = Metastasis in 2–3 regional lymph nodes; N1c = Tumor deposit(s) in the subserosa, mesentery, or nonperitonealized pericolic or perirectal tissues without regional nodal metastasis; N2 = Metastasis in 4 or more regional lymph nodes; N2a = Metastasis in 4–6 regional lymph nodes; N2b-metastasis in ≥7 regional lymph nodes. M (Distant Metastasis): M0 = No distant metastasis; M1 = Distant metastasis; M1a = Metastasis confined to one organ or site; M1b = Metastasis in more than one organ/site or the peritoneum.

Source: American Committee on Cancer (2010), pp. 174–198.

6.2.3. Strategies for Treating CRC

A general description of the treatment strategies for colon and rectal cancer is provided below.

6.2.3.1. Surgery

Surgery is the primary strategy to treat CRC. Even if the person has metastatic disease, the primary colorectal tumor will be removed because of the high risk of bleeding or morbidity due to blockage. The standard operation is to remove the portion of the colon or rectum containing the tumor and then to reattach the remaining sections. This procedure is termed a segmental or a wedge resection. Because the malignant cells typically invade through the colorectal walls, this is deemed the best way to prevent local spread. In rectal cancer, it may be a more difficult surgical procedure because the rectum is wedged up against the pelvic bone (making it harder to obtain clear margins) and because it is important to avoid damaging the sphincter muscles (which control continence). If the neoplasm is small or the malignant cells are fully contained within a polyp, then it may be possible to excise the tumor without taking the segment of normal tissue. Regional lymph nodes are almost always sampled when malignant colorectal cells are identified. The surgical removal of the entire colon and rectum is termed a colectomy. A colectomy may be recommended if:

- the tumor is especially large or aggressive
- there are two or more primary colorectal tumors
- it is not possible to obtain clean margins
- the person has a genetic predisposition to CRC

Following a colectomy, the waste products that would normally pass through the colon and rectum are redirected to an internally constructed pouch (ileo-anal pouch or j-pouch) or to a small sack outside the body (colostomy bag). A colostomy may also be performed as a temporary measure to allow the tissue to heal.

6.2.3.2. Radiation

Radiation therapy is used to shrink tumors and reduce the likelihood of local spread. Radiation therapy is frequently used to treat rectal cancer, which has a higher rate of local recurrences than colon cancer. Radiation therapy is rarely used in the treatment of colon tumors. One exception may be cecal cancers (occurring at the juncture of the small and large intestines); radiation is sometimes given to reduce the risk of recurrence. Radiation can be dispensed in discrete doses via external beams or can be given continuously by using radioactive "seeds" and placing them in the rectum. Radiation therapy can also be used to treat localized metastatic disease or for palliative purposes in order to relieve pressure on nerves or bones.

6.2.3.3. Chemotherapy

Adjuvant chemotherapy is necessary if any malignant cells have spread through the colorectal wall or to the lymph nodes, or if the tumor has characteristics making it a high metastatic risk (such as large size). The main chemotherapeutic agent used to treat colorectal cancer is 5-FU (fluorouracil), although its effectiveness in treating MSI-high tumors is still being debated. Other chemotherapeutic agents include leucovorin, irinotecan, levamisole, oxaliplatin, and floxuridine. Chemotherapy can be administered by pill form, by injection into the vein or muscle, or by placing it directly into the abdomen near the cancer site. Chemotherapy agents can also be used to shrink a tumor prior to surgical resection or for palliative purposes to relieve pressure on nerves or bones.

6.2.3.4. Biological Therapy

Biological agents include cancer vaccines, monoantibody-based agents, and inhibitors of tumor angiogenesis. Many of these therapies are still investigational. One example of an investigational biological agent used in CRC is MOAB 17-1A, which targets a cell surface antigen expressed by many colorectal carcinomas.

6.2.4. CRC TREATMENT BY STAGE

6.2.4.1. Stage 0

In situ colorectal tumors may not require any treatment beyond surgical removal of the tumor and normal margins (at least 5 cm on either side of the tumor). Pedunculated colon tumors can generally be removed with a snare, while sessile tumors and low-lying rectal tumors may require more extensive procedures. Adjuvant therapy is not typically necessary for these early-stage malignancies. The 5-year survival rate with Stage 0 tumors is 95% or better.

6.2.4.2. Stage I

The standard treatment for Stage I CRC is the surgical removal of the tumor and normal margins. This procedure can be done transanally or transabdominally depending on where the tumor is located. Although the cancer cells have begun to spread, they have not gone beyond the mucosal layer of the colorectal wall. Adjuvant or neoadjuvant therapy is not typically necessary for Stage I colon tumors. Neoadjuvant radiation therapy may be used to shrink Stage I rectal tumors to provide better surgical options. Depending upon the characteristics of the tumor, regional lymph nodes may also be sampled. The 5-year survival rate with Stage I tumors is about 90–95%.

6.2.4.3. Stage II

Surgery remains the primary treatment strategy for Stage II tumors. In Stage II CRC, the malignant cells have begun to spread beyond the mucosal lining, but have not reached the lymph nodes. The standard surgical procedure is a segmental colectomy and excision of neighboring lymph nodes (which are negative by definition). Adjuvant or neoadjuvant chemotherapy and radiation are generally given to patients with rectal cancer. Adjuvant chemotherapy may be given to patients with colon cancer if the risk of relapse is considered to be high based on the size, characteristics, or initial spread of the tumor. Adjuvant radiation therapy may be used in cases of cecal cancer that have begun to spread. The 5-year survival for CRC is about 80–85% for Stage IIA cancers and about 65–70% for Stage IIB cancers. In general, the survival rates associated with colon cancer are a bit higher than the rates with rectal cancer. MSI-high tumors also seem to have better prognoses.

6.2.4.4. Stage III

In Stage III CRC, the malignant cells have spread locally and to the lymph nodes but have not shown up in distant organs. The standard therapy is segmental resection followed by chemotherapy. Biological agents may also be given. The 5-year survival rate for Stage III CRC is between 20–60% depending on the extent of local spread and the number of positive lymph nodes. The prognosis seems to be better for MSI-high tumors.

6.2.4.5. Stage IV

In Stage IV malignancies, the cancer cells have metastasized to distant organs (typically the liver and lungs). Therefore, the focus of treatment is on systemic interventions, such as chemotherapy and biological treatments. Individuals with isolated liver metastases may undergo surgery to excise these tumors. The 5-year survival rate for Stage IV CRC is about 5–10%, with better prognoses in MSI-high tumors. Individuals with isolated metastases generally have higher survival rates (20–25%). The most common cause of death for people with metastatic CRC is liver failure.

6.2.4.6. Recurrent Disease

Individuals with recurrent disease may be given chemotherapy and radiation treatments. The focus of these treatments is generally on the sites of metastases. Surgery may also be done to treat local recurrences, isolated metastases, or for palliative purposes.

6.3. CRC SYNDROMES

Colon cancer syndromes are categorized as either polyposis or nonpolyposis syndromes. The major polyposis syndromes are Familial Adenomatous Polyposis (FAP) syndrome, Juvenile Polyposis syndrome (JPS), MYH-Associated Polyposis (MAP), and Peutz–Jeghers syndrome. The major nonpolyposis syndrome is Lynch syndrome. In these five syndromes, CRC and polyps are major features. Additional hereditary cancer syndromes that confer heightened risks of CRC are listed in Table 6.5.

TABLE 6.5. HEREDITARY CANCER SYNDROMES THAT HAVE INCREASED RISKS OF CRC

CRC is a major feature in:
- FAP
- JPS
- Lynch syndrome
- MAP syndrome
- Peutz–Jeghers syndrome

CRC is a minor feature in:
- Bloom syndrome
- GIST, familial
- Hereditary diffuse gastric cancer syndrome
- Li–Fraumeni syndrome

Sources: Kohlmann and Gruber (2006); Lindor et al. (2008).

This section provides information about tumor characteristics, family history assessment, and management recommendations for FAP syndrome, JPS, Lynch syndrome, and MAP. (See Section 5.3.4 for similar information about Peutz–Jeghers syndrome.)

6.3.1. FAP SYNDROME

FAP accounts for less than 1% of total CRC cases. The hallmark feature of FAP is the carpeting of precancerous polyps along the walls of the colon and rectum.

Very few hereditary cancer syndromes are associated with 100% risks of cancer, but FAP is one of them. Men and women with FAP have virtually 100% risks of developing CRC unless they undergo total colectomies. (See Section 4.10 for additional information about FAP.)

6.3.1.1. Tumor Types

- *Adenocarcinoma*—FAP-associated carcinomas arise from the mucosal layer of cells lining the organs of the GI tract, including the colon, rectum, small intestine, ampulla of Vater, bile duct, stomach, or pancreas. The colorectal adenocarcinomas are more likely to be mucinous or signet ring subtypes.

- *Brain tumors*—Individuals with FAP are at increased risk for developing brain tumors. Most FAP-associated brain tumors are medulloblastomas. However, other types of brain tumors, such as ependymomas and gliomas, can also occur. (An individual with colorectal polyposis and a brain tumor has Turcot syndrome, which is a subtype of FAP.)

- *Desmoid tumors*—Desmoid tumors develop from soft tissue cells that form tendons and ligaments. Desmoids are rarely malignant, but can be difficult to eradicate or control. FAP-associated desmoid tumors typically occur in the abdomen rather than the external limbs. Desmoids are associated with the Gardner subtype of FAP and represent the highest cause of mortality in FAP patients who have had colectomies.
- *Polyps*—Individuals with classic FAP will have hundreds or thousands of adenomas lining the colorectal walls. These adenomas can be tubular, villous, or a combination of the two (tubulovillous). Many of the colorectal adenomas are sessile in shape, although pedunculated polyps may occur as well. Adenomas can also develop in the small intestine, especially at the ampulla of Vater, which is the juncture of the small and large intestines. FAP-associated polyps that develop in the stomach tend to be fundic gland polyps (hamartomas), which have a low likelihood of malignant transformation. Gastric adenomas may also occur.
- *Additional tumors*—Other tumors associated with FAP include:
  - Epidermal cysts and other benign skin lesions
  - Hepatoblastoma
  - Lipoma
  - Osteoma (benign bony growth)
  - Pancreas cancer (islet cell tumors)
  - Thyroid cancer (nonmedullary)

6.3.1.2. Family History Assessment

Classic FAP is defined as the presence of 100 or more adenomas carpeting the walls of the colon and rectum. Therefore, the clinical diagnosis of classic FAP is fairly straightforward. The main diagnostic challenges occur when an individual has developed between 10 and 100 adenomas. Clinicians will want to evaluate whether the individual could have the attenuated form of FAP, MAP syndrome, or an unusual presentation of Lynch syndrome.

APC mutations are more likely in personal or family histories with colorectal polyposis or cancer, hepatoblastoma, desmoid tumors, fundic gland polyps, osteomas, sebaceous or epidermoid cysts, dental abnormalities, and congenital hypertrophy of the retinal pigment epithelium (CHRPE). About 25% of *APC* mutations occur as *de novo* genetic events so an affected individual may have a completely negative family history.

6.3.1.3. Management Recommendations

Table 6.6 outlines the clinical recommendations for people with FAP. Individuals with classic FAP need to undergo colectomies to remove the

TABLE 6.6. MANAGEMENT RECOMMENDATIONS FOR INDIVIDUALS WITH FAP

- Recommend flexible sigmoidoscopy or colonoscopy annually beginning at age 10–12 years. Once polyps begin to emerge, then colonoscopy (rather than sigmoidoscopy) should be performed annually.
- Once the adenomas have begun to emerge, then recommend the surgical removal of the colon via proctocolectomy or colectomy.[a] The timing of the colectomy is dependent on several factors, including the advent and extent of polyp development.[b]
- If an ileal pouch was created from the colectomy, then recommend that follow-up endoscopic surveillance of the ileal pouch be performed every two years.
- If the rectum has been retained post-colectomy, then recommend that follow-up sigmoidoscopies be performed every year.
- If the rectum has been retained post-colectomy, then consider the use of non-steroidal anti-inflammatory drugs (NSAIDs) to reduce the polyp burden.
- Recommend upper endoscopy exam every 1–3 years starting at age 25–30 years or following the surgical removal of the colon (whichever comes first).
- Recommend clinical thyroid exam annually starting by age 18 years.
- Recommend that abdominal palpation be performed annually following the colectomy procedure.
- Consider recommending the use of abdominal and pelvic computerized tomography (CT) or MRI every 3 years, especially if the patient has a family history of desmoids.
- Consider adding small bowel visualization to the abdominal and pelvic CT or MRI scan, especially if the patient has a family history of small bowel cancer.
- Consider recommending screening for hepatoblastoma, including liver palpation, abdominal ultrasound and measurement of alpha-fetoprotein, every 3 to 6 months, from birth to age 5 years.

Source: Burt and Jasperson (2008) and National Comprehensive Cancer Network (NCCN), Familial Adenomatous Polyposis. v.1.2010 http://www.nccn.org.

Source: National Comprehensive Cancer Network (NCCN), v.1.2010 http://www.nccn.org/professionals/physician_gls/f_guidelines.asp.

[a]The surgical options for patients with FAP are as follows: total abdominal colectomy with ileorectal anastomosis (TAC/IRA), total proctocolectomy with anal ileostomy (TPC;/EI), or total protctocolectomy with ileal pouch anal anastomosis (TPC/IPAA).

[b]For patients with classic FAP, colectomy is typically performed between ages 15 and 25 years. However, for patients with attenuated FAP, the timing of the colectomy may be delayed by several years.

entire colon and possibly the rectum as well. This surgery is typically per-formed prior to age 25 and is often performed during adolescence. The timing of the prophylactic surgery is based on the onset of polyps, the family history of polyposis and CRC, and the genotype information. While some individuals with attenuated FAP can be successfully followed with annual colonoscopies, others will require colectomies (albeit at older ages than those with classic FAP).

Individuals with FAP who retain their rectum are still at high risk for developing polyps in the remaining epithelial cells. The use of NSAIDs, such as sulindac or celecoxib, has been found to slow or reduce the development of polyps. It is important to note that the use of NSAIDs does not replace the need for colectomy in a person with classic FAP.

Because of the risk-reducing prophylactic colectomies, individuals with FAP are more likely to die from extracolonic malignancies than from CRC. One of the most challenging FAP-associated tumors to treat is the abdominal desmoid tumor. Desmoid tumors are extremely difficult to manage and surgical resection may actually stimulate the growth of the tumor. Therefore, clinicians are advised to take a conservative approach toward using surgery in the management of FAP-associated desmoid tumors.

6.3.2. JUVENILE POLYPOSIS SYNDROME

JPS is a rare hereditary cancer syndrome that accounts for less than 1% of colon cancer cases. The diagnosis of JPS rests on the presence of five or more juvenile polyps.

Individuals with JPS have a greater than 90% likelihood of developing the characteristic polyps in their colon, rectum, and in other organs of the GI tract. CRC is most common malignancy associated with JPS. The lifetime risk of cancer in JPS may be as low as 10% and as high as 50%. (See Section 4.14 for additional information about JPS.)

6.3.2.1. Tumor Types

- *Colon cancer*—Individuals with JPS are at increased risk for developing colorectal adenocarcinomas. The CRCs in JPS do not appear to be a specific morphology or histology type. It is postulated that most of the JPS-associated CRCs arise from adenomatous polyps rather than from juvenile polyps.

- *Juvenile polyps*—Juvenile polyps, which are classified as a type of hamartoma, have a different histology and pathology from other types of GI polyps. As described by Joy Haidle and James Howe, "Juvenile polyps show a normal epithelium with a dense stroma, an inflammatory infiltrate, and a smooth surface with dilated, mucus-filled cystic glands in the lamina propria. Muscle fibers and the proliferative characteristics of adenomas are typically not seen in juvenile polyps" (2008, p. 2). The juvenile polyps can be sessile or pedunculated in shape and can develop throughout the GI tract, especially in the small intestine, stomach, colon, and rectum. Most of the polyps are benign with a low (but not zero) potential of becoming malignant. Juvenile polyps can occur at various ages from infancy to adulthood, although most juvenile polyps occur in children or adolescents.

- *Additional tumors*—Individuals with JPS are also at increased risk for developing cancers of the stomach and small intestine.

6.3.2.2. Family History Assessment

The pathognomonic feature of JPS is the presence of juvenile polyps. Most individuals with JPS have developed at least one of these characteristic polyps by age 20. Therefore, a key element in the diagnosis of JPS is a careful review of the polyp(s) by a skilled pathologist.

SMAD4 and *BMPR1A* mutations account for about 40% of JPS cases. These mutations can occur as *de novo* genetic events, so the family history may be completely negative. Individuals with *SMAD4* mutations also exhibit features of Hereditary Hemorrhagic Telangiectasia (HHT). Thus, they may report histories of frequent nose bleeds, small broken blood vessels on the face or fingers (telangiectasia), and/or arteriovenous malformations (AVMs).

6.3.2.3. Management Recommendations

Individuals with JPS need to have careful regular surveillance of their colon and stomach. (See Table 6.7.) Some people with JPS develop multiple polyps and require a partial or complete colectomy or gastrectomy. However, most individuals with JPS can be effectively managed with serial upper and lower endoscopy procedures.

On average, individuals with JPS start having upper and lower endoscopy exams at 15 years of age. These exams should be initiated at earlier

TABLE 6.7. Medical Management Recommendations for Individuals with JPS

- Recommend a baseline colonoscopy at about age 15 or earlier if there are symptoms. Recommend follow-up colonoscopy every year if polyps are found and every 2–3 years if no polyps are found.
- Recommend a baseline upper endoscopy at about age 15 or earlier if there are symptoms. Recommend follow-up endoscopy every year if polyps are found and every 2–3 years if no polyps are found.
- Discuss the option of prophylactic colectomy or gastrectomy if the polyp burden becomes difficult to manage.

Source: Haidle and Howe (2008) and National Comprehensive Cancer Network (NCCN), Juvenile Polyposis syndrome, v.1.2010 http://www.nccn.org.

ages if the child is experiencing any abnormal GI symptoms or if any of the child's family members developed polyps at an earlier age. Follow-up endoscopy exams should be performed every 2–3 years if no polyps are identified, and annually if polyps (of any type) are identified.

Some clinicians recommend performing blood tests (CBCs) every few years to look for signs of possible internal bleeding.

6.3.3. Lynch Syndrome

Lynch syndrome, defined as hereditary deficiency of mismatch repair protein, accounts for 2–3% of all colorectal cancers and 2% of all endometrial cancers. (See Section 4.17 for more information about Lynch syndrome.)

Individuals with Lynch syndrome are at 70–85% risk for developing colorectal cancer and 30–60% risk for developing endometrial cancer. The risk of a second colorectal primary tumor is 30–50%. There are also increased risks for developing other malignancies of the gastrointestinal, reproductive, and urinary tracts. The cancer risks in Lynch syndrome may differ depending on one's gender, ethnicity, or geographic region. For example, in parts of Asia, it is gastric cancer that is most prevalent.

6.3.3.1. Tumor Types

- *CRC and polyps*—Individuals with Lynch syndrome are at increased risk for developing one or more colorectal adenocarcinoma(s). Lynch syndrome-associated colon cancers are more likely to develop in the ascending (right-sided) colon than sporadic tumors. In addition, Lynch syndrome-associated carcinomas are more likely to be poorly differentiated, have mucinous or signet ring histology, and to demonstrate MSI and the absence of one or more of the mismatch repair proteins (e.g., MSH2, MLH1 MSH6, and PMS2) by IHC. Adenomas that develop in people with Lynch syndrome tend to be larger with more dysplastic features than adenomas found in the general population. The Lynch syndrome-related polyps are also more likely to be sessile (flat), making them harder to identify and remove. In addition, the malignant transformation from an adenoma occurs more frequently and in a shorter time span in people with Lynch syndrome compared with the general population.
- *Uterus*—Women with Lynch syndrome are at increased risk for developing endometrial adenocarcinomas. There is a risk of developing synchronous or metachronous tumors. Some of the endometrial carcinomas display MSI and absent mismatch repair proteins by IHC analysis. Some researchers have suggested that, in comparison to sporadic uterine cancer, Lynch syndrome-related uterine tumors are

more likely to contain tumor-infiltrating lymphocytes, display tumor heterogeneity, and involve the lower uterine segment.

- *Skin*—Individuals with Lynch syndrome are also at increased risk for developing unusual skin lesions, such as keratoacanthomas, epitheliomas, sebaceous adenomas, and sebaceous carcinomas.

- *Additional tumors*—Lynch syndrome associated malignancies also include:
    - biliary tract cancer
    - glioblastoma and possibly other brain tumors
    - ovarian cancer
    - small bowel cancer (especially at the ampulla of Vater)
    - stomach cancer
    - urinary tract cancer (especially transitional cell cancer)

6.3.3.2. Family History Assessment

Lynch syndrome is one of a handful of hereditary cancer syndromes that has clear-cut diagnostic criteria for identifying families and offering genetic testing.

Individuals who meet Amsterdam II criteria for Lynch syndrome (refer to Section 4.17.2) should be offered DNA testing and tumor block analysis (MSI and IHC). These tests can be done simultaneously; DNA testing may still be recommended even if the tumor block results are normal. DNA testing generally starts with a comprehensive analysis of the *MLH1, MSH2,* and *MSH6* genes to look for both mutations and deletions. If these initial DNA tests are negative, then clients can consider being tested for mutations in the *EPCAM (TACSTD1)* gene and/or the *PMS2* gene if the IHC results suggest a mutation in either of these genes or if there is no tumor block available for analysis.

Individuals who meet Bethesda criteria should be offered MSI and IHC analyses of a tumor block. If the tumor block results are abnormal, then DNA testing should also be offered. If the tumor block results reveal stable MSI and intact proteins by IHC, then, in most cases, no further genetic testing is indicated.

Pedigrees of families with Lynch syndrome tend to include early-onset colorectal cancer (especially the signet-ring type), fewer than 10 adenomatous polyps, sebaceous skin lesions, multiple primaries, and cancers of the endometrium, ovary, stomach, small intestine, Ampulla of Vater, kidney, or ureter. Some families will display less striking histories, hence the utility of tumor testing. Newly available computerized risk models, such as PREMM and MMRpro, can also assess the likelihood of a mismatch repair defect.

TABLE 6.8. MEDICAL MANAGEMENT RECOMMENDATIONS FOR INDIVIDUALS
WITH LYNCH SYNDROME

- Recommend colonoscopy every 1–2 years starting at age 20–25 years or 10 years prior to the youngest age at diagnosis in the family (whichever is earlier).
- Recommend endoscopic rectal exam every 1–2 years starting at age 20–25 years.
- If any polyps are found, then the polyps should be removed via endoscopic polypectomy followed by careful pathologic review of the polyps.
- Recommend complete colectomy following a diagnosis of colorectal cancer.
- Recommend routine annual physical examinations, including neurological and skin exams.
- Discuss the option of colectomy if there are adenomas that are either difficult to resect or have high grade dysplasia.
- Discuss any clinical screening studies designed for patients with Lynch syndrome.
- Provide patient education regarding the signs and symptoms of Lynch-syndrome related cancers.
- Consider recommending upper gastrointestinal (GI) endoscopy including side-viewing examination every 1–3 years starting at age 2-5-30 years, especially if there is a family history of gastric or small bowel cancer.
- Consider recommending that female patients be referred to a gynecologic oncologist in order to be screened for gynecologic cancers, especially endometrial cancer.
- Consider recommending that female patients undergo prophylactic total abdominal hysterectomy and bilateral salpingo-oophorectomy upon menopause or the completion of child-bearing.
- Consider the use of annual urinalysis to check for urothelial cancer.

Source: Kohlmann and Gruber (2006) and National Comprehensive Cancer Network. (NCCN) Lynch syndrome, v.1.2010 http://www.nccn.org.

6.3.3.3. Management Recommendations

See Table 6.8 for a list of the medical management recommendations for people with Lynch syndrome. Individuals with Lynch syndrome need to have annual colonoscopy exams beginning at ages 20–25. The malignant transformation of colorectal polyps can be more rapid in people with Lynch syndrome so the interval between colonoscopy procedures should not extend beyond 12 months. In addition, the polyps are more likely to be sessile (i.e., flat) making them more difficult to detect; all detected polyps should be removed and sent to pathology for review. People with Lynch syndrome can also consider prophylactic colectomy if the clinician is concerned about the development of an interval CRC or if the patient is extremely anxious about developing CRC or has a hard time with the frequent screening.

Individuals with Lynch syndrome-related colon cancer are at increased risk to develop a second colon cancer within 10 years of the initial diagnosis. For this reason, it is recommended that individuals with Lynch syndrome who are diagnosed with colon cancer undergo partial or total colectomies rather than a simple resection of the malignant tumor.

Upper endoscopy exams to screen for gastric and ampullary neoplasms are also recommended, although it is not clear how often this procedure should be performed in people with Lynch syndrome. The use of a capsule endoscopy can be used to look for cancer of the small bowel; however, the effectiveness of this procedure has not been demonstrated.

Women with Lynch syndrome should also undergo screening for endometrial cancer. However, clinicians acknowledge that the current screening for endometrial cancer—which consists of transvaginal ultrasound, pelvic exam, and endometrial biopsies—is decidedly poor at detecting early-stage uterine cancer. Therefore, women with Lynch syndrome may want to consider having a complete hysterectomy, which involves removal of the uterus and ovaries once their families are complete.

People with Lynch syndrome may also be at increased risk for developing lesions of the skin, including skin cancers. Therefore, it makes sense for at risk individuals to undergo regular skin examinations.

6.3.4. *MYH*-ASSOCIATED POLYPOSIS SYNDROME

MAP syndrome is a recessive genetic disorder. It is estimated that MAP syndrome accounts for less than 1% of total CRC cases. Although biallelic *MYH* mutations appear to be rare, monoallelic *MYH* mutations may occur in as many as 1% of the general population.

Individuals with biallelic *MYH* mutations appear to have an 80% risk of developing CRC and perhaps an equally high risk for developing adenomatous polyps. Individuals with monoallelic *MYH* mutations may have slightly increased risks for developing CRC or polyps. (See Section 4.21 for detailed information about MAP.)

6.3.4.1. Tumor Types

- *Adenocarcinomas*—People with MAP syndrome are at increased risk to develop adenocarcinomas of the colon, rectum, and the duodenal section of the small intestine. These carcinomas tend to be MSI stable, but do not seem to display any other characteristic pathology or histology.

- *Polyps*—Individuals with MAP syndrome typically develop colorectal adenomatous polyps, but the number of polyps can range from a few to hundreds. Most people with MAP syndrome develop 15 or more colorectal adenomatous polyps over their lifetime. People with

MAP syndrome can also develop adenomas in the small intestine and fundic gland polyps in the stomach.

6.3.4.2. Family History Assessment

Individuals with multiple adenomatous polyps (15 or more) and/or a diagnosis of MSI-stable CRC under age 50 should be offered *MYH* genetic testing.

MAP syndrome is an autosomal recessive condition; therefore, individuals are more likely to have affected siblings than parents or children. Similar to other recessive conditions, there may be consanguineous matings or the client may have no family history of the disorder.

MAP syndrome is a rare, newly described hereditary cancer syndrome. Therefore, the features of the syndrome and associated risks of cancer are still being characterized. At this time, it appears as though families with MAP syndrome may have features that are reminiscent of other CRC syndromes, such as:

- 100 or more colorectal adenomas, fundic gland polyps, CHRPE, osteomas, and dental cysts (similar to FAP)
- Between 10 and 100 colorectal adenomas (similar to attenuated FAP)
- CRC, a few colorectal adenomas, and cancer of the small intestine (similar to Lynch syndrome)
- Multiple hyperplastic polyps of the colon or rectum (similar to Hyperplastic Polyposis syndrome)

Thus, the identification of a family with MAP syndrome often starts by ruling out FAP or Lynch syndrome.

6.3.4.3. Management Recommendations

The clinical management of people with MAP syndrome is largely driven by the individual's development of polyps. (See Table 6.9.) Individuals with no polyps (and this can be the case) should be followed with colonoscopy exams every 3–5 years. Individuals who develop multiple adenomatous polyps should be followed with annual colonoscopy exams and may need to consider the option of subtotal or total colectomy depending on the size or characteristics of the polyps. Individuals who develop a carpeting of adenomatous polyps (polyposis) need to be managed similarly to those with FAP, that is, they are recommended to undergo total colectomies followed by close surveillance of the remaining rectal tissue.

Individuals with MAP syndrome should also have upper endoscopy exams every 3–5 years beginning at ages 30–35 to look for signs of polyps or cancer in the stomach or duodenum. The use of a side-viewing duodenoscope may provide an enhanced view.

TABLE 6.9. MEDICAL MANAGEMENT RECOMMENDATIONS FOR INDIVIDUALS
WITH MAP

For individuals with bi-allelic *MYH* mutations and no polyps:
- Recommend baseline colonoscopy at age 25–30. If no polyps are found, then continue performing follow-up colonoscopies every 3–5 years. If polyps are detected, then recommend follow-up colonoscopies every 1–2 years.
- Consider recommending upper endoscopy and side viewing duodenoscopy every 3 to 5 years starting at age 30–35 years.

For individuals with bi-allelic MYH mutations and polyps:
- Recommend baseline colonoscopy at age 25–30. If polyps are detected, then recommend follow-up colonoscopies every 1–2 years. If no polyps are found, recommend follow-up colonoscopies every 3–5 years.
- Consider recommending upper endoscopy and side viewing duodenoscopy every 3–5 years starting at age 30–35 years.
- Discuss the option of subtotal colectomy or proctoocoloectomy if, over time, the colorectal adenomas become too numerous or too difficult to resect.
- If colorectal adenomatous polyposis develops, then follow recommendations for FAP. (See Table 6.6.)

For individuals with mono-allelic *MYH* mutations:
- Consider recommending colonoscopy every 5 years starting at age 40.

Source: Lindor et al. (2008) and National Comprehensive Cancer Network (NCCN), MYH-Associated Polyposis, v.1.2010 http://www.nccn.org.

6.4. FURTHER READING

Adrouny, AR. 2002. Understanding Colon Cancer. University Press of Mississippi, Jackson, MS.

American Cancer Society. 2011. ACS Guidelines for the early detection of cancer. http://www.cancer.org/healthy/findcancerearly/cancerscreeningguidelines/american-cancer-society-guidelines-for-the-early-detection-of-cancer.

American Joint Committee on Cancer. 2010. Cancer Staging Handbook, 7th edition. Springer, New York.

Burt, RW, and Jasperson, KW. 2008. APC-associated polyposis conditions. Gene Reviews. http://www.genetests.org.

Cho, E, and Smith-Warner, S. 2004. Alcohol intake and colorectal cancer: a pooled analysis of 8 cohort studies. Ann Intern Med 140:603–613.

Dixon, S. 2007a. How is colon cancer diagnosed? About.com: Colon Cancer http://www.coloncancer.about.com.

Dixon, S. 2007b. What are the symptoms of colon cancer? About.com: Colon Cancer http://www.coloncancer.about.com/od/coloncancerbasics/a/colcansymptoms.htm.

Haidle, JL, and Howe, JR. 2008. Juvenile Polyposis syndrome. Gene Reviews. http://www.genetests.org.

Kohlmann, W, and Gruber, SB. 2006. Hereditary non-polyposis colon cancer. Gene
    Reviews. http://www.genetests.org.
Lindor, NM, McMaster, ML, Lindor Carl, J, and Greene, MH. 2008. Concise Handbook
    of Familial Cancer Susceptibility Syndromes, 2nd edition. JNCI Monogr,
    38:1–93.
Markowitz, S, and Bertagnolli, M. 2009. Molecular basis of colorectal cancer. NEJM
    361:2449–2460.
Myers, D. 2008. Top 10 colon cancer prevention tips. About.com: Colon Cancer
    http://www.coloncancer.about.com.
Schneider, K, and Garber, J. 2010. Li-Fraumeni syndrome. Gene Reviews. http://
    www.genetests.org.
Tsong, W, and Koh, W. 2007. Cigarettes and alcohol in relation to colorectal cancer:
    the Singapore Chinese health study. Br J Cancer 95:821–827.

COLLECTING AND INTERPRETING CANCER HISTORIES

> I view a pedigree like a quilt, stitching together the intimate and colorful scraps of medical and family information from a person's life. Familial pedigree patterns are the clinician's matrix for providing pedigree risk assessment as well as clinical and diagnostic recommendations. Yet just as the quilter takes artistic liberty with tried-and true patterns to make each quilt a unique work of art, each pedigree has a unique human story behind it.
>
> (Bennett, 2010a, p. 9)

The careful collection and interpretation of the client's personal and family history of cancer forms the foundation of the cancer counseling session. This chapter provides strategies for collecting a comprehensive cancer history and describes challenges that can arise in the process. This chapter also discusses ways to assess and classify cancer histories and ends with three case examples.

7.1. COLLECTING A CANCER HISTORY

Taking a comprehensive cancer history involves asking clients a systematic series of questions to gather relevant personal and family medical information. Being able to take an accurate and complete family history is considered one of the most important skills acquired by genetic counselors. This section begins with the definition and purpose of a pedigree, describes the key elements of taking a cancer history, including helpful tips for gathering this information, and ends with ways to confirm the cancer diagnoses.

Counseling About Cancer, Third Edition. Katherine A. Schneider.
© 2012 Wiley-Blackwell. Published 2012 by John Wiley & Sons, Inc.

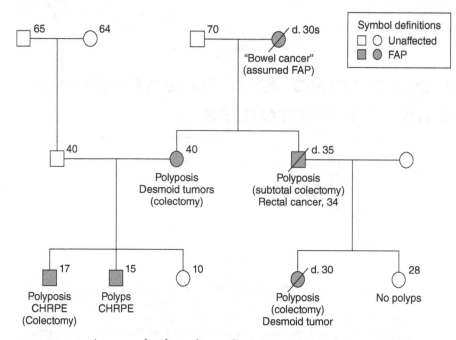

FIGURE 7.1. An example of a pedigree illustrating a family history of FAP.

7.1.1. THE DEFINITION AND PURPOSE OF THE PEDIGREE

Genetic counselors collect relevant family history information from their clients and convert the information into pictorial form by the construction of a pedigree. A pedigree is a diagram of standardized lines and symbols that demonstrates the biological relationships, medical conditions, and other pertinent information within a family. (See Fig. 7.1) Please refer to Appendix B for a review of the basic pedigree symbols. Figure 7.2 describes the basic pedigree system used in the Cancer Genetics and Prevention Center at the Dana-Farber Cancer Institute.

The collection of the family history involves asking a series of open-ended and targeted questions and then carefully listening to and recording the client's responses. Creating a family pedigree serves many purposes for genetic counselors as presented in the succeeding sections.

7.1.1.1. Identify a Cancer Syndrome

The main purpose of gathering personal and family history information during a cancer counseling session is to determine whether a client could have a specific hereditary cancer syndrome. Clinical criteria have been established for a number of the hereditary cancer syndromes, which can be useful

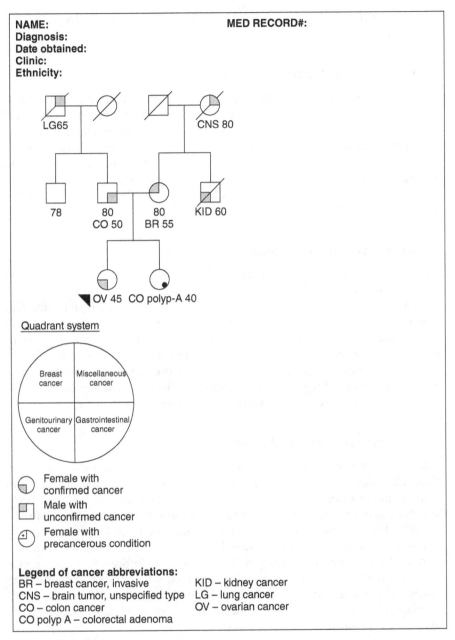

FIGURE 7.2. An example of the cancer pedigree quadrant system (This template form has been provided courtesy of Dr. Judy Garber, Director of the Cancer Genetics and Prevention Center, Dana-Farber Cancer Institute, Boston, MA).

in formulating targeted questions to ask clients. (Refer to syndrome entries in Chapter 4.)

7.1.1.2. Determine the Need for Genetic Testing

Individuals who meet clinical criteria for a hereditary cancer syndrome will be offered DNA testing (if available) to confirm the clinical diagnosis and identify the underlying gene mutation in the family. Individuals who have a moderate or high likelihood of having a hereditary cancer syndrome are typically offered DNA testing as well. Genetic testing may also be used to reassure people who are at low risk for having a hereditary cancer syndrome and to clarify the risk status of individuals who have incomplete or indeterminate family histories.

7.1.1.3. Assist with Management Recommendations

In making decisions about managing individuals at high risk for inherited cancers, clinicians need to be guided by the person's own family history as well as any published data (scarce as they are) regarding early detection and prevention. Even in hereditary cancer syndromes with established medical management guidelines, clinicians should also consider the specific pattern of cancer in the client's family. For example, female *BRCA* carriers are advised to initiate breast imaging studies at age 25, but a young woman with a *BRCA1* mutation whose mother developed breast cancer at age 28 will likely be advised to initiate breast screening at a younger age.

7.1.1.4. Uncover Other Syndromes

Almost all cancer genetic counselors have had the experience of clients (or their physicians) indicating a specific syndrome on the initial intake form only to find out upon taking the family history that the client has an entirely different genetic condition. For example, a woman who has been referred for *BRCA* testing because of a striking family history of breast cancer may actually turn out to have Li–Fraumeni syndrome or PTEN Hamartoma syndrome. In addition, collecting the family history information may reveal features of other noncancer genetic disorders, which would benefit from further discussions or referrals. Examples include striking histories of miscarriages, birth defects, mental illness, cardiac or respiratory problems, or Alzheimer's disease.

7.1.1.5. Identify the Disorder's Inheritance Pattern and Other Relatives at Risk

A cancer pedigree typically contains information about affected and unaffected individuals over three or more generations. Thus, the pattern of the disorder—as well as the biological relationships—in a family can be quickly and accurately assessed by glancing at a single page. This information may be useful in determining the likelihood of a dominant or recessive single-gene disorder. For example, three brothers with multiple colon adenomas are more likely to have an autosomal recessive polyposis syndrome than a family in which the adenomas have occurred in a grandfather, father, and son. A completed pedigree can also delineate the blood relatives who are potentially at risk for inheriting a cancer predisposition gene and should be offered genetic counseling and testing.

7.1.1.6. Develop a Useful Counseling Aid

The completed pedigree can be used to illustrate various points during the discussions about risk and testing, including:

- The inheritance pattern of a hereditary cancer syndrome
- The associated malignancies and other features of a cancer syndrome
- The specific relatives who are potentially at risk for having the condition

7.1.1.7. Create an Important Clinical Record and Research Tool

A pedigree is a valuable record of family history information that can be reviewed or updated over time. The use of the pedigree's standardized format and symbols also makes the information accessible to cancer genetic colleagues and other clinicians. Clinical programs often rely on computerized pedigree drawing programs, such as Progeny Softwave, LLC (http://www.progenygenetics.com), to create a standardized pedigree. Another advantage to using a computerized pedigree program is that it becomes a stored database of all the family history information, which can later be sorted or searched. For example, a cancer genetics program can search their pedigree files for the number of families who have pancreatic cancer and have been found to carry *BRCA* mutations. Thus, pedigree data can help guide clinical policies and formulate ideas for clinical research.

7.1.1.8. Become Aware of Family Dynamics and Level of Support

A pedigree indicates important relationship information, including the client's degree of relatedness to affected relatives, the number and gender of relatives in each generation, and whether relatives are living or deceased. This information can lay the foundation for obtaining a psychosocial assessment either informally during the collection of the family history or formally with a specialized assessment such as a genogram or colored eco-genetic relationship map (CEGRM). (See Sections 10.2.3 and 10.2.4 for more information on these psychosocial tools).

7.1.1.9. Hear the Client's Family Stories

Hearing the details about the downward spiral of a relative with advanced cancer may not have relevance for the identification of a cancer syndrome, but it has a great deal of relevance for counseling the client. Listening to the family stories may provide counselors with a great deal of information about their clients in regard to:

- Their purpose for seeking genetic counseling or testing
- Their thoughts about what is important or relevant
- Their use of magical thinking or family myths to explain the cancer in the family
- Their knowledge of the cancer history and awareness of a genetic link
- Their readiness to hear that they are at risk
- Their reactions and emotions brought up by telling the stories
- Their level of trust in the medical system and in cancer screening regimens
- Their attitudes toward genetic testing

7.1.1.10. Assess the Client's Emotional State

Clients may present to the cancer counseling session with a variety of different emotions, including fear, confusion, anger, determination, or eagerness. The range of emotions and reactions observed during the recounting of family stories are helpful to the genetic counselor in ascertaining the client's level of distress and any potential vulnerability. This awareness will help the counselor to determine how best to broach or discuss certain issues during the ensuing genetic counseling discussion.

7.1.1.11. Set the Tone for the Session

Clients are frequently nervous or tense at the beginning of the cancer genetic counseling session. The systematic—yet friendly—question-and-answer format of the family history interview can help put people at ease. In addition, listening with interest and empathy to the client's responses can establish a level of trust and rapport that is critical to the work that goes on later in the session.

7.1.2. KEY ELEMENTS OF A COMPREHENSIVE CANCER HISTORY

Collection of the family history information typically occurs near the beginning of a cancer genetic counseling session. Most genetic counselors open the discussion by briefly describing the overall nature and purpose of the family history questions. The counselor then gathers information about the client's cancer diagnosis or current health status, and goes on to ask a similar set of questions regarding each of the client's:

- Children
- Siblings
- Nieces and nephews
- Parents
- Maternal aunts, uncles, and grandparents
- Maternal first cousins
- Paternal aunts, uncles, and grandparents
- Paternal first cousins
- Great-aunts, great-uncles, or great-grandparents (if information is available)
- Distant cousins (if information is available)

The exact order in which information is collected differs from counselor to counselor. However, it is best to ask questions in a systematic manner rather than skipping around to different relatives in an erratic fashion (although sometimes this is how the clients report the information!). The major pieces of information to collect during a cancer family history intake are described below. (Also see Table 7.1.)

7.1.2.1. Cancer Diagnosis

The main focus of the family history intake is to learn which individuals in the family have had cancer. Since hereditary cancer syndromes tend to be associated with specific tumor types or histologies, the more specific the information, the better. Ideally, a client would be able to provide precise information, such as, "My mother was diagnosed with a serous ovarian adenocarcinoma at age 51 and she died at age 55." Realistically, a client is more likely to say something like, "My mother had ovarian cancer in her early 50s and died a few years later." Sometimes the client has only vague information about the diagnosis, such as: "My mother had some type of female reproductive cancer and died in her 50s." Clients should be encouraged to bring in written documentation of the cancer diagnoses in their

TABLE 7.1. SAMPLE CANCER HISTORY QUESTIONS TO ASK

- Is your relative still living?
  - If yes: How old is your relative now?
  - If no: At what age did your relative pass away? Do you know what year that was? What did your relative die of?
- Did your relative ever have cancer?
- Do you know what type of cancer your relative had?
  - Do you know where (in what organ) the cancer started?
  - Do you know the exact name of the cancer?
  - Would it be possible for you to obtain the medical records report (pathology report) on the relative's cancer?
- How old was your relative when diagnosed with cancer?
  - Do you know what year that was?
- Do you know what kind of cancer treatments your relative had?
  - Where does your relative live?
  - Do you know the name of the hospital where your relative was treated?
- Did your relative ever have genetic testing?
  - If yes: Do you know what type of genetic testing your relative had? Do you know what the results were? Would it be possible for you to ask your relative for a copy of the genetic test results?
  - If no: Do you know if your relative was ever offered genetic testing? Did your relative ever meet with a genetic counselor?
- Was your relative exposed to any harmful agents that might have caused the cancer?
  - Did your relative smoke cigarettes?
  - What did your relative do for work?
  - Did your relative's physician ever say what might have caused the cancer?

---

family. (Section 7.1.4 discusses strategies for confirming pedigree information.) If a client mentions that a relative had two or more types of cancer, it is important to determine whether the malignancies represent separate primaries or metastatic disease. Lastly, depending on the type of cancer mentioned, other features (e.g., bilateral disease or the presence of certain tumor markers) may be important as well.

7.1.2.2. Ages and Dates

The age at which an individual was diagnosed with cancer is one of the key elements in determining the likelihood of a hereditary cancer syndrome. It is conventional to note the age that the cancer was formally diagnosed, not the age at which symptoms began. Other useful ages and dates to obtain include:

- The approximate date (year) that the cancer was diagnosed
- The current age and date of birth of the client

- The current ages of living relatives; include dates of birth if available
- The age of death for deceased relatives
- Dates of birth for close relatives
- Dates of death (approximate) for affected relatives

The client's date of birth will be recorded in his/her medical chart, but it is worth rechecking this information at the time of the visit. The client's age is an important factor in determining appropriate medical management once the risk assessment has been completed and may also raise or lower the risk of developing a specific cancer. Clients may be more likely to remember a relative's age at the time of death than time of diagnosis. If this is the case, it may be helpful to ask if the relative was diagnosed within a few years of his/her death or was diagnosed many years earlier. The dates of cancer diagnoses or death may be helpful in efforts to obtain a pathology report or death certificate. In addition, it may be possible to obtain tumor specimen blocks for individuals who died within the past 10–20 years, which can be used for tumor confirmation or genetic studies.

7.1.2.3. Cancer Treatment and Follow-Up

Standard methods to treat cancer include surgery, chemotherapy, and radiation. Counselors may want to ask a few questions about the treatment that clients and relatives have undergone (or are still going through). This information may be helpful in assessing the risks of subsequent cancers. For example, children with hereditary retinoblastoma have increased risks of sarcoma; these risks are magnified if they underwent radiation treatments. It may also be helpful to learn whether recommendations have been made regarding future cancer monitoring. If the client is unsure about a particular cancer diagnosis or is using unusual terminology, then learning some details about the treatment and follow-up may help clarify the nature of the diagnosis.

7.1.2.4. Current Status and Prognosis

In discussing plans to obtain additional family history information or undergo genetic testing, it is important to be aware of the current cancer status and short-term prognosis for the affected client or relative. This is also useful information to know, because individuals in active treatment will likely have different motivations and concerns than those who are long-term survivors or those with recurrent disease. If the affected relative is overwhelmed with the current treatment regimen or is terminally ill, then it is helpful to ask the client to identify another family member who might be able to help coordinate obtaining documentation or specimens for genetic studies. The counselor can also consider whether it would be better to hold off on pursuing documentation or specimens for genetic testing until the family expresses that they are ready to continue with these efforts.

7.1.2.5. Current Surveillance Practices

In many families, clients and relatives will have had some type of baseline screening. In fact, they may even be following a high-risk surveillance regimen. For clients who have had specific monitoring tests, it is useful to obtain the following information:

- types of screening tests performed
- dates of the screening tests
- results of the screening tests
- planned frequency of the screening tests

Whenever possible, obtain a written copy of the client's screening test results. If the family turns out to have a hereditary cancer syndrome, this information may be useful in determining the client's risk status. In addition, these screening tests can be used as baseline practices that may need to be altered, depending on the genetic test results, pattern of cancer in the family, and the client's other risk factors. It may also be helpful to obtain information about the client's close relatives and their screening regimens, especially if any of the tests yielded abnormal results.

7.1.2.6. Presence of Noncancerous Features

During the family history intake, counselors should ask about other medical conditions and benign lesions. Some hereditary cancer syndromes are associated with observable physical features or other conditions. Examples include:

- *Associated benign lesions*—such as sebaceous cysts with Gardner's syndrome
- *Physical features*—such as café au lait spots with neurofibromatosis
- *Medical conditions*—such as high blood pressure with pheochromocytomas
- *Behavioral or learning problems*—such as autism with PTEN Hamartoma syndrome
- *Birth defects*—such as aniridia with familial Wilms' tumor

It is important to record other significant medical conditions and benign lesions when collecting the family history, especially if the features appear to be tracking with the cancer occurrences in the family. If the condition in question hinges on a careful physical exam or diagnostic tests, then clients should be referred to a physician who specializes in cancer genetic syndromes.

7.1.2.7. Unaffected Relatives

Looking for evidence of an inherited cancer syndrome relies on assessing the number of at-risk relatives who have gone on to develop cancer. However, a completed pedigree should also include information about the relatives who have not had cancer. A family that includes two siblings with cancer may seem significant until learning that they are part of a sibship of 12. In addition, it is important to document both sides of the family even if it seems obvious which side of the family has the cancer predisposition. Sometimes it turns out that the less interesting side of the family is actually the one that has the hereditary cancer syndrome. For unaffected relatives, it is useful to obtain the following information:

- The relative's current age or, if deceased, the relative's age at the time of death and the major cause of death
- Whether the relative has had any relevant cancer screening tests or surgeries that might impact risk.
- Whether the relative might have had any significant, noncancerous features associated with the syndrome in question

7.1.2.8. Other Cancer Risk Factors

There are several established environmental risk factors that can increase the risks of specific forms of malignancy (refer to Table 1.15). The main environmental risk factors are sun exposure, alcohol, and tobacco use. Depending on the pattern of cancers in the family, it may be useful for the counselor to ascertain whether an exposure to a particular carcinogen could have contributed to the development of cancer. Examples of environmental risk factors that may cause cancer include:

- *Lifestyle habits*—such as cigarette smoking, which is linked with lung cancer
- *Medical conditions*—such as Crohn's disease, which is linked with colorectal cancer
- *Viruses*—such as the human papillomavirus (HPV), which is linked with cervical cancer

- *Job-related carcinogens*—such as asbestos exposure in shipyards or carpentry, which is linked with mesothelioma
- *Environmental carcinogens*—such as sprayed pesticides or toxic dumping, which are linked with clusters of cancer that occur in certain neighborhoods or towns

7.1.2.9. Psychosocial Factors

A client's interpretation of risk and decisions about genetic testing are greatly influenced by a variety of psychosocial factors. Therefore, genetic counselors might find it beneficial to gather information about family dynamics, the family's communication style, and the amount of contact and supportiveness of various relatives. (See Section 10.2 for more detailed information about this topic.)

7.1.2.10. Ethnic Background

It is important to obtain the client's ethnicity (country of origin, nationality, and/or religious affiliation) for each side of the family. Many individuals in the United States have mixed ancestry and it may be useful to correlate the ethnicity with the pattern of cancer in the family. This information can help determine the most appropriate genetic tests to order. For example, individuals of Eastern European (Ashkenazi) Jewish ancestry who have any history of breast and ovarian cancer should typically be offered genetic testing for the three *BRCA* founder mutations.

Cancer history pedigrees typically extend for four generations (grandparents, parents, clients, and children). If the pattern of cancer in the family is suggestive of a particular hereditary cancer syndrome, then the counselor will want to follow up with a series of targeted questions regarding a specific cancer diagnosis (see Table 7.2) or to look for other features suggestive of certain hereditary cancer syndromes (see Table 7.3). To complete the family history intake, counselors may want to ask a short series of general questions such as those listed in Table 7.4.

7.1.3. ADDITIONAL STRATEGIES AND HELPFUL HINTS

Genetic counselors will develop their own methods for collecting family history information. This section presents some additional strategies and helpful hints for counselors. These suggestions are geared toward newer genetic counseling colleagues and are not specific to the collection of cancer family histories per se.

TABLE 7.2. SAMPLE FOLLOW-UP QUESTIONS ABOUT A BREAST CANCER
DIAGNOSIS

"You mentioned that several people in your family have had breast cancer. Let's
focus on your sister's recent diagnosis of breast cancer."

- Is the cancer in one breast or both breasts?
- Where in the breast did the cancer originate—in the ducts or the lobules?
- How was the breast cancer staged?
- Is the tumor estrogen or progesterone receptor positive? Is your sister planning
  to take tamoxifen?
- Does the tumor have the growth factor called Her2/neu?
- Did your sister's physician mention that there was anything unusual about the
  tumor?
- How was your sister's breast cancer found? Did she have any symptoms?
- What is the plan for treating your sister's cancer?
- How is your sister doing? How is the rest of the family dealing with it? How
  are you doing?
- Had your sister ever had any prior problems with her breasts?
- Does your sister have any other major health problems?
- Was your sister ever exposed to a lot of radiation? Does she smoke cigarettes or
  drink a lot of alcohol? Could she have been exposed to any harmful agents
  (carcinogens) at work or at home?

7.1.3.1. Learn the Art and Skill of Collecting a Family History

There is both an art and skill to effectively collecting the family history intake
and creating an accurately drawn pedigree. Helpful hints for collecting an
effective and accurate history are listed in Table 7.5. The counselor's choice
of words is important; tread gently with topics and terms that may be distressing to clients. It is also a good idea to avoid medical jargon unless the
client is a health-care professional and to start the family history intake by
asking easy questions rather than going right to the hard ones. Shortcuts are
permissible if there are time constraints and the client either reports no
history of benign or malignant tumors in that branch of the family or the
client has no information about those relatives. Most importantly, always
treat clients in a respectful and kind manner.

7.1.3.2. Respond to Client Stories in an Empathetic Manner

In the process of sharing their family history, clients may tell you about an
important event that has occurred in their lives. In some cases, these events
will be germane to the discussion, such as a distressing experience with a
screening test, a recent cancer diagnosis, or a relative's cancer-related death.
In other cases, the events are completely unrelated to the cancer discussion.

TABLE 7.3. SAMPLE FOLLOW-UP QUESTIONS TO LOOK FOR OTHER FEATURES ASSOCIATED WITH HEREDITARY BREAST CANCER

"Some families have an inherited predisposition to breast cancer. This series of questions will help me figure out if your family could have one of the hereditary breast cancer conditions."

- Has anyone in your family had ovarian cancer?
- Has anyone in your family had pancreatic cancer?
- Has anyone in your family had prostate cancer?
- Has anyone in your family had two separate cancer diagnoses, like bilateral breast cancer or breast and ovarian cancer?
- Have any men in your family been diagnosed with breast cancer?
- Does anyone in your family have any unusual skin lesions? Any birthmarks? Any moles that had to be removed?
- Does anyone in your family have a large-sized head?
- Has anyone in your family had any fatty tumors (lipomas) removed?
- Has anyone in your family had thyroid cancer? Has anyone had a goiter? Has anyone had thyroid surgery?
- Has anyone in your family been diagnosed with autism?
- Does anyone in your family have high blood pressure that has been difficult to control by medication?
- Has anyone in your family died unexpectedly from a stroke? On the operating table? In childbirth?
- Are there any children in your family who have been diagnosed with cancer?
- Were there any children in your family who died at young ages? Do you know what they died of?
- Has anyone in your family had cancer of the bone or soft tissue (muscle)?
- Has anyone in your family had a brain tumor?
- Has anyone in your family had cancer that was diagnosed under age 45?
- Has anyone in your family had colon cancer? Anyone have cancer of the rectum, small intestine, or stomach?
- Has anyone in your family been found to have a noncancerous growth (a polyp) in their colon or rectum? Any polyps found elsewhere in the digestive tract?
  - If yes: Do you know what types of polyps were found? Would you be able to obtain a copy of the pathology report on the polyps? When was your relative told to have another colonoscopy?
  - If no: Has anyone in the family had colon cancer screening with a sigmoidoscopy or colonoscopy?

Examples include a wedding, a new baby, a graduation, a divorce, or even bankruptcy. Upon hearing the client's news, counselors need to acknowledge the impact of the event for the client by providing some type of empathetic comment or reaction. These empathetic responses convey the impression that the counselor is seeing the clients and their families as people rather than as a collection of diagnoses. Even if clients do not wish

TABLE 7.4. EXAMPLES OF GENERAL QUESTIONS TO ASK TO COMPLETE A CANCER PEDIGREE

- Are there any other relatives who had cancer that I did not ask about?
- Are there any children in the family who were born with serious birth defects or who died young?
- Has anyone in the family had skin cancer?
- Are you having any type of cancer screening?
  - If yes: What types of tests were performed? What were the dates of your most recent screening tests? What were the results of these screening tests? Can you obtain copies of these results and send them to me? When are you scheduled to have these tests performed again?
  - If no: Have you spoken to your physician about being screened? At what age are you planning to initiate screening?
- Do you have any major medical conditions or problems?
- What is the ethnicity of your mother's family? What is the ethnicity of your father's family?
- Is there any chance that you could be of Eastern European (Ashkenazi) Jewish ancestry?
- Is there any chance that you and your husband might be related to each other?
- Is there any chance that your parents or grandparents might be cousins (or other types of relations) who married?
- Is there anything I did not ask about that you think I should include in the family tree?

TABLE 7.5. HELPFUL HINTS FOR COLLECTING A FAMILY CANCER HISTORY

- Keep your questions simple and specific
- Ask one question at a time in a systematic fashion
- Watch your terminology; avoid medical jargon
- Use open-ended, follow-up questions
- Know the purpose of each question in case clients want to know why you are asking
- Adapt your questions to clients' needs and cultural backgrounds
- Avoid "why" questions that may be viewed as judgmental
- Know when it is appropriate—and not appropriate—to use shortcuts
- Gently control or guide the process; manage the time effectively
- Listen to the clients' answers and ask them to clarify their responses if you are not sure what they are talking about
- Avoid interrupting client answers, but allow clients to interrupt you
- Allow for moments of silence during the process; don't fill with unnecessary questions
- Acknowledge recent events that have occurred in the client's family; this will humanize the client's story

Sources: Veach et al. (2003, pp. 75–78); Schuette and Bennett (2009, p. 53).

to delve further into the matter, they will usually appreciate the effort. It also makes the family history discussion appear less like a formal medical intake and more like the give and take of normal conversation.

7.1.3.3. Use Standardized Pedigree Nomenclature

Constructing a cancer pedigree is like cursive handwriting; there is a correct form to follow, but everyone has their own style. (Refer to Appendix B for a review of the standardized pedigree nomenclature.) Some cancer risk programs use a specific quadrant system or different types of shading to denote different types of cancer (see Fig. 7.2 for the system used at the Dana-Farber Cancer Institute). High Risk Programs may want to install computerized pedigree drawing software, which utilizes a standard set of genetics nomenclature. Programs should also decide how to delineate other features, such as confirmed tumors and genetic test results.

7.1.3.4. Adhere to Confidentiality Practices

A pedigree is a record of sensitive information and it needs to be treated accordingly. Cancer risk programs will need to decide upon the types of information that will or will not be included on the pedigree. This might include full names of relatives, genetic test results, and other potentially sensitive information (such as adoption status, mental illness, suicidality, alcoholism, or HIV status). If in doubt, ask clients whether certain ancillary information should be included on the finalized form of the pedigree. Although a copy of the pedigree can (and in my opinion, should) be placed in the client's permanent medical record, names of relatives should not be included since they have not consented to the posting of their private information. Pedigrees forwarded to other institutions or physician's offices should also omit names and other identifying information for the client and relatives unless you have permission to release this information.

7.1.3.5. Consider the Accuracy of the Historian

Clients are more likely to accurately report a cancer diagnosis in first-degree relatives than diagnoses that have occurred in more distant relatives. This is hardly surprising since clients are more apt to be directly involved in the care of a close family member. The site of cancer may also influence accuracy rates. While reports of breast cancer, prostate cancer, and melanoma tend to be quite accurate, reports of other forms of cancer have much lower rates of accuracy. This is especially true for the following types of cancer:

- Cancers of the gastrointestinal tract
- Cancers of the female reproductive tract

- Tumor that are common sites of metastases
- Tumors that are rare or have lengthy names

Counselors need to become savvy at determining when the cancer history information is less likely to be accurate. If the family history information may not be accurate, then the counselor should encourage the client to verify the facts by checking with other relatives or by obtaining written documentation. Obviously this type of request needs to be made tactfully. It is especially important for counselors to ask clients to confirm their personal or family histories of cancer in the following situations:

- *The client provides different information to various staff members.* A client may tell his physician that three relatives died from brain tumors but at the genetic counseling visit, he states that only one relative had a brain tumor (and two relatives died from strokes). Sometimes the altered information can reflect new or confirmed information that the client has obtained and other times it means that the client is confused or simply guessing.

- *The client provides different information than another family member has provided.* A client may relate that three relatives had kidney cancer, while the client's first cousin insists that these relatives had colorectal cancer or nonmalignant kidney disease. In this type of situation, the counselor's task is to determine which of the two relatives is more likely to be the accurate historian.

- *The client provides information about a cancer diagnosis that does not seem realistic in terms of the reported treatment or the survival time.* As examples, genetic counselors may wish to question clients further if they relate that a family member had a solid tumor that required no surgical intervention or that a relative is a long-term survivor of a particularly aggressive cancer (such as pancreatic or gastric cancer).

- *The client provides other information that suggests the reported diagnosis is not accurate.* For example, a client might report that her cousin gave birth to a baby several years after being diagnosed with uterine cancer (which typically results in a hysterectomy).

- *The client provides family history information that includes the presence of less commonly occurring tumors on both sides of the family.* Excluding situations of consanguinity, it would be unusual to see cases of rare tumors, such as gastrointestinal stromal tumors (GIST), in both a paternal uncle and a maternal grandparent.

- *The client provides family history information that includes multiple relatives who have developed cancer at exactly the same age.* Clients may latch onto a specific age due to their own diagnosis or that of a close relative and then report that all other relatives were diagnosed at similar ages.

7.1.3.6. Work within Existing Family Relationships

The counselor is dependent upon the client's ability and willingness to obtain a comprehensive family history. But counselors should recognize that obtaining this information can be quite time consuming, and, in some cases, it is an emotional land mine. It may be helpful for counselors to suggest ways to obtain information with a minimum of effort or involvement by other family members. For example, a client may not feel comfortable contacting a distant cousin about his newly diagnosed cancer, but perhaps an aunt would either know the information or be willing to obtain it on behalf of the client.

7.1.3.7. Use Family History Intake as a Counseling Tool

In addition to eliciting the pattern of cancer in the family, the family history discussion can provide information about relationships with other family members, the clients' perceptions of risk, and even attitudes toward cancer monitoring or genetic testing. In addition, counselors should note the points at which the client becomes emotional or quiet; these "triggers" may be important clues for how the client is dealing with personal or family issues. If the counselor notices that a client seems distressed when talking about a specific issue, the counselor should respond in an empathetic manner. Then, depending on the circumstances, the counselor can proceed in one of the following ways:

- Maintain a few moments of silence to allow the client to regroup and then resume the family history intake.
- Avoid references to the topic if it is not germane to the discussion at hand.
- Decide that the issue needs to be addressed either at this point or later in the session. Be especially tactful and gentle during the discussion since this seems to be an emotionally distressing issue for the client.
- Collect more detailed information about the client's emotional wellbeing. Depending on the assessment, it may be appropriate to refer the client to a mental health provider. If the client is already in the care of a therapist, then it may be helpful for the counselor to speak directly to the therapist, especially if the client wants to have genetic testing.

- Determine that the topic is such a powerful emotional trigger for the client that any further discussion of it would be beyond the scope of the average genetic counseling visit. Following the session, the counselor should consult with a mental health provider on staff regarding any concerns about the client's safety or for suggestions on how to proceed during future interactions with the client.

7.1.3.8. Consider the Use of a Family History Questionnaire

Collecting the family history information can take up much of the allotted visit with the client. Therefore, counselors may find it beneficial to use a preliminary family history questionnaire. Several groups have looked at ways to expedite the process of gathering the family history and also as a way of increasing the number of appropriate genetic counseling referrals. In addition to the many pen-and-paper family history intake forms that have been developed, there are also family history questionnaires that are computerized or Web based.

7.1.4. WAYS TO CONFIRM PEDIGREES

It is crucial for pedigrees to reflect the most accurate information that is possible. However, even clients who are good historians can provide inaccurate or incomplete information. This is why obtaining confirmation of the diagnosis, in the form of a pathology report or physician's note, remains the gold standard. Unfortunately, the process of obtaining the necessary documentation can be incredibly time consuming and frustrating for both the client and the counselor. And sometimes, even with the best of intentions, it is not possible to obtain the needed records. Thus, it may be more feasible to focus efforts on documenting the diagnoses that are germane to interpreting the cancer history rather than attempting to confirm each and every cancer diagnosis in the family. For example, to determine whether a client's family has a hereditary colorectal cancer, the counselor can focus on documenting the cases of colorectal cancer or polyps and other related cancers, such as uterine cancer.

The confirmation process involves obtaining prior permission from the relative in question (or if deceased, the designated next of kin). The following information is usually needed: the relative's full name (including maiden name), the relative's date of birth, the approximate date of diagnosis (or death), and the name of the hospital where the cancer was diagnosed or autopsy performed.

If the counselor is planning to assist the client in obtaining medical records documentation, then he or she should make sure to obtain the names of the hospitals where the client has been treated. A lack of precise information can make the task of confirming information even more tedious, and much less likely to be successful.

Sometimes, clients are stymied about how to go about obtaining documentation. The red tape involved in obtaining copies of a medical record can be daunting to individuals who are unfamiliar with hospital procedures, and they may be intimidated by the thought of contacting a physician's office or hospital. Counselors should provide clients with general instructions for how to obtain documentation and they may even want to assist families with these efforts.

The various ways to confirm a cancer history are described below.

7.1.4.1. Verbal Confirmation

Collecting a comprehensive cancer history may require conversations with more than one family member. Reviewing the pedigree with additional family members allows counselors to verbally confirm the information already obtained and also to learn new information. Speaking directly with the relatives who have had cancer tends to be the most useful. If this is not possible, then it is helpful to ask to speak with the person's spouse or another close relative. Counselors need to keep in mind that relatives may not share the same knowledge base or interest in these issues as the client. Given the stringent rules about patient privacy, it may work best to ask that the relative(s) be the ones to initiate the contact if they are willing to discuss these issues.

7.1.4.2. Pathology Report

Obtaining the pathology report is the best method of documenting the tumor. The diagnosis of cancer almost always involves an analysis of the malignant cells, which results in a written pathology report. The pathology report generally includes:

- The patient's full name and hospital identification number
- The patient's date of birth and current age
- The date of the analysis
- The name of the tumor and site of origin
- The histology, pathology, and grade of the tumor

Reviewing pathology reports should be done in conjunction with a physician (preferably an oncologist or pathologist). Pathology reports are typically part of the individual's medical record; however, it may be easier to obtain a copy directly through the hospital's pathology department.

7.1.4.3. Genetic Test Results

If the client reports that someone in the family underwent genetic testing, the counselor should request a copy of the test result. This is especially important if the client is interested in having targeted genetic testing or if the client is making medical decisions based on the verbally reported genetic test result. It may turn out that the positive result is actually a variant of uncertain significance or that a negative result is less than reassuring because the wrong test was ordered or the wrong person in the family was tested. It may also be possible to offer additional genetic testing options to the family since genetic testing technologies are constantly evolving.

7.1.4.4. Hospital Summary Notes

If the pathology report is not accessible, another option is to obtain and review other entries in the medical record, such as surgical records, hospitalization discharge notes, or summaries of outpatient visits. Counselors should look for records close to the time of diagnosis, which may include the most accurate and detailed information.

7.1.4.5. Autopsy Report

If an autopsy has been performed, it may contain information regarding the presence of a malignancy or other syndromic features. This report is typically included in the deceased individual's medical record.

7.1.4.6. Death Certificate

Another possible source of confirmation is the death certificate. The death certificate typically lists the individual's cancer diagnosis if it is considered the primary cause of death. If the cancer is considered a contributing factor (secondary diagnosis), then it might also be included in the death certificate. However, family members who were long-term cancer survivors and died of other causes are less likely to have the diagnosis listed on the death certificate. The death certificate usually indicates whether an autopsy has been performed (which is more likely to mention the prior cancer diagnosis). Death certificates are a matter of public record and should be obtainable provided the client has sufficient information to locate it. Required information typically includes where the person died (city and state) and date of death. It may also be helpful to have the individual's date of birth, name of spouse, and name of parents.

7.2. CHALLENGES TO COLLECTING AN ACCURATE HISTORY

Counselors depend upon clients to provide accurate and complete family histories. Yet cancer family histories can be notoriously inaccurate. This can occur because clients have lost touch with some of their relatives or because they are confused about the actual diagnosis. Perhaps most challenging are the clients who report specific cancer diagnoses that later turn out to be false. This section discusses reasons why the cancer history might be inaccurate and offers strategies that counselors can use to elicit better histories.

7.2.1. THE FAMILY HISTORY INFORMATION IS INCOMPLETE

Some clients are much better at recounting their family histories than others. In some cases, the problem lies in the client's skill as a historian. Clients may be poor historians for the reasons presented in the succeeding sections.

7.2.1.1. Family Members Live Far Away

It is rare these days to find an extended family that has remained in the same city or region. Much more frequently, members of a family have scattered to different parts of the country and may only get together on special family occasions, if at all. As a result, some clients may be unaware of the medical histories of entire branches of the family. Alternatively, they may have heard about the diagnosis from an indirect (and potentially unreliable) source. Also, clients may feel awkward about asking for more detailed family history information from relatives whom they barely know. Even among family members with solid relationships, clients may hesitate to ask too many questions. They may be concerned that raising the topic will cause their relatives to be sad, worried, or even angry.

7.2.1.2. Clients Are Not Prepared to Answer Questions

Clients may not be good at remembering dates and are hazy about who died from what. For this reason, it is helpful to have alerted clients beforehand about the types of questions they will be asked to provide during the genetic counseling visit. It may also be the counseling session itself that has hampered the client's ability to recall detailed information. Questions about the family history may cause some clients to feel put on the spot or swamped with emotional memories; neither is conducive to providing accurate information.

7.2.1.3. Cancer Is Not Discussed in the Family

A generation ago it was not unusual to call cancer "the big C," as though saying the word itself was too frightening. Although it is now more common for people to talk about their cancer diagnoses, some individuals remain fiercely private about their medical problems. Clients may have been rebuffed in their efforts to obtain family history information or they may want to honor their relatives' wishes that they "don't want to talk about it." The lack of discussion about cancer may also reflect a lack of opportunity. If clients only see their relatives on festive occasions, it may be awkward to discuss details about their cancer diagnoses.

In the above scenarios, clients may not be aware of their family histories but probably do have access to the information. In collecting a cancer history, counselors may want to utilize the following strategies:

- Ask specific questions about each family member to help jog the client's memory.
- Link ages or dates with other family events or special occasions.
- Help the client to identify relatives who might have the needed information and help clients think about how best to broach the topic with these relatives.
- Review with the client exactly what information is needed. Be specific.
- Reassure clients that it is okay for them not to have all the family history information at the first visit. (Otherwise, they may not return.)

7.2.2. THE FAMILY HISTORY INFORMATION IS NOT AVAILABLE

In certain situations, the family history information may simply be unobtainable. This can occur because of the situations presented in the succeeding sections.

7.2.2.1. Relatives or Records Are Lost

Family members who live far apart may, over time, lose contact with one another. Clients may have little awareness of the current health status of certain relatives and may not even have current contact information for them. The death of key relatives can also lead to a loss of contact with entire branches of the family. This is especially true if a parent has died young and the other parent ended up remarrying. Even if the client is in contact with the affected relative, the confirmatory medical records may no longer be available; physicians retire, hospitals are demolished, and stored records may be discarded or misplaced.

7.2.2.2. Estrangement from Family

Familial relationships may be full of conflict or practically nonexistent; in either case, clients may have less than complete information about their relatives' cancer histories. Sometimes, even family members who live in the same city have not spoken to each other in years. There may be complicated reasons for the estrangement due to desertion, sexual or physical abuse, use of drugs or alcohol, or family rifts. Sometimes, in the tradition of Hatfield and McCoy type family feuds, it is not the client who has broken off contact with others, but someone from a previous generation. Individuals who are estranged from affected family members will have no way of obtaining documentation of their cancer diagnoses or genetic test results. In fact, the clients may be missing information about entire branches of the family.

7.2.2.3. Adoption or Donor Eggs/Sperm

Individuals who were adopted as infants or young children generally have limited information about their biological relatives. The following information is typically included on birth certificates:

- Name of the biological mother
- The name of the biological father (if available)
- The date and time of birth
- Race and age of the mother (and possibly father)

At the current time, most adoptions are arranged privately rather than through an adoption agency and the amount of shared personal information varies widely from case to case. As adults, some adoptees do reconnect with biological relatives, allowing them to obtain some medical information. Individuals or couples may also utilize donor eggs or sperm to become parents. Agencies that arrange these procedures generally collect some medical information about the donors. However, most of the time, clients who were adopted or conceived with donor eggs or sperm will have limited information about their biological relatives.

In the above listed situations where access to information may be limited, counselors can consider utilizing the following strategies:

- Focus on the information that is currently available, which at a minimum includes the client's personal history.
- In cases of lost contact or estrangement, discuss alternative ways of obtaining this information, such as contacting other relatives or friends of the family who might have the needed information.
- In cases of adoption or donor eggs/sperm, explore whether the client has any options—and any interest—for trying to obtain information about biological relatives.

- Accept that there are situations in which it is not possible to obtain any more information and reassure clients that this is okay.

7.2.3. THE REPORTED HISTORY IS FALSE

The most challenging counseling situations can occur when clients provide information about their family histories that turns out to be inaccurate. These types of situations can occur when clients are mistaken or confused about the cancer diagnosis, or are deliberately fabricating history.

7.2.3.1. The Clients Are Mistaken About the Cancer Diagnosis

Cancer diagnoses among relatives may turn out to be benign lesions that have been biopsied or removed. The relative may have undergone surgery for reasons that were unrelated to a cancer diagnosis. For example, the client's aunt may have had a hysterectomy because of a benign uterine fibroid, not uterine cancer. Relatives may also be assumed to have cancer if they have a medical condition that leads to invasive procedures or treatment. Examples include gastric ulcers and inflammatory bowel disease.

7.2.3.2. The Clients Are Confused About the Diagnosis

Clients may be making assumptions about the site or type of cancer among relatives or may be confused about which relatives had which cancers. They may know, for example, that the relative had colon polyps, but not that the polyps were hamartomas. In addition, clients frequently do not distinguish between the primary site of cancer and sites of metastatic disease. In fact, it may be the metastatic cancer that is more likely to be remembered as it is probably what led to the relative's death. Clients may also have little knowledge of anatomy or medical terminology. Thus, "stomach cancer" may mean any malignancy in the abdomen and "uterine cancer" may be a euphemism for any female reproductive cancer. Vague reports of a "brain tumor" can also be problematic, as it can be used for anything from a benign cyst to a hemangioblastoma or malignant astrocytoma.

7.2.3.3. The Clients Are Deliberately Fabricating History

It is rare that clients deliberately falsify their family histories of cancer, but when it occurs, it creates a difficult and awkward counseling dilemma. Clients might provide fabricated histories because they want to ensure that they will be monitored closely or have access to prevention options, such as prophylactic surgery. In addition to providing fabricated cancer histories, clients may also falsely claim that there is a deleterious gene mutation in the family. Sometimes, it is not the client who has fabricated the history, but rather another relative. Clients or relatives may also fabricate their cancer histories because they are seeking sympathy or attention. This type of behavior can also indicate the presence of an emotional disorder termed Münchausen syndrome. Individuals with Münchausen syndrome, which has been observed more frequently among women, are hypochondriachal and may actually seek out painful, invasive procedures.

Falsely provided information, whether deliberate or not, can wreak havoc on the interpretation of the family history. Counselors can employ the following strategies to help ensure that the recounted history is correct:

- Encourage clients to confirm the history with other family members rather than making assumptions about the diagnoses.
- Obtain documentation of cancer diagnoses, especially if key to the interpretation of the family history.
- Diagnoses that appear questionable should be explored further, but in a respectful and gentle manner.
- If there is evidence that the history has been fabricated, carefully consider the potential ramifications if this information is shared with the client. Unless the corrected information is germane to the risk assessment, it might be best not to challenge the claims of the relative or client.

7.3. INTERPRETING A CANCER HISTORY

Once the cancer history information has been collected and the pedigree has been drawn, it is time to assess the pattern of cancer in the family for the likelihood that the client could have a hereditary cancer syndrome. This section describes the major features of hereditary cancer syndromes and discusses possible ways to classify the patterns of cancer within families.

7.3.1. FEATURES OF INHERITED CANCERS

As the family history information is being gathered, counselors should be on the lookout for certain "red flags." This section describes eight pedigree features that, if present, raise the likelihood that the client's family has a hereditary cancer syndrome. These features are also listed in Table 7.6. A pedigree that is suggestive of a hereditary cancer syndrome tends to display at least some of the features presented in the succeeding sections.

7.3.1.1. Several Relatives with the Same or Related Cancers

The first and foremost feature of a family with hereditary cancer is the presence of cancer. In general, families in which three or more blood rela-

TABLE 7.6. Main Features of Hereditary Cancer Syndromes

- Several relatives with the same or related cancers
- Younger age of onset than is typical
- Autosomal dominant pattern of cancer
- Presence of rare cancers
- Excess of multifocal or bilateral cancers
- Excess of multiple primary cancers
- Presence of other nonmalignant features
- Absence of environmental risk factors

tives have developed similar cancers may have a hereditary cancer syndrome. This is especially true if the client is closely related to the affected relatives. Thus, clients who have a sibling, mother, and maternal aunt with similar cancers are at greater risk for having an inherited predisposition to cancer than clients who have three maternal great-aunts with cancer. The greater the number of family members with cancer, the stronger the likelihood there is a genetic predisposition. In families with a highly penetrant cancer syndrome such as familial adenomatous polyposis (FAP, as depicted in Fig. 7.1), it is not unusual for there to be five or more affected individuals. However, the presence of the same type of cancer in a few relatives is more striking than multiple family members with a variety of cancers. Cancer susceptibility genes are typically associated with specific forms of cancer. An important part of assessing the pattern of cancer in the client's family is to determine which diagnoses could be due to the same underlying gene mutation. It is important for counselors to become familiar with the spectrum of cancers that could be linked to the same underlying genetic factor. For example, hereditary ovarian cancer can be associated with:

- Cancers of the peritoneum, fallopian tube, breast, pancreas, and prostate (which are all features of Hereditary Breast–Ovarian Cancer syndrome).
- Cancers of the uterus, colon, rectum, small intestine, stomach, kidney, and ureter (which are all features of Lynch syndrome).

7.3.1.2. Younger Age of Onset Than Is Typical

Inherited forms of cancer typically have earlier ages of onset than sporadic tumors. In fact, younger than usual age at diagnosis is one of the strongest predictors of inherited risk. Inherited childhood cancers are more likely to occur months or years earlier than sporadic cases and are also more likely to occur during the first 12 months of life. In adult-onset cancer syndromes, the associated malignancies can occur years or decades earlier than is seen in the general population. Therefore, the occurrence of early-onset cancer in one or more family members is strongly suggestive of an inherited form of cancer. However, malignancies occurring at later ages should not be completely dismissed; it is the overall pattern of cancer that is important to assess. Also, there are certain tumors that are significant regardless of the age of onset, such as ovarian cancer, male breast cancer, paragangliomas and other less commonly occurring neoplasms.

7.3.1.3. Autosomal Dominant Pattern of Cancer

Most hereditary cancer syndromes identified to date follow autosomal dominant inheritance patterns. Thus, the pattern of cancer should present as a vertical pattern, occurring over two or more generations in certain branches of the family. In other words, the presence of cancer in a grandparent, parent, and child is more compelling evidence of an inherited syndrome than cancer among cousins in the same generation. However, a dominant pattern of inheritance is sometimes subtle due to variable penetrance, small family size, or young ages of the majority of family members. Cancers that are sex limited (e.g., ovarian or prostate) or sex influenced (e.g., breast) may also be more difficult to track through a family.

7.3.1.4. Presence of Rare Cancers

A cluster of tumors that occur rarely in the general population is more difficult to explain by chance alone and provides evidence for an inherited basis. While two siblings with colorectal cancer may have been caused by shared multifactorial factors or random chance, two siblings with cancer of the duodenum almost certainly have some type of underlying genetic predisposition. Pedigrees suggestive of inherited forms of cancer may also include malignancies that have developed in an unusual subgroup. Examples include men with breast cancer, teenagers with colorectal cancer, and African Americans with melanoma.

7.3.1.5. Excess of Multifocal or Bilateral Cancers

Most tumors are monoclonal, meaning that the population of malignant cells has arisen from a single cancer cell. Individuals with inherited forms of cancer more frequently present with malignancies that are multifocal (more than one tumor within the same organ) or bilateral (tumors that have occurred in both paired organs).

7.3.1.6. Excess of Multiple Primary Cancers

Cancer survivors who have an inherited susceptibility to cancer are at substantially increased risks for developing additional malignancies. These second primaries may be synchronous (diagnosed at the same time as the initial cancer) or metachronous (diagnosed at a different time). Although all cancer survivors have small increased risks for developing a second cancer, the risk is exponentially higher for people with hereditary cancer syndromes. For example, the risk of contralateral breast cancer may be as high as 65% for female breast cancer survivors who carry *BRCA* mutations, which is a much higher risk than for those who have sporadic breast cancers.

7.3.1.7. Presence of Other Nonmalignant Features

Certain hereditary cancer syndromes are associated with benign tumors or other physical characteristics. Examples include the very large head size associated with PTEN Hamartoma syndrome, the distinctive eye finding termed congenital hypertrophy of the retinal pigment epithelium (CHRPE) associated with FAP, and the rare types of polyps found in Juvenile Polyposis and Peutz–Jeghers syndrome. Table 7.7 lists some of the nonmalignant features that are associated with one or more hereditary cancer syndromes. Appendix A, which lists inherited cancer syndromes by tumor type, includes some of the relevant nonmalignant features.

7.3.1.8. Absence of Environmental Risk Factors

It is also important not to forget potential environmental causes of tumors. This is especially true for cancers commonly associated with carcinogenic exposures such as mesothelioma (asbestos) and lung cancer (tobacco) or viral exposures, such as cervical cancer (HPV) or stomach cancer (*Helicobacter pylori*). In addition, some forms of cancer are associated with preexisting

TABLE 7.7. Examples of Nonmalignant Features in One or More Hereditary Cancer Syndromes*

Type	Features
Congenital defects	Ureter–renal defects, absent thumbs, aniridia
Dental problems	Absent teeth, supernumerary teeth
Eye findings	CHRPE, hemangioma, droopy eyelids
Neurological problems	Seizures, ataxia, autism, intellectual impairments, compulsive overeating
Polyps	Adenomas, hamartomas, hyperplastic polyps, juvenile polyps
Skeletal findings	Doliencephaly, scoliosis, rib defects, butterfly rash
Skin lesions	Café au lait spots, dysplastic nevi, palmer pits, sebaceous adenomas, trichilemmomas, poikiloderma

Source: Lindor et al., 2008.

*See Appendix A for syndrome associations.

medical conditions. Examples include lymphoma and Kaposi's sarcoma in individuals with HIV, colon cancer in those with ulcerative colitis, and testicular cancer in men born with undescended testes. Although there are towns that have been documented to have higher cancer rates due to contaminated well water, paper-making mills, or manufacturing plants, true cancer clusters of this kind are uncommon, or at least they are difficult to prove.

7.3.2. WAYS TO CLASSIFY FAMILY HISTORIES OF CANCER

Cancer can cluster in families due to a variety of factors including inherited factors, shared exposures to carcinogens, or simply random chance ("bad luck"). Even if the family does not have a hereditary cancer syndrome, family members might still have some level of increased risk.

Once the family history has been collected and reviewed, genetic counselors will determine how best to classify the cancer history.

The pattern of cancer in a family can be classified in the following ways, which are presented in the succeeding sections.

7.3.2.1. Hereditary Cancer Syndrome

Pedigrees of families with hereditary cancer typically exhibit one or more of the features listed in Table 7.6. In simplistic terms, families with dominantly inherited hereditary cancer syndrome are more likely to have patterns of cancer that follow the 3–2–1 rule:

- 3 individuals with similar or related cancers,
- 2 generations of cancer cases, and
- 1 person diagnosed at an unusually young age (e.g., <age 50 for adult-onset cancers).

In addition, the pedigree should display distinctive features that are consistent with or highly suggestive of a specific hereditary cancer syndrome. Clients who are found to have a hereditary cancer syndrome are at greatly increased risk for developing the associated malignancies even if these cancers have not occurred in the family.

7.3.2.2. Familial Cluster of Cancer

Clients may have a familial cluster of cancer if they have two or more relatives who have developed similar cancers, but the family does not have any other features suggestive of a hereditary cancer syndrome. Familial clustering of cancer is more likely caused by multifactorial factors, that is, a combination of genetic factors and environmental agents. Clients with a familial cluster of cancer may have increased risks for developing similar types of cancer, but the associated cancer risks tend to be lower (and less predictable) than in families with hereditary cancer syndromes.

7.3.2.3. Environmentally Caused Cluster of Cancer

In some cases, members of the same family have developed similar cancers because of exposures to the same carcinogenic agent. If an exposure is shared by several members of a family, then the incidences of cancer may resemble a familial pattern. Examples include:

- *Carcinogenic agents in a family business*—such as dry cleaners, mill workers, farmers, and construction workers
- *Lifestyle habits*—such as dietary preferences and the use of tobacco or alcohol
- *Broad exposures to carcinogens*—such as excessive sun exposure or toxic well water

Individuals in families with environmentally caused clusters of cancer are only at increased risk for developing cancer if they share the carcinogenic exposure. For example, a male client might report that several of his relatives developed lung cancer after being long-term cigarette smokers. Given this family history, the client's risk of lung cancer is only increased if he himself smokes cigarettes.

7.3.2.4. Sporadic Forms of Cancer

It is important to keep in mind that most cases of cancer occur randomly without an obvious underlying risk factor. In fact, it is seldom possible to identify the main cause for why a specific person developed cancer. Thus, a pattern of cancer in a family may very well represent multiple sporadic cases that have happened to occur in the same family. This is especially true if family members have developed commonly occurring cancers at standard ages or if the cancer types are diverse and are not typically linked by a common gene mutation or carcinogenic agent.

7.3.3. HIGH, MODERATE, LOW, AND UNCERTAIN RISK CATEGORIES

Another way to classify cancer histories is by the likelihood that the family could have a hereditary predisposition to cancer. Distinguishing between "high-risk" and "low-risk" families will impact the remainder of the counseling discussion, from the discussion of genetic testing options to offering medical management recommendations. The classification of risk, in terms of the likelihood of having a hereditary cancer syndrome are presented in the succeeding sections.

7.3.3.1. Family at High Risk

The pedigree of a family at high risk shows strong evidence for having an inherited predisposition. The pattern of cancer in the family is consistent with or highly suggestive of a specific hereditary cancer syndrome. Family members should be counseled that they fit criteria for the syndrome, even if genetic testing is not informative. In other words, an indeterminate negative test result will not change the fact that the family has the syndrome. Figure 7.3 shows a family with hereditary retinoblastoma.

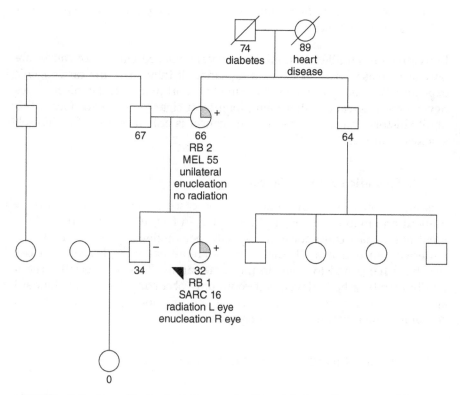

FIGURE 7.3. A pedigree depicting a family with hereditary retinoblastoma. MEL = melanoma; RB = retinoblastoma; SARC = sarcoma.

7.3.3.2. Family at Moderate Risk

A family at moderate risk for having a hereditary predisposition has some features suggestive of a cancer syndrome. However, the family may not quite meet criteria for the syndrome or the family may have certain features that are inconsistent with the syndrome. As an example, see Figure 7.4. In this pedigree, the client has a finding (two renal cysts) that can be associated with von Hippel–Lindau (VHL) syndrome. Although her first-degree relatives show no signs of VHL, she has a paternal uncle with renal cell carcinoma; a cardinal feature of VHL. So, in assessing this family, the genetic counselor might list those features that are/are not suggestive of VHL.

- Features in pedigree suggestive of VHL:
  - Client has two renal cysts
  - Uncle with renal cell carcinoma
- Features not suggestive of VHL:
  - Client does not have other manifestations of VHL
  - Father (presumed obligate carrier) had no signs of VHL

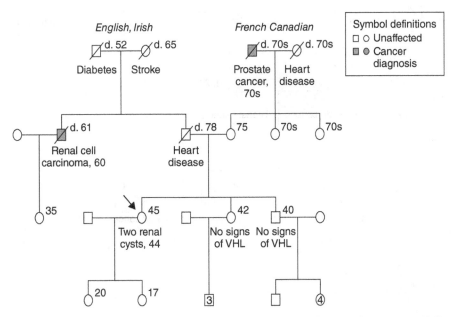

FIGURE 7.4. A pedigree depicting a client at moderate risk for having VHL syndrome.

7.3.3.3. Family at Low Risk

A family at low risk for having a hereditary cancer syndrome has a negative or noncontributory history of cancer. Figure 7.5 shows an example of a low-risk pedigree. Although there are several cases of cancer in the family, the cancer types are ones that frequently occur among older individuals. This pattern of cancer is therefore unlikely to be due to a common inherited factor. Low-risk families typically include the following features:

- Few, if any, first- or second-degree relatives with cancer
- Cancer(s) that are not usually associated with a hereditary syndrome
- Cancers that have occurred at typical ages
- Cancers that occur commonly in the general population
- No cancers among sibling pairs or parent–child pairs
- No unusual tumor characteristics or other physical findings

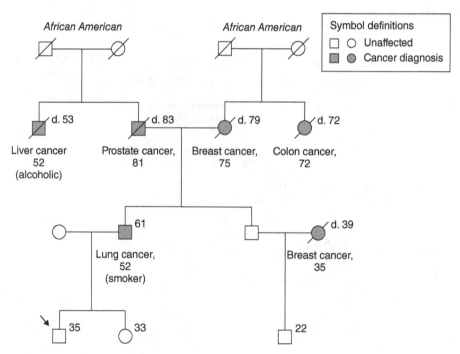

FIGURE 7.5. A pedigree depicting a client at low risk for having a hereditary cancer syndrome.

7.3.3.4. Family at Uncertain Risk

Even the most skilled genetic counselor will not be able to provide a meaningful cancer risk assessment for every client. As discussed previously in Section 7.2, some clients are better historians than others. There may be key information missing from the family history or there may be doubts about the accuracy of the verbal history given. In some cases, the counselors may need to delay the assessment of the client's pedigree until additional information and/or documentation has been obtained. If the client is not able to obtain any further information, counselors can either say to clients that it is not possible to interpret the pedigree or can offer the range of possible interpretations.

7.4. Case Examples

The following three case examples illustrate some of these challenges involved in collecting and interpreting cancer family histories.

Case 3: "Men in our family don't make it to 50."

When the genetic counselor asked Mike why he was here today, he gestured over at his wife and said, "Ask her." While the wife explained that their internist had raised concerns about the amount of cancer in Mike's family, the counselor took note of the fact that Mike kept staring at his shoes like a student hoping the teacher won't call on him.

Noticing Mike's T-shirt of the local sports team, the counselor said, "Well Mike, I see you like the hometown team; we have that in common. Do you think we have a chance to win the next game?" As they chatted about sports, Mike visibly relaxed and became more attentive to the discussion.

The counselor then transitioned to collecting the family history information. Mike, age 46, was in good health, as were his 8-year-old twin sons. Mike's only brother was 3 years younger, also in good health. Their mother was cancer free at age 72, but their father had died from a sudden heart attack a few months before his 50th birthday. The father's autopsy, which Mike had brought to the session, revealed that the father had widely metastatic cancer (of unknown primary) at the time of his death. No cancer history was reported for the mother's family, so the counselor focused on collecting information about the paternal relatives.

With a lot of help from his wife, Mike related that his paternal aunt was cancer free at age 80, but that his paternal uncle had died from cancer in his forties.

"Do you know what type of cancer your uncle had?" asked the counselor.

"It was somewhere in his body. I think it was in one of his organs." Mike replied earnestly.

The counselor wondered if he was trying to make a joke, but decided that he wasn't and continued on. "Did this uncle have any children?"

"Yeah, he had three kids—Lisa, Alan, and Matt." replied Mike.

"Has Lisa ever had cancer?"

"Yeah, she got diagnosed with cancer last month. She is the same age as me."

"Do you know what type of cancer your cousin Lisa has?" asked the counselor.

"Uhhh, maybe lung cancer?" he guessed. His wife interjected, "No, it was something else. But I don't know the name of it. It was something rare, I remember her saying that."

The counselor wrote "cancer—type unknown, rare cancer" by Lisa's name on the pedigree.

"Okay, what about your cousin, Alan?" asked the counselor.

"Alan died from cancer. He had cancer in his neck." said Mike. "That's right," agreed his wife. "It went to his brain. He was gone in about 2 months. It was awful."

"It sounds awful," agreed the counselor. "And it sounds like Alan was fairly young when he died. Do you remember the age he was when he died?"

"Well, let's see, his son was still in high school," said Mike. "And it was right after we took that cruise," added his wife.

The counselor's pen hovered over Alan's name on the pedigree but she wasn't sure what to write. She decided to try a different tactic. "Mike, you said that Lisa was about your age. Was Alan older or younger than the two of you?"

"Oh, he was older by 2 or 3 years."

"So do you think that Alan might have been in his early forties when he died?"

"Yeah, that sounds about right. Men in our family don't make it to 50."

"Oh, don't talk like that," frowned his wife. "I don't like it when you talk about having some kind of family curse."

Mike shrugged his shoulders. "Well there's nothing we can do about it. Only seems to happen to the men. Well at least that's how it seemed until Lisa got cancer. Now I don't know what to think."

"Well, looking at how much loss there has been in your family, I can see why you might think there is some kind of curse going on. Some families that have lots of cancer turn out to have an inherited predisposition to cancer that is being passed on through the family like other family traits." The genetic counselor paused and then asked, "What would it be like to hear something like that?"

Mike thought about it for a few minutes. "Well I guess it depends on what you tell me. But I think it's important to find out what's going on. I mean, I do have two sons and I am worried about them."

"That's understandable. And I'm sure you would like to be around to watch them grow up! One of the advantages of knowing that you are at certain risks of cancer is that you may be able to have better screening options. Let's take another look at your family tree to see what it can tell us."

The genetic counselor reviewed the initial pedigree (see Fig. 7.6), noting that four closely related individuals had developed cancer under the age of 50, definitely a worrisome cluster of cancer. However, it was a cluster of unknown types of cancer, which meant it could be anything—or nothing. This lack of information made it impossible for the counselor to provide any type of meaningful risk assessment. The first order of business was to discuss ways to obtain more information about the cancers in the family.

The genetic counselor explained what she had been thinking about and then said, "You're here for answers, but I'm afraid I need more information from you before I can be more helpful to you. We need to find out what types of cancer that your uncle and cousins had. Can you think of anyone in the family who might have this information?"

"Well, my mother would know. She kept track of all that stuff," said Mike.

"Would you feel comfortable asking your mother for this information?" asked the counselor.

"Sure, but it wouldn't do me any good now; she's got dementia." Mike said matter-of-factly.

"Oh dear, I'm sorry to hear that," responded the counselor. "That's got to be tough on all of you."

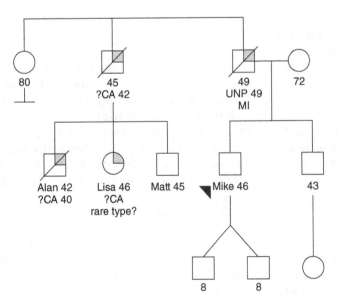

FIGURE 7.6. Mike's initial pedigree, which cannot be assessed due to missing information. (See the text for further discussion of this case.) CA = cancer; ?CA = cancer, type unknown; MI = myocardial infarction; UNP = primary of unknown origin.

"Yeah, what are you gonna do?" Mike shrugged, clearly uncomfortable with this line of conversation.

The counselor tactfully resumed discussing the topic at hand, "Well, the best person to talk to about the cancer diagnoses would be your cousin, Lisa. Do you ever talk to her?"

"Well I see her at family events, weddings, birthdays, things like that. I haven't seen her in quite awhile," said Mike.

"Would you feel comfortable contacting her to find out more about the cancers in the family?" asked the counselor.

"I don't know," said Mike hesitantly. "She's going through so much right now. I'd hate to bother her." He then gestured over at his wife. "But you could do it—you're good at bothering people."

The wife and counselor both laughed at this. Then the wife said, "Well, in a way he's right. I do tend to be the one who calls everyone in his family to organize the get-togethers. I'd be happy to call Lisa."

"Are you sure that you are okay with this?" asked the counselor. "Do you think Lisa would be willing to talk to you or might the questions be upsetting to her?"

"Oh, I think Lisa is fine talking about this stuff. She's a nurse and the whole family badgers her with their medical questions. Besides, she has kids of her own and she's probably worried about them getting cancer," said Mike's wife.

The genetic counselor wrote out a list of questions to ask the cousin—if it seemed appropriate to do so. She also scheduled a follow-up visit with Mike and his wife to resume discussions about the family history once they had more information.

At the second counseling visit, Mike's pedigree looked very different. (See Fig. 7.7.) According to Lisa—and confirmed with medical records— her father had died from clear cell renal carcinoma and her brother Alan had died from a malignant paraganglioma. Lisa's tumor was a benign pheochromocytoma. This pattern of tumors is highly suggestive of either Herediary Paraganglioma–Pheochromocytoma syndrome or von Hippel Lindau syndrome. The genetic counselor is arranging genetic testing for the family.

Case 3 wrap-up: This case illustrates possible methods for dealing with clients who have incomplete (but possibly worrisome) family histories.

Case 4: "I don't want to make this a big deal, but I don't want to ignore things, either."

"It's good to finally meet you in person," said the genetic counselor as she greeted her next client, Emma. Emma had rescheduled her appointment in the High-Risk Clinic at least three times before actually making it in.

Emma smiled back and said that she was glad too. As a theater major, it was difficult for her to make time for medical appointments in between classes and rehearsals. Emma, age 22, had spiky short dark hair and wore a

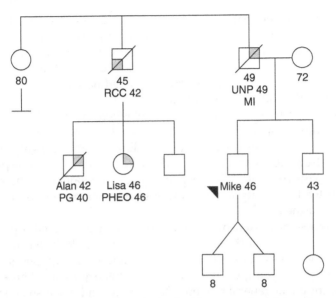

FIGURE 7.7. Mike's final pedigree, which is highly suggestive of pheochromocytoma–paraganglioma syndrome. (See the text for further discussion of this case.) MI = myocardial infarction; PG = paraganglioma; PHEO = pheochromocytoma; RCC = renal cell carcinoma; UNP = primary of unknown origin.

long glittery scarf wrapped several times around her neck. She sat down in the chair near the counselor's desk, curling her legs underneath her.

The genetic counselor pulled out the handwritten pedigree that she had jotted down during their earlier phone conversations.

"So maybe we should start from the beginning, just to make sure I have the right information," began the counselor.

Emma plunged right into her story: "Alright, here's the deal: My parents adopted me when I was 3 days old. That was 22 years ago. About 3 months ago, out of the blue, I got a message on Facebook asking if I had been born in Allentown, Pennsylvania to a woman named Nicollette Raines. I said yes and we started chatting online. It turns out she is my sister—or my half-sister anyway. Her name is Krystal, and she is like 17 years old. I have a couple of half-brothers too, but I don't know anything about them. Nicollette—everyone called her Nicki—had a lot of problems with alcohol and all the kids got taken away by the state, but Nicki sort of kept in contact with Krystal. According to Krystal, Nicki finally got her act together and sobered up, but then she got really bad breast cancer and died. She was only 38 years old. Totally sad, huh?"

The counselor agreed that it was a very sad story. She asked if it was hard for Emma to talk about it.

Emma shook her head and gave a nervous giggle. "Not really, I mean I never knew her. It's like I'm telling a story about a stranger."

The counselor wondered if there was more to this than Emma was letting on or was even aware of, but continued collecting the family history information—as limited as it was. Having noted how Emma referred to her birth mother, the counselor did likewise.

"Are you pretty sure that Nicki was 38 when she died?"

"Yes, I am. I searched the Web and found her obituary notice in a local newspaper. I made a copy of it; wait a sec." Emma leaned down and grabbed her wallet from her purse. She pulled out a folded-up piece of paper and handed it to the counselor. "It tells people to donate money to a breast cancer charity instead of giving flowers and it also mentions her sister who took care of her at the end."

The counselor looked over the obituary, which featured a picture of a young woman with short dark hair and a bright smile. The counselor was not sure exactly how best to respond, but felt as though she should say something before going on with the family history intake. She settled on making a couple of general remarks. "It's always sad when someone dies at such a young age. It sure is a nice picture."

"It is a nice picture, isn't it? She looks a lot like me, doesn't she?" Emma beamed.

"Yes I definitely see a resemblance," the counselor agreed with a smile.

"You should see the picture of Krystal. Oh my god, she could be my twin. It's totally weird."

"I can imagine," said the counselor. "Can you say more about how it's weird?"

"I don't know—it just feels strange knowing there is someone out there that looks exactly like me. I mean, she is my sister and everything, but at the same time, she is like a total stranger to me. It's all kinda weird," explained Emma.

"Do you wish she hadn't contacted you?" asked the counselor gently.

"Oh no, I'm glad she did. It's just a matter of getting used to it, that's all."

"You are dealing with some big things right now. Sometimes this kind of situation can bring up a lot of different feelings. Do you have anyone that you can talk to about it?" asked the counselor.

"Well I've talked a little bit about it with my friends, but mainly I talk to my mom about it. She has been great. In fact, Krystal and I are talking about getting together in a few weeks and my mom is fine with that; in fact, she wants to meet her too at some point. That would be an interesting meeting, huh?" Emma smiled and rolled her eyes.

"Sounds like your mom is very supportive of you," observed the counselor.

"Yes she is. Of course, right now she is freaking out about me getting breast cancer. She really wanted to come with me today, but she couldn't get out of work."

"So it was your mother who encouraged you to come in to talk to us?" asked the counselor.

"Actually it was my gynecologist who first suggested it. She thought it would be a good idea for me to have the genetic test. I mean, I don't want to make this a big deal, but I don't want to ignore things, either. You know what I mean?" said Emma.

"Yes I do, that makes a lot of sense. Well, before we talk about the genetic test, let's see what more we can learn from the family tree. Has Krystal mentioned anyone else in the family who has had breast cancer?" asked the counselor.

"Oh yeah, I forgot to mention it before. She said that her grandmother had breast cancer too—that's Nicki's mother."

"Do you know old Nicki's mother was when she got cancer?" asked the counselor.

"Nope, that's all I know," said Emma.

"Have you heard about anyone else in the family who had cancer?"

Emma shook her head. "Nope, that's it."

"Alright, we know that Nicki had at least one sister. Do you know whether she had any other brothers or sisters?" asked the counselor.

"I haven't heard about any other brothers or sisters, but I haven't really asked." admitted Emma. "Is it important?"

"Well in general, the more information we have, the better. But it is not a big deal. If you learn of any more relatives, I can always add them later to the family tree. And if you are not able to get any more information, that is okay too," reassured the counselor. She did not want Emma feeling obligated to discuss her biological relatives before she was ready.

"Now, I know that your real father is the man who raised you, but do you know anything about your biological father?" asked the counselor.

"I don't know anything about him; not even his name. I do know that Krystal and I have different fathers, but she doesn't know anything about her father either."

The counselor looked at the completed pedigree (Fig. 7.8) and discussed with Emma the possibility that her biological mother could have had a *BRCA* mutation, given her early age at diagnosis. Nicki's excessive use of alcohol almost certainly contributed to her development of breast cancer, but it didn't rule out the possibility of an inherited predisposition.

The counselor discussed the process of genetic testing, including the risks and benefits and the types of results it could give her. The counselor also encouraged her to take a little time to think it over first, because she thought it might be helpful for Emma to have a little more time to process everything. Emma seemed relieved not to proceed right to testing (although

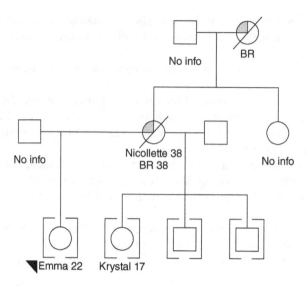

FIGURE 7.8. Emma's pedigree, which may be suggestive of hereditary breast–ovarian cancer syndrome. (See the text for further discussion of this case.) BR = breast cancer, invasive.

that might have been because of her squeamishness about having blood drawn).

The genetic counselor arranged for Emma to return to the High-Risk Clinic in about 1 month to discuss testing further and also to meet with the program breast oncologist to discuss appropriate breast cancer monitoring. The counselor also gave Emma written information about the *BRCA* genetic test. Emma was eager to share the information with her mother and planned to bring her to the next set of appointments.

Case 4 wrap-up: This case demonstrates ways to collect family history information, which is incomplete and potentially emotionally charged.

Case 5: Will the real historian please stand up?

Kim Tatro, age 38, launched into a speech before the genetic counselor had completely entered the room.

"My mother had cancer and so did all her brothers and sisters. Now my sister has cancer too. I know I'm next. I have terrible heartburn and I'm always getting stomach cramps; aren't those both signs of cancer?"

The genetic counselor took a deep breath and tried to figure out where to start. He assured Kim that she was in the right place to get some answers. He also explained that she would be meeting with one of the oncologists who would take the client's medical history and could provide advice about any symptoms she was having. "Would it be alright to wait with those questions until you meet with the doctor?"

"I guess that's okay. But what are we going to talk about?"

"Well, my role is to focus on the family history to see how that might impact on your risk of developing cancer. It sounds like there is quite a bit of cancer in your family. May I ask you some questions about the family history?"

"Sure. There've been a lot of medical problems in my family. Lots of mental problems too, if you really want to know," said Kim as she launched into stories about her "crazy uncle" and "paranoid sister."

Taking the family history was a challenge. Kim was quite anxious and also excessively chatty—a combination that was difficult to manage effectively. She offered all kinds of information that did not contribute to the pattern of cancer—incidences of asthma, diabetes, and hernia operations—but responded vaguely to queries about the cancer diagnoses. She said that she was not on good terms with her five siblings, but heard from her younger sister, Julie, "once in awhile."

Kim reported that her oldest sister, Elizabeth, had been diagnosed with ovarian cancer last year at age 47 and that two of their maternal aunts had developed breast cancer in their forties ("I'm very sure about one of them and not so sure about the other one"). She also mentioned that a maternal uncle had died recently from lung cancer at about age 70. As far as Kim was aware, none of her maternal cousins had developed cancer. Her father had died from a stroke at age 65 and there was no history of cancer on the father's side of the family.

The counselor paused to review the pedigree (see Fig. 7.9) and decided that the family might have an increased likelihood of having a BRCA mutation if the patient's sister really had ovarian cancer.

"How sure are you that your sister Elizabeth had ovarian cancer?" queried the counselor.

"I'm fairly certain it was ovarian cancer. I mean she had a hysterectomy and everything. Of course, I don't talk to her directly. This is just what I've heard from other family members. My sister is totally secretive about any kind of medical stuff. One time she was hospitalized with pneumonia for an entire week and didn't tell anyone."

Before the client launched into yet another family story, the counselor redirected the conversation back to the cancer history, "It would really be helpful to confirm exactly what type of cancer your sister had. Plus there are different types of ovarian cancer. Some are linked with hereditary breast cancer and some are not. Is there any possibility that you could get written confirmation of your sister's ovarian cancer?"

"Not a chance. We haven't spoken to each other since our father died about 5 years ago." said Kim, looking expectantly at the counselor to ask the source of their quarrel.

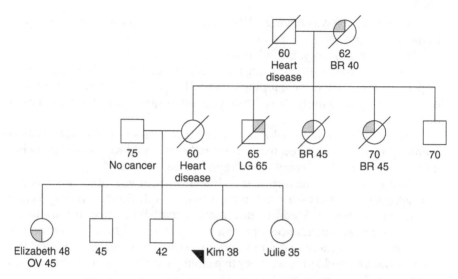

FIGURE 7.9. Kim's version of the Tatro family history, which is suggestive of hereditary breast–ovarian cancer syndrome. (See the text for further discussion of this case.)
BR = breast cancer, invasive; LG = lung cancer; OV = ovarian cancer.

The counselor said, "You and your family have certainly been through
a lot. I appreciate the stories that you have shared with me about your family.
I don't mean to cut the story short, but the physician is going to start wondering where you are! So we had better try to wrap this up in the next 15
minutes or so. Is that okay with you?"

"Absolutely. I have a lot of questions for the doctor." said Kim. The
counselor made a mental note to warn the physician that it would not be a
quick visit.

"Well, it would be helpful to find out exactly what type of cancer your
sister had. Is there anyone else in the family who might have more information about it?" asked the counselor.

"I don't think so. Like I said, she doesn't talk to anyone about her
medical issues."

The genetic counselor then explored the possibility of documenting the
two breast cancer diagnoses in her aunts. Unfortunately, both aunts were
deceased and Kim was not in touch with any of her cousins.

Given the family history of breast and ovarian cancer, it was appropriate
to discuss *BRCA* testing with Kim. As the counselor began to talk about the
option of genetic testing, Kim interrupted him. "Oh yeah, my sister Julie had
that test. It didn't find anything."

"Do you think that you could get a copy of your sister's results? It would
be helpful to review the results." asked the counselor.

Kim said that she would arrange for her sister's results to be faxed to the counselor's office. Kim also granted permission for the counselor to share the pedigree and test result with her sister's genetic counselor.

The counselor discussed the importance of reviewing her sister's test results but also explained that a negative *BRCA* result in the sister would not eliminate the possibility that Kim could have an inherited susceptibility. Kim seemed to understand this reasoning and wanted to proceed with testing that day. The counselor asked if testing might exacerbate Kim's worries about cancer but Kim disagreed. "I know I'm a worrier but having my results would help me to be monitored more closely. Not being tested would stress me out even more."

The genetic counselor spoke to the medical oncologist and they agreed that it was reasonable (though not ideal) for Kim to be tested that day. The counselor was relieved that his next client was late due to traffic, because his usual 45-minute session had turned into a much longer one.

Kim's *BRCA* results were negative. That same week, the counselor received the pedigree and test results from Julie's counselor (see Fig. 7.10). Julie's test results were negative for mutations in *MSH2*, *MLH1*, and *MSH6*, not *BRCA*. The two genetic counselors compared notes and discussed possible strategics for determining which client (if either) had reported the family history accurately.

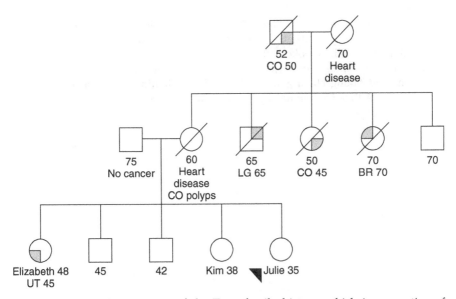

FIGURE 7.10. Julie's version of the Tatro family history, which is suggestive of Lynch syndrome. CO = colon cancer; LG = lung cancer; BR = breast cancer; UT = uterine cancer.

Kim returns next week to discuss her genetic test results and the information from her sister's genetic consultation. The genetic counselor anticipates another very long counseling session.

Case 5 wrap-up: This case illustrates the challenges of conflicting, and most likely, not confirmable family history information.

7.5. FURTHER READING

Armel, SR, McCuaig, J, Finch, A, et al. 2009. The effectiveness of family history questionnaires in cancer genetic counseling. J Genet Couns 18:366–378.

Bennett, R. 2010a. The language of the pedigree. In The Practical Guide to the Genetic Family History, 2nd edition. Wiley-Blackwell, Hoboken, NJ, 1–17.

Bennett, R. 2010b. Using a pedigree to recognize individuals with an increased susceptibility to cancer. In The Practical Guide to the Genetic Family History, 2nd edition. Wiley-Blackwell, Hoboken, NJ, 177–219.

Bennett, R. 2010c. Medical verification of family history, and resources for patients to record their genetic family histories. In The Practical Guide to the Genetic Family History, 2nd edition. Wiley-Blackwell, Hoboken, NJ, 220–229.

Dominguez, FJ, Lawrence, C, Halpern, EF, et al. 2007. Accuracy of self-reported personal history of cancer in an outpatient breast cancer. J Genet Couns 16:341–345.

Lindor, NM, McMaster, ML, Lindor, CJ, et al. 2008. Concise handbook of familial cancer susceptibility syndromes, 2nd edition. J Natl Cancer Inst Monographs 38:1–93.

Schuette, JL, and Bennett, RL. 2009. The ultimate genetic tool: the family history. In Uhlmann, WR, Schuette, JL, and Yashar, BM (eds), A Guide to Genetic Counseling. Wiley-Blackwell, Hoboken NJ.

Veach, PM, LeRoy, BS, and Bartels, DM. 2003. Gathering information: asking questions and taking client genetic history. In Facilitating the Genetic Counseling Process: A Practice Manual. Springer, New York, 73–92.

8

CANCER RISK COMMUNICATION

> Genetic counselors assess, explain and discuss risks with their patients through-
> out the entire genetic counseling process. Risk communication does not center
> exclusively on the statistical likelihood of the patient having a genetic condition.
> It also involves feelings, beliefs, and reactions to the overall concept of risk.
>
> *(Dixon and Konheim-Kalkstein, 2010, p. 67)*

In many ways, risk communication *is* genetic counseling. Cancer genetic
counselors deal with the various aspects of risk communication throughout
the counseling and testing process. This chapter provides background information about genetic counseling sessions and risk communication, offers
strategies for effective discussions about risk, and describes counseling techniques specific to families at low, moderate, and high risk for having a
hereditary cancer syndrome. The chapter ends with three case examples.

8.1. GENETIC COUNSELING AND RISK PERCEPTION

8.1.1. ELEMENTS OF CANCER GENETIC COUNSELING SESSIONS

Risk communication influences all of the components of a cancer genetic
counseling session, from the initial setting of goals with clients to discussing
genetic test results and options for cancer surveillance. To put the topic of
risk communication into proper perspective, this section provides an overview of a typical cancer genetic counseling session.

Counseling About Cancer, Third Edition. Katherine A. Schneider.
© 2012 Wiley-Blackwell. Published 2012 by John Wiley & Sons, Inc.

TABLE 8.1. MAJOR ELEMENTS OF AN INITIAL CANCER GENETIC COUNSELING
SESSION

- Setting goals for the session
- Collecting a cancer family history
- Conducting a risk assessment
- Communicating risk information
- Discussing and arranging genetic testing
- Discussing options for medical management
- Exploring psychosocial issues
- Making appropriate referrals
- Agreeing on plans for follow-up

The main elements of a cancer genetic counseling session are presented
in the following sections (also see Table 8.1).

8.1.1.1. Setting Goals for the Session

The goal-setting process has two major components:

- *Counselor goals*—Genetic counselors generally have an educational
  or information-oriented goal for the session. Counselors can say to
  clients: "In this visit, we will review your family history to determine
  if you could have an inherited predisposition to cancer" or "I will
  describe the pros and cons of genetic testing so you can decide if
  this is something you would like to do." The counselor should also
  indicate whether the stated goals are likely to be reached within the
  one session. Counselors may also wish to describe the elements of
  the counseling session to clients so that they will know what to
  expect.

- *Client goals*—Client goals can be quite broad, such as "I am here to
  get some general information" or "What can you tell me about
  genetic testing?" Other clients may have very specific goals in mind,
  such as "I need to know what to tell my 16-year-old daughter about
  the *BRCA* mutation in the family" or "Based on the family history,
  how often should I be having colonoscopies?" Counselors should
  listen carefully to the client's goals and alter the plans for the session
  accordingly. In a few cases, the counselor may realize that the client's
  goals cannot be met during the session. Clients may have erroneous
  ideas of what genetic counseling or testing can tell them or they may
  be better served by meeting with a different health-care provider. In
  these instances, the counselor should reaffirm what he or she can do
  for the client and then either mutually agree on different goals for

the session or arrange for the client to be seen by a more appropriate provider.

8.1.1.2. Collecting a Cancer Family History

Counselors typically gather family history information for three or more generations and construct a pedigree that can then be altered or expanded over time. Some high-risk programs request the family history information prior to the counseling session. This can be accomplished by use of family history surveys or intake telephone calls. Having the information prior to the visit can help with case preparation and may save time during the session, although the family history should always be reviewed during the session. It is important to collect as much detailed information as possible about each case of cancer in the family, including the exact diagnosis and the age at diagnosis. Cancer diagnoses should be confirmed with medical records documentation whenever possible. (Refer to Section 7.1 for more specific information about collecting a cancer family history.)

8.1.1.3. Conducting a Risk Assessment

Once the family history information has been collected, the counselor will assess the family's pattern of cancer to determine whether the family could have a specific hereditary cancer syndrome. In some cases, the identification of a cancer syndrome may require further information about the cancer diagnoses, additional diagnostic tests, or genetic tests. (Refer to Section 7.3 for more specific information about conducting a risk assessment from the client's pedigree.)

8.1.1.4. Communicating Risk Information

The genetic counselor will inform clients about the probability of having a hereditary cancer syndrome and developing cancer. The counselor and client will then have a dialogue about the risk information in order to clarify any misunderstandings and to help the client make decisions about cancer genetic testing or medical management. (See Sections 8.2 and 8.3 for more specific information about risk communication.)

8.1.1.5. Discussing and Arranging Genetic Testing

Many cancer genetic counseling clients will be given the option of genetic testing. Initial discussions about genetic testing can include the appropriateness of testing, possible genetic test results, limitations of testing, risks and benefits of testing, and logistics of the testing process. (See Section 9.2 for more specific information about pretest genetic counseling.)

8.1.1.6. Discussing Options of Medical Management

The purpose of cancer monitoring is to detect tumors *prior* to the onset of symptoms. Monitoring strategies can include imaging studies, endoscopes, blood tests, urinalysis, or random biopsies. These procedures include standard screening tests (like mammograms), which may be initiated at earlier ages and more frequent intervals, as well as less commonly used screening procedures (like magnetic resonance imaging [MRI]) targeted at those considered to be high risk. Clients need to be warned that none of these screening tests are 100% effective in detecting tumors. These screening tests also carry a risk of identifying a questionable finding that requires follow-up tests. Counselors can provide clients with appropriate referrals and can help empower them to be evaluated at more frequent intervals or to seek medical attention in the event of any symptoms.

8.1.1.7. Exploring Psychosocial Issues

The exploration of psychosocial issues is the "counseling" portion of the genetic counseling session. It involves an assessment and discussion of the client's emotional state, reactions, and feelings about the risk information and decisions about genetic testing or medical management. To enhance the counselor–client rapport, the counselor needs to provide information in a professional and compassionate manner and also to listen carefully and empathetically to all client responses and questions. (See Section 10.2 for more specific information on the psychosocial aspects of counseling.)

8.1.1.8. Making Appropriate Referrals

Some clients may benefit from referrals to other health-care providers. This can include referrals to a medical geneticist, oncologist, gastroenterologist, dermatologist, or surgeon. It may also become clear that the client could use another type of specialist, such as a mental health therapist, grief counselor, psychologist, or social worker. The genetic counselor can talk to clients about the possible benefits of meeting with additional providers and can also help facilitate the referrals.

8.1.1.9. Agreeing on Plans for Follow-Up

At the end of the genetic counseling session, the counselor and client should agree on the plans for how to proceed. This can include any need for medical records as well as setting up additional appointments for testing or follow-up. Genetic counselors typically dictate a note of the visit into the client's medical chart and often send detailed letters to clients following the counseling session. These client letters may summarize the counseling discussions, the family history information, and/or the genetic test results. Clients should also be encouraged to recontact the genetic counselor if there are any questions about the issues that were discussed or if they learn of any new cancer diagnoses in the family.

8.1.2. TYPES OF CANCER GENETIC COUNSELING VISITS

Clients who go on to have genetic testing are often scheduled to have two or three genetic counseling appointments. (See Fig. 8.1; refer also to Chapter 9, which discusses the genetic testing process in greater detail.) As described below, the counseling goals and discussions differ at each of these visits.

8.1.2.1. Risk Assessment Visit

At the initial genetic counseling visit, the primary goals of the session are to collect a detailed family history and to determine the client's risk for having a specific hereditary cancer syndrome. It has also become routine to discuss and arrange genetic testing at the initial counseling visit. However, not all clients will be ready to be tested at this time; some will require insurance preauthorization and others will have medically or emotionally based concerns about testing. If clients are missing key family history information at the initial risk assessment visit, then it may be necessary to schedule follow-up visits in order to complete the assessment of risk and discuss genetic testing options.

8.1.2.2. Genetic Testing Visit

The primary goals of this counseling visit are to obtain informed consent and specimens for genetic testing. Often the testing and risk assessment visits are combined. The informed consent process involves a detailed discussion about the possible test results, limitations, risks and benefits, and the logistics of testing, including any costs associated with the testing process. Clients also need to be told how they will receive their results (e.g., at a follow-up visit or by telephone) and approximately how many weeks it will take to obtain their results. Clients should always be given the option of deferring the test or electing not to receive their results.

8.1.2.3. Results Disclosure/Follow-Up Visit

At this point, cancer genetic test results are often disclosed via telephone conversations with follow-up visits scheduled for some or all clients. Generally, clients who receive positive or variant test results are asked to

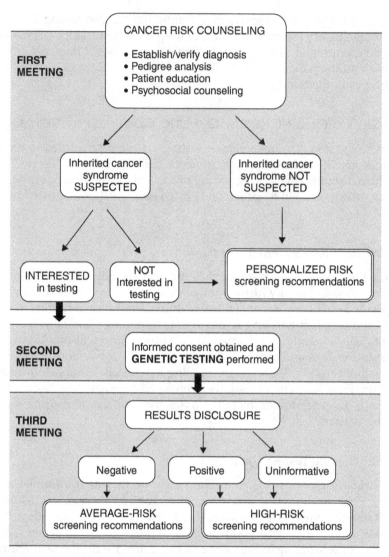

FIGURE 8.1. A schema depicting the main objectives of the risk assessment, testing, and follow-up visits. Source: Yelland (2004, p. 31). Reproduced with permission by Springer.

return for follow-up sessions. The main goals of the results disclosure/ follow-up visits are to answer questions about the genetic test result and to discuss the medical and emotional implications of the test result for the client and other relatives. For clients with positive results, it is a good idea to have a physician at this visit, because the majority of questions will be about medical management.

8.1.3. THE DEFINITION AND GOAL OF RISK COMMUNICATION

Risk is defined as the probability that a certain event will happen. The term "risk" also implies that there is some uncertainty as to what the outcome will be and implies that at least one possible outcome is undesirable.

The main goal of cancer risk communication is to provide clients with sufficient information so that they can make decisions about genetic testing and/or medical management. Clients may also be seeking the risk information on behalf of their children or other relatives.

A successful dialogue about risk may give clients:

- An increased sense of control or security
- Reduced anxiety and/or better coping skills
- More realistic expectations regarding their risks

In cancer genetic counseling, the communication of risk involves the dissemination of factual information and statistical probabilities regarding the client's risks of cancer and likelihood of having a hereditary cancer syndrome. Therefore, counselors must be cognizant of the current, relevant, and accurate risk information that is available, and must be able to effectively communicate that information to their clients.

A cancer counseling session may include the following types of risk information:

- The risk that the client or family has a specific hereditary cancer syndrome
- The clinical features of a hereditary cancer syndrome, including its penetrance, expressivity, and inheritance pattern
- The estimates of cancer risk associated with a specific hereditary cancer syndrome
- The risks, benefits, and limitations of genetic testing
- The sensitivity and specificity of the genetic analysis
- The likelihood of obtaining a positive, negative, or variant genetic test result
- The risk of an inherited versus *de novo* germline mutation
- The risks, benefits, and limitations of cancer surveillance and risk reduction strategies
- The risks to other relatives if the client tests positive for a specific hereditary cancer syndrome
- The psychosocial issues relating to the client's perception of risk or discussion of risk

8.1.4. THE CLIENT'S PERCEPTION OF RISK

The term "risk perception" refers to the way in which clients react to, comprehend, and assimilate the information about their personal risks. Genetic counselors need to be aware that clients filter the factual risk information through their personal lens of experiences and knowledge. Clients may view their personal risks differently over time or following a major life event. For example, clients who profess little concern about the family's risks of cancer may feel quite differently about these risks when they become parents or they receive abnormal cancer screening test results.

To be effective, genetic counselors need to recognize how the clients perceive the risk information and be able to adjust the discussions accordingly. Clients' perceptions of risk may also influence how they use the risk data to make decisions. For example, the way in which clients perceive their cancer risks may be more predictive of whether or not they will undergo genetic testing than the clients' actual risk estimates.

The factors presented in the succeeding sections can contribute to a client's perceptions of risk (see Table 8.2).

8.1.4.1. Cognitive Functioning

Clients' perceptions of risk may be influenced by their grasp of statistical concepts, ability to think abstractly, comfort with mathematical concepts, and/or familiarity with medical terminology. The client's learning style may also influence how well he or she understands risk.

8.1.4.2. Cultural or Ethnic Identity

The ways in which clients view health, illness, genetic testing, or the medical care system in general can be heavily influenced by their ethnic or cultural

TABLE 8.2. FACTORS THAT IMPACT A CLIENT'S PERCEPTION OF RISK

- Cognitive functioning
- Cultural or ethnic identity
- Emotions and coping styles
- Family interactions
- Heuristics
- Other sources of information
- Perceived burden of outcome
- Personal attributes and health status
- Personal experiences with the condition
- Personality types
- Spirituality

Sources: Veach et al. (2003); Baty (2009).

identities. For example, clients who grew up in China may have very different attitudes toward their risks of cancer (and how to manage these risks) than clients of Chinese ancestry who grew up in the United States. Genetic counselors also need to be careful not to assume that all individuals within a certain cultural or ethnic group hold similar views.

8.1.4.3. Emotions and Coping Styles

When contemplating their personal risks, clients may experience feelings of fear, stress, vulnerability, guilt, grief, anger, or shame. All of these emotions can affect a client's understanding of the risk information and can strongly influence how that risk is perceived. Although clients often seek risk information in order to combat feelings of vulnerability and fear, clients who experience overwhelming feelings of distress may shut down and may be incapable of proceeding with the discussion (at least temporarily). A client's emotional response to risk may also impact the client's ultimate decisions regarding genetic testing or medical management. In general, the more a potential outcome is feared, the less a person is willing to risk it. Since cancer is a greatly feared outcome, it is not surprising that some clients may insist on having genetic testing (which they see as proactive care) even though they have a low likelihood of a meaningful result. The complex emotions engendered by risk can also lead to a variety of coping strategies, some of which may also affect how risks are perceived. (See Sections 10.1.1 and 10.1.2 for more information about clients' emotional responses and coping strategies.)

8.1.4.4. Family Interactions

The ways in which clients view risk are often strongly influenced by their family's attitudes and responses toward risk. Other factors that can contribute to a client's response to risk include the family's communication style, value system, and level of supportiveness. The family's ethnicity and geographic proximity may also help determine the involvement of other relatives. Some clients rely heavily on input from their relatives when making health-related decisions, while other clients appear to be acting much more autonomously.

8.1.4.5. Heuristics

Heuristics are those fascinating shortcuts that the brain takes when it seeks to reconcile new information with prior knowledge and experiences. Examples of heuristics that can influence clients' perceptions of risk include:

- Knowing several individuals with the disorder or feeling as though the disorder is "everywhere"

- Having multiple and/or negative experiences with the disorder in the past
- Identifying with or feeling similar to the affected relative in some way
- Being convinced that one's personal risk is high prior to the counseling session

8.1.4.6. Other Sources of Information

Clients may have gleaned risk information from a variety of other sources, including their personal physician, relatives, friends, and Internet resources. The more that the clients trust the source of their information, the more likely it is that they will accept it as fact (and the harder it will be for the counselor to dislodge any fallacious information). Heightened media attention on a specific disorder may also cause clients to feel more vulnerable to the threat of the disease.

8.1.4.7. Perceived Burden of Outcome

The seriousness of the disorder in question may also influence the client's response to risk. Clients may have a more difficult time accepting that they are at increased risk for disorders that have high rates of mortality and/or morbidity. Clients may also be less likely to risk the occurrence of a "high-burden" disease (such as cancer) compared with the risk of a "low-burden" disease (such as the common cold).

8.1.4.8. Personal Attributes and Health Status

Men and women can differ in their perceptions of risk and may place different values on the risk information. For example, clients in their twenties are likely to perceive their risks very differently than clients who are in their sixties. The client's current health status is also important. For example, clients undergoing cancer treatments may feel ill or worn-down, making it harder for them to concentrate on or cope with the information.

8.1.4.9. Personal Experience with the Condition

Clients who have had some type of personal experience with the disorder tend to use their experiences as frames of reference for interpreting their own risks. For example, clients whose relatives have died from cancer may view their own personal risks with greater trepidation than clients whose affected relatives have all survived. Clients who have some type of personal experience with the disorder may overestimate their own risks. The timing of the counseling session in relation to the cancer experiences may also impact a client's risk perception. For example, clients who are newly diagnosed with cancer may have very different reactions to the news than clients who are cancer free or long-term cancer survivors.

8.1.4.10. Personality Types

A client's personality type can also influence his/her perception of risk. Most of the major personality types are relatively stable, although a person's experiences can certainly affect one's view toward risk. For example, a client who feels chronically unlucky may not be surprised by a positive genetic test result, but might feel even more vulnerable to cancer than the risk estimates suggest. The following personality types might affect clients' perceptions of risk:

- Achievement oriented versus failure threatened
- Optimistic versus pessimistic
- Information seeking versus information avoiding
- Risk taking versus risk avoiding

8.1.4.11. Spirituality

Clients' religious beliefs and connection with a religious community may impact their perceptions of risk and subsequent decisions. A client's religious beliefs may provide an important source of support, or, in other cases the religious beliefs may exacerbate feelings of guilt or shame.

8.1.4.12. Impact of Risk Perception on Client Reactions

A client's perceptions of risk can hamper the client's ability to understand or accept the risk information. As genetic counselors discuss cancer risk information, here is what clients may be thinking:

- I don't get all these "ifs" and "maybes"; either it will happen or it won't (difficulty with concepts of probability or abstract thinking).
- Oh man, I never understand what these medical people are trying to say (not good with medical terminology, not an auditory learner).
- I know I'm going to get cancer like my mother because I look just like her (heuristics, pessimism).
- I watched my two sisters get cancer. I know everything I need to know about this stupid gene (personal experience, anger).
- Hmm, that's not what my physician told me (other sources of information, trust).
- Yikes, I don't want to hear all this stuff, it's too much (fear response, information avoider).

- I haven't thought about my father's death in years but talking about it brings it all back; it makes me so sad (grief response, personal experience).

- These risk figures may be true for most people but I don't think they pertain to me (heuristics, coping style, personality style).

- Whatever happens, happens. I'm leaving everything in God's hands (fatalism, spirituality).

8.2. THE COMMUNICATION OF RISK

The communication of risk is an important aspect of cancer genetic counseling. In addition to providing the numerical risk information, counselors should also discuss the accuracy, limitations, relevance, and psychosocial aspects of the information. This section describes strategies for providing both quantitative and qualitative data and provides additional suggestions for effective risk communication and counseling.

8.2.1. PRESENTING RISK INFORMATION

The presentation of risk in cancer genetic counseling often involves complicated statistical concepts filled with ambiguities and caveats. Concepts of probability are a source of confusion to many clients. Certain statistics like 50/50, zero, and 100% are easy to convey because people tend to understand "all-or-nothing" situations. Unfortunately, the statistics used in clinical cancer genetics are rarely this straightforward, hence the need for so many different ways to describe risk.

Cancer genetic counselors have an array of numerical estimates to choose from when they impart cancer risk information to clients. Counselors can present risk statistics in a variety of ways, including percentages, odds, and ranges. Keep in mind that a single approach will not work with every client. Risk estimates can be presented in different ways, as described in the succeeding sections (and shown in Table 8.3).

8.2.1.1. Number

Counselors will usually provide some type of numerical risk estimate to clients. For example, the counselor might say, "One out of four women with this syndrome will develop breast cancer."

8.2.1.2. Percentage

Percentages are often used in genetic counseling sessions. However, counselors should be cautioned that some clients may have difficulty interpret-

TABLE 8.3. FORMATS FOR PRESENTING RISK INFORMATION

- Number
- Percentage
- Range
- Proportion
- Gambler's odds
- Ratio
- Qualitative description
- Comparison with another disorder or event
- Comparison with population risks
- Personalized or framed risk

ing percentages. (The classic example is that even educated people do not always recognize that 1 in 100 = 1%.) However, many of the published risk estimates are reported in a percentage format, making it a popular one to use during cancer risk counseling sessions. The counselor can say, "Women with this syndrome have a 25% chance of developing breast cancer."

8.2.1.3. Range

Providing a range of risk allows the counselor to use both minimum and maximum risk estimates. This technique is especially useful in situations where there is disparate information about risk estimates or if the currently available risk estimates are based on a small number of families. Providing a range of risk can also convey the fact that the associated cancer risks are increased but not definite. The counselor can say, "Women with this syndrome have a 15–25% chance of developing breast cancer."

8.2.1.4. Proportion

A proportion compares the number of people with a specific disorder to the total number of people who are at risk. The counselor can say, "If you consider 100 women with this syndrome, 25 of them will develop breast cancer."

8.2.1.5. Gambler's Odds

The use of gambler's odds (also called "odds against") seems to be an effective way to present risk data. In fact, it may be easier for clients to grasp gambler's odds than percentages or fractions. The counselor can say, "In this syndrome, the odds against breast cancer are 3 to 1," meaning it is 3 times more likely that breast cancer will *not* occur.

8.2.1.6. Ratio

In general, ratios are not as useful in cancer risk counseling sessions as other approaches. Clients seem to have a difficult time grasping ratio figures and may be more likely to overestimate their risks if a ratio is used rather than a percentage or number. To present the information as a ratio, the counselor might say, "Women with this syndrome are about two times more likely to develop breast cancer than the average woman."

8.2.1.7. Qualitative Description

The use of a word qualifier such as "high," "moderate," or "low" may help clients to remember their risk estimates. However, counselors should be cautioned that clients may interpret these risk qualifiers quite differently than the counselors intend. For example, clients may interpret a high risk as an inevitable outcome while the counselor is actually saying that the high risk translates to a 40% risk. Therefore, it may be helpful to provide the numerical risks before labeling them with word descriptors. The counselor might say, "As I said earlier, women with this syndrome have a 25% chance— or a moderate risk—of developing breast cancer." Clients may also shy away from accepting risk data that are at either end of the risk spectrum (either very high or very low).

8.2.1.8. Comparison with Another Disorder or Event

Sometimes it is helpful to compare the risk estimate to another disorder or event. For example, the counselor might say, "Women with this syndrome have about a one in four chance of developing breast cancer. This risk is lower than the risk of developing gastrointestinal (GI) polyps, which is the main risk associated with this syndrome."

8.2.1.9. Comparison with Population Risks

Comparing the syndrome-related cancer risks with the risks in the general population helps to put the risk information into the appropriate context. It also reminds clients that all people are at risk for developing cancer. The counselor might say, "The lifetime risk of breast cancer is one in four for women with this syndrome compared to one in nine for women in the general population."

8.2.1.10. Personalized or Framed Risk

In this approach, the counselor discusses reasons why the client's actual risk may actually be a bit higher or lower than the published risk estimates. For

TABLE 8.4. Strategies for Presenting Risk Information Effectively

- Start with what the client knows
- Present both quantitative and qualitative data
- Focus on the most relevant facts and figures
- Present both sides of the risk figures
- Provide absolute risks rather than relative risks
- Explain the limitations of the risk data
- Stress that risk numbers are not guarantees of outcome
- Describe the features of the cancer syndrome
- Discuss the certainty of the diagnosis
- Keep your language simple
- Use visual images
- Be flexible
- Match patient preferences

Sources: Weil (2000); Veach et al. (2003); Baty (2009); Uhlmann (2009).

example, the counselor can say, "Women with this syndrome have a 25% chance of developing breast cancer. But this risk estimate does not take into account that you will be carefully monitored and offered strategies to help reduce the risk of breast cancer."

8.2.2. Effective Strategies for Presenting Risk Information

There are many different ways to present and discuss the risk information. This section offers some specific strategies to help genetic counselors effectively present risk information to clients (see Table 8.4).

8.2.2.1. Start with What the Client Knows

One effective counseling technique is to ask clients to state their risks and then to use this information as a starting point in the discussion. Clients will vary in terms of their understanding of cancer terminology and their personal risks. Some clients have long been aware that there is an inherited predisposition to cancer in the family while others may be shocked to learn this information. In addition to assessing the extent of the client's knowledge about their cancer risks, it may also be useful to determine the source of their information.

8.2.2.2. Present Both Quantitative and Qualitative Data

When presenting risk information, counselors are encouraged to present both a numerical value and some type of qualifying text. The use of a combined quantitative and qualitative approach appears to maximize the client's understanding of risk and may increase the client's recall of risk.

8.2.2.3. Focus on the Most Relevant Facts and Figures

Being an effective risk communicator begins with the selection of which facts and figures to share with clients. Clients rarely need to be told every available fact and figure; in fact, quoting multiple statistics may overwhelm or confuse them. Counselors may want to start the conversation with the most important risk estimates and gauge the client's interest and understanding before providing more complex or nuanced statistical information. Another strategy is to end the session by reiterating the most important take-home messages.

8.2.2.4. Present Both Sides of the Risk Figures

It may seem redundant to state both the likelihood that an event will occur *and* the likelihood that an event will not occur, but this technique appears to be an effective one. It also appears to be a more value-neutral way to present the information. Thus, counselors should get in the habit of saying, "You have a 50% chance of having the altered gene and you have a 50% chance of *not* having the altered gene."

8.2.2.5. Provide Absolute Risks Rather Than Relative Risks

Although textbooks are fond of using relative risks, these can provide the wrong impression. To state that one has a 200-fold increased risk of a certain cancer might translate into an actual risk of 6%. The former statistic is certainly more dramatic, which is why it shows up in media reports, but it may be alarming and misleading to use these types of figures with clients.

8.2.2.6. Explain the Limitations of the Risk Data

Risk estimates associated with cancer syndromes that are rare or newly described may be overinflated (because it is the most striking families that are written up in case reports) or based on a very small series of cases. Over time, the cancer risks associated with a specific cancer syndrome are likely to change. There may be additional cancers that are not currently recognized as part of the syndrome, or the risk estimates may fluctuate as additional families with the syndrome are identified. The wise genetic counselor, therefore, always qualifies the risk estimates given.

8.2.2.7. Stress That Risk Numbers Are Not Guarantees of Outcome

The risk estimates used in cancer genetic counseling allow clients to make informed decisions about genetic testing and medical management. However, the counselor should remind clients that these risk numbers are not a guarantee of any specific outcome. Cancer risk estimates are helpful pieces of data when making health-related decisions, but they are not a crystal ball; they do not predict the future for any particular client.

8.2.2.8. Describe the Features of the Cancer Syndrome

Discussions about the syndrome should begin with naming it. This includes providing correct pronunciation and spelling of the syndrome, as well as its standard abbreviation (e.g., Familial Adenomatous Polyposis or FAP). The description of the cancer syndrome should include the condition's mode of inheritance, penetrance and variable expressivity, as well as the range of tumors and other features associated with the syndrome.

8.2.2.9. Discuss the Certainty of the Diagnosis

In a subset of cases, the diagnosis of an inherited cancer syndrome is unequivocal. More typically, there will be a certain level of uncertainty that needs to be addressed. Counselors should describe those features that are consistent and inconsistent with the syndrome. If the family history raises the possibility of more than one cancer syndrome, then each syndrome should be described.

8.2.2.10. Keep Your Language Simple

One of the genetic counselor's tasks is to take the complicated scientific and statistical information and to find a way to present the information in a way that is free of medical jargon yet retains the original meaning. In general, the simpler the counselor can keep the explanations, the more likely it is that the clients will comprehend the information.

8.2.2.11. Use Visual Images

The phrase "A picture is worth a thousand words" is an appropriate one for cancer genetic counselors. The use of visual aids to illustrate probability concepts can be extremely helpful. Suggestions include the use of drawings, diagrams, newspaper illustrations, or the ever popular Greenwood flipchart. Analogies can also be useful to describe some of the basic concepts such as the two-hit hypothesis (see Section 3.2.2) or the risk of inheriting a familial gene mutation. For example, a mutation in a cancer susceptibility gene can be compared to:

- A misspelled word in a book
- An error in a computer software program
- A differently colored bead in a necklace
- A set of faulty brakes in a car
- A green sock in a drawer full of white socks

8.2.2.12. Be Flexible

As with all aspects of genetic counseling, using the same risk communication approach will not work with every client. It is important for counselors to assess the client's level of understanding, need for detail, and types of emotional reactions and then to present the information accordingly.

8.2.2.13. Match Client Preferences

Counselors should try to match their risk presentations to the preferences of their clients. For example, clients who are not mathematically savvy may become overwhelmed or confused if presented with an array of numbers. Conversely, clients who are seeking such figures will become increasingly frustrated with and even suspicious of counselors who avoid the use of hard data. However, it is not always easy to discern how clients would like the information presented. Even asking clients for their preferences is not a guarantee; clients may not articulate a preference or they may give you the answer they think you want to hear.

8.2.3. ADDITIONAL COUNSELING STRATEGIES AND TIPS

Risk communication involves much more than the presentation of relevant facts and figures. It is a process that encompasses the clients' perceptions of risk and the decisions that they make to better clarify or manage these risks. This section describes some additional strategies for counselors to counsel clients effectively about risk (see Table 8.5).

8.2.3.1. Be Adequately Prepared for the Session

Counselors need to make sure that they have all the necessary facts and figures prior to the cancer counseling session. Case preparation includes knowing the reason for the referral, the features and inheritance pattern of the hereditary cancer syndrome in question, genetic testing options, risks and benefits of testing, and the possible medical management strategies. It

TABLE 8.5. STRATEGIES FOR COUNSELING EFFECTIVELY ABOUT RISK

- Be adequately prepared for the session
- Be consistent with your verbal and nonverbal cues
- Be mindful of word choices
- Avoid being excessively reassuring
- Be aware of your own biases
- Check in frequently with the client
- Pay attention to how the client perceives the risks
- Be sensitive to cultural differences
- Accept and validate the client's experiences
- Discuss the client's emotional reactions
- Encourage questions
- Admit when you don't know the answer
- Manage the time wisely
- Provide resources to clients

Source: Weil (2000); Veach et al. (2003); Baty (2009); Uhlmann (2009).

is also important to ascertain the accuracy and sources of the currently available risk figures. During case preparation, counselors can also consider the types of questions and issues that might arise during the discussion of risk. For example, a long-term cancer survivor may be more concerned about whether his or her children have increased cancer risks while a client with newly diagnosed cancer may be more focused on whether a genetic test result would alter plans for treatment or follow-up.

8.2.3.2. Be Consistent with Your Verbal and Nonverbal Cues

It is important for the counselor's demeanor, posture, tone of voice, and inflections to match the nature of the discussion. Counselors who are inconsistent with these verbal and nonverbal cues can cause confusion in their clients. For example, the client may understand the high-risk numbers being presented, but may subconsciously assume that the situation is not as bad as the numbers imply given the counselor's overly cheerful demeanor. Conversely, clients may interpret a low-risk situation as more worrisome than the risk numbers suggest if it is presented in an overly somber manner.

8.2.3.3. Be Mindful of Word Choices

The purpose of sharing risk data with clients is to provide information, not advice. Counselors need to make sure that their presentation of risk is performed in a nondirective and nonjudgmental manner. In addition, counselors need to be sensitive to the fact that certain words or phrases might be distressing or offensive to certain clients. It may be necessary to define certain terms or to find different word choices that are more acceptable. For example, clients with brain tumors or ductal carcinoma *in situ* may become upset to hear their diagnoses referred to as "cancer." Acknowledging and mirroring the client's terminology may help genetic counselors to build rapport with clients.

8.2.3.4. Avoid Being Excessively Reassuring

It is natural for counselors to want to comfort tearful clients who are distressed by the discussion of risk. However, it is important to allow clients the time and space to express their emotions and reactions. It is also important to recognize that the emotional impact of the information is not something that counselors can take away nor should they try. Overly reassuring clients by telling them "not to worry" or that "it's not that bad" can be seen as patronizing or insincere. Instead, genetic counselors should acknowledge the difficulty of the news, offer support and information as needed, and help explore ways to help the client adjust to the news.

8.2.3.5. Be Aware of Your Own Biases

Motherless daughters, dying patients, children with cancer, a newly diagnosed patient—all of these situations can tug at the counselor's heartstrings, making it difficult to provide objective informational-based counseling. Then there are the clients who are contentious, demanding, or overly dramatic, which can push different buttons in counselors. Lastly, there may be certain types of cases that hit too close to home, causing the counselor to identify too strongly with the client or situation. It is important for counselors to know their own biases so that they can keep their own emotions and biases out of the genetic counseling discussions. Genetic counselors should always be self-introspective about cases that trigger intense emotional reactions in themselves. It may also be helpful to discuss these types of cases with other colleagues or in a genetic counseling supervision group.

8.2.3.6. Check In Frequently with the Client

It is not enough for counselors to try and guess when clients are struggling with a certain aspect of the risk dialogue. Counselors should check in with clients frequently during the session. This may involve asking questions regarding the client's understanding, perception, or reactions to the risk information. It may also be helpful to simply pause during the discussion to allow clients an opportunity to process the information and ask questions. These questions may be satisfied with a simple information-oriented response or may lead to a more in-depth conversation about a certain aspect of risk.

8.2.3.7. Pay Attention to How the Client Perceives the Risks

One challenge to providing numerical risks is that different clients will interpret the same numbers differently. For example, some clients given a 5% risk
of carrying an altered gene will feel optimistic about the low risk, while
others will consider a 5% risk to be alarmingly high. The factors that influence clients' perceptions of risk include their previous life experiences, their
coping styles, and the nature of the perceived threat. (See Section 8.1.4 for
more information about risk perception.) It is important to recognize that a
client's perception of risk represents a subjective and personal viewpoint,
not a wrong answer that needs correction.

8.2.3.8. Be Sensitive to Cultural Differences

When sharing risk information with clients of different ethnicities, counselors need to be sensitive to possible cultural factors that may influence the
risk discussion. Word choices, verbal and nonverbal cues, rapport, and even
the way in which questions are asked may be influenced by the client's
cultural background. While it is important not to assume that every person
of a certain ethnicity will hold similar values, it is useful to recognize that
the counselor's interpretation of clues may be "off" given the cultural differences. For example, the inclination to ask questions or the extent of
showing emotion may vary across cultures. The use of an interpreter during
the session also adds a layer of complexity to the dialogue and rapport with
clients. It is also important to recognize that there may be cultural differences
beyond the client's ethnicity or country of birth. The client may identify
with a specific community, which may also influence the perceptions of
illness, health, and risk. Examples include communities that center on religious beliefs (Buddhists, Christian Scientists, Hassidic Jews) or sexual identity (gays, lesbians, or transgendered individuals). As genetic counselors are
well aware, all clients need to be treated in a humanistic and respectful
manner.

8.2.3.9. Accept and Validate the Client's Experiences

Genetic counselors need to consider the client's experiences and the role that
these experiences may play in their perception of risk. For example, clients
may also have family stories for why cancer cases occurred, from exposures
to chemicals to eating the wrong types of food. Counselors can sometimes
get sidetracked into trying to "correct" a client's impression of an experience
or perception of risk, a strategy that seldom works. Instead, counselors
should accept these impressions and perceptions and consider them as the
discussion proceeds. By accepting these stories as part of the client's experiences (rather than simply dismissing them), clients are more likely to listen

to your explanation that the malignancies might be due to an underlying inherited gene mutation.

8.2.3.10. Discuss the Client's Emotional Reactions

Clients may be alarmed that their cancer history is being taken so seriously or annoyed that they are considered to be "low risk" despite the family history of cancer. Any strong emotional reaction can influence how the client listens to and processes the information. Exploring reactions to the words "cancer" and "syndrome" may also be appropriate. (See Section 10.2.2 for tips on how to provide effective psychosocial cancer counseling.)

8.2.3.11. Encourage Questions

Clients should be encouraged to ask questions throughout the genetic counseling session. This helps the interaction to become a true dialogue rather than a lecture. It also allows clients to become active participants in the conversation rather than passive listeners. Counselors need to recognize that some clients will feel inhibited or shy about interrupting the counselor or asking for clarification and thus may need to be encouraged to ask questions. Whenever possible, counselors should answer the clients' questions as soon as they are asked—even if it means switching topics. It is also important to gauge whether the client is genuinely interested in learning the answers or is peppering the counselor with questions out of fear or agitation. Keep in mind that continued questions about statistical minutia or non sequiturs might be masking the client's underlying feelings of fear or helplessness. Exploring these underlying feelings may be the better counseling strategy.

8.2.3.12. Admit When You Don't Know the Answer

Genetic counselors need to be honest with clients if they do not know the answer to a specific question. Newer counselors may worry that this admission will diminish their credibility with clients, but there is evidence that the opposite is true. Clients appreciate this type of candor and it may lead to a greater level of trust and respect in the counselor. Counselors can suggest ways for clients to find out the answers or they can offer to find out the information for the clients.

8.2.3.13. Manage the Time Wisely

Genetic counselors need to have sufficient time to explain and explore the implications of the risk information with clients. Counselors who feel pressured to rush through each topic in order to cover everything in the allotted time are not doing themselves or their clients any favors. First of all, this is a very stressful way to counsel! Second, it is much more difficult to gain rapport, assess psychosocial factors, and encourage client questions if the counselor's main focus is on the clock. In the event of a severe time constraint, it is far better to let clients know about the time constraints at the beginning of the session and to prioritize together how to best utilize the time. Counselors may be able to eliminate or minimize certain topics that are less relevant to the client's situation or they can arrange to continue the discussion via a follow-up visit or telephone call. For clients who are especially chatty or are easily distracted, it is perfectly acceptable for counselors to be mindful of the time and to redirect clients back to the topic at hand.

8.2.3.14. Provide Resources to Clients

Counselors typically impart a great deal of information to clients, which they may want to revisit after the session. Clients can be encouraged to take notes during the discussion, and counselors should also provide them with some adjunct materials. These resources can help to affirm the information that was given and allow clients to review the information, perhaps in a different format. Useful client resources can include brochures, fact sheets, medical articles, Web site links, support group information, and personalized summary letters. In addition, the questions and needs of clients often differ over time. For example, clients with FAP who are planning a family may want to know about the risks to offspring and possible options of prenatal and preimplantation testing, but in the future their questions may center on having their children tested or screened. Counselors should always encourage clients to recontact them if issues come up in the future, but should also provide clients with alternative resources.

8.3. COUNSELING CLIENTS AT VARIOUS RISKS

This section describes the major discussion points for clients categorized at high, moderate, or low risk for having a hereditary cancer syndrome. (Refer to Section 7.3.3 for a more information of these risk categories.) These discussion points include the likelihood of the cancer syndrome, the risks of cancer, the risks for other family members, the option of genetic testing, and monitoring recommendations. As these sections demonstrate, discussions of risk vary for clients at the different categories of risk.

8.3.1. CANCER RISK ASSESSMENT: LOW RISK

Clients at low risk for having a hereditary cancer syndrome may be quite relieved to learn that their risks of cancer are not as high as expected. Although the main focus of a clinical program is to identify clients at high risk, providing reassurance to individuals at low risk also serves an important purpose.

8.3.1.1. Likelihood of Cancer Syndrome

Clients at low risk can be told that there is very little evidence that they have a hereditary cancer syndrome. The counselor can explain how this conclusion was reached by pointing to why the pattern of cancer in the family is not suggestive of a cancer syndrome. Figure 8.2 depicts a client assessed to be at low risk for a hereditary cancer syndrome. In this instance, the counselor could explain to the client, "Yes, it's true that your mother had ovarian cancer and your great-aunt had breast cancer, but both women were in their eighties when diagnosed. Plus, no one else in your mother's family has been diagnosed with cancer. This makes it much less likely that mother's ovarian cancer was caused by an underlying inherited risk factor."

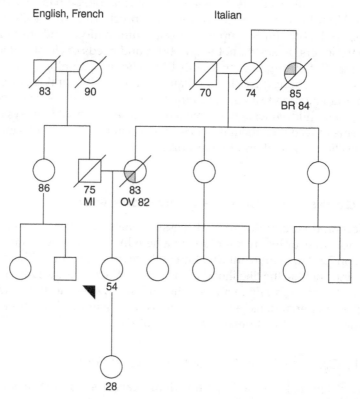

FIGURE 8.2. Pedigree depicting a client at low risk for having HBOCS. BR = breast cancer, invasive; OV = ovarian cancer; MI = myocardial infarction.

8.3.1.2. Risk of Developing Cancer

Clients at low risk can generally be quoted general population risks of cancer. This type of information is available through the American Cancer Society (http://www.cancer.org) and the National Cancer Institute (http://www.cancer.gov). Having a single first-degree relative with a certain form of cancer may increase the client's risks by two- to threefold and therefore it might be appropriate to discuss possible increased risks of cancer based on shared genetic and environmental factors. For example, a woman in the United States has a 1.5% lifetime risk of developing ovarian cancer. If her mother has been diagnosed with ovarian cancer (and the remainder of the family history is basically negative), then the woman's risks of ovarian cancer might be increased to 6–9% over her lifetime.

8.3.1.3. Risks for Other Family Members

Sometimes clients have sought genetic counseling because of concerns about other family members, especially offspring and siblings. Clients at low risk can usually be reassured that other family members are unlikely to be at increased risk. Referring again to Figure 8.2, the client's daughter is even less likely to have an inherited predisposition to ovarian cancer, especially if the client remains cancer free.

8.3.1.4. Option of Genetic Testing

Genetic testing is not typically indicated for clients at low risk because of the extremely low likelihood of a meaningful, positive result. Such testing is unlikely to be beneficial and, similar to other medical tests, contains a risk of identifying an uncertain result (such as a variant of uncertain significance) that could lead to unnecessary medical screening and increased client anxiety. In most cases, clients at low risk will be relieved to learn that they do not meet criteria for genetic testing, as long as the rationale for the decision is explained. However, there may be certain clients who insist upon being tested regardless of their low *a priori* risks. If the client depicted in Figure 8.2 insists on having *BRCA1* and *BRCA2* genetic testing, then she would need to be informed that insurance might not cover the cost of the genetic analysis given the lack of other significant family history.

8.3.1.5. Monitoring Suggestions

It is generally appropriate for clients at low risk to follow standard guidelines for cancer screening. The American Cancer Society, National Cancer Institute, and the National Comprehensive Cancer Network (http://www.nccn.org) have excellent resources regarding cancer screening recommendations for individuals at low risk (as well as those at high risk). Although clients may be at low risk for developing an inherited form of cancer, they may have other significant cancer risk factors that need to be considered. Thus, clients should be encouraged to speak to their physicians before making any changes in their cancer monitoring regimens.

8.3.2. CANCER RISK ASSESSMENT: MODERATE RISK

Clients at moderate risk for having a hereditary cancer syndrome may be among the most challenging to counsel. In moderate-risk families, the pattern of cancer could turn out to be hereditary or due to multifactorial causes. The challenge to the genetic counselor is to identify the small subset of moderate risk families who have an inherited cancer syndrome.

8.3.2.1. Likelihood of Cancer Syndrome

Clients at moderate risk range from those whose histories suggest a specific syndrome to others in which a cancer syndrome is unlikely but cannot be completely ruled out. See Figures 8.3 and 8.4 for two examples of moderate risk pedigrees. Note that the pedigree in Figure 8.3 almost meets Amsterdam

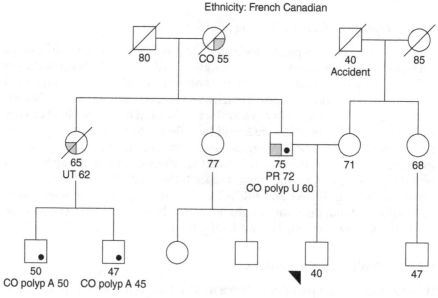

FIGURE 8.3. Pedigree depicting a client at moderate risk for having Lynch syndrome (also termed hereditary nonpolyposis colorectal cancer syndrome). Note that the pattern of cancer in the family almost meets clinical criteria for Lynch syndrome (Refer to Section 4.17.2.). CO = colon cancer; CO polyp A = colorectal adenoma; CO polyp U = colon polyp, type unknown; PRO = prostate cancer.

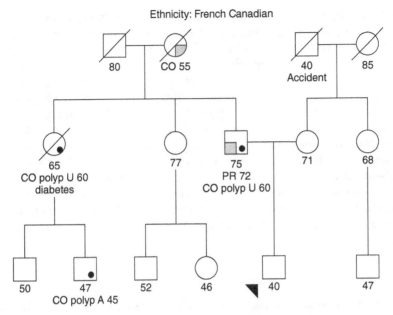

FIGURE 8.4. Pedigree depicting a client at moderate risk for having Lynch syndrome (hereditary nonpolyposis colorectal cancer syndrome). Note that the pattern of cancer in this family is less striking than the pattern of cancer in the family in Figure 8.3; however, Lynch syndrome cannot be completely ruled out. CO = colon cancer; CO polyp A = colorectal adenoma; CO polyp U = colorectal polyp, type unknown; PRO = prostate cancer.

II criteria for Lynch syndrome (also termed Hereditary Nonpolyposis Cancer syndrome). In contrast, the family depicted in Figure 8.4 is much less likely to have Lynch syndrome, although it cannot be completely ruled out. Counselors should be cautious in ruling out cancer syndromes if there are few at-risk relatives or if the client has limited information about the family history. Clients at moderate risk should be given some information about the possible cancer syndrome. This discussion might elicit additional information from the client that helps confirm or rule out the cancer syndrome in question. Diagnoses should be confirmed with medical records whenever possible and clients should be encouraged to recontact the counselor if any new tumor diagnoses occur in the family. If the family does have a hereditary cancer syndrome, then additional cancer diagnoses will almost certainly occur over time. If no new tumors occur over the next several years, then the family is less likely to have a hereditary cancer syndrome.

8.3.2.2. Risk of Developing Cancer

The level of increased risk will depend upon the pattern of cancer in the family. Clients with pedigrees that come close to meeting criteria for a known hereditary cancer syndrome (as in Fig. 8.3) can be counseled about the syndrome-related cancer risks. Counselors should be clear that the client's cancer risks *may be* as high as the syndrome-related risks, but that the risks might also be much lower. Counselors can either provide a range of risks or quote two sets of risks given the two separate scenarios (e.g., family does/does not have Lynch syndrome). Clients with pedigrees that have only a few features suggestive of a hereditary cancer syndrome (as in Fig. 8.4) may also be counseled with a range of risks. However, in this type of counseling situation, it may be appropriate to stress that the client is unlikely to have the maximum risks quoted. Counselors who tell clients that they "probably" or "probably do not" have a cancer syndrome need to be certain that these conclusions are based on concrete evidence, that is, a documented pedigree, not because of pressure from clients to interpret their risks in a certain way or a desire to reassure them.

8.3.2.3. Risks for Other Family Members

If clients are assessed to have moderately increased cancer risks, then it is possible that the risks are increased for other family members as well. In some cases, relatives will be at potentially higher risk than your client. For example, in Figure 8.3, the patient's two cousins who had adenomas may be at higher risk than the client. For this type of moderate-risk family, it may be more appropriate to provide general information rather than a numerical value and to focus on strategies for better refining the cancer risks for the entire family.

8.3.2.4. Option of Genetic Testing

Moderate-risk families are perhaps the most benefited by genetic test results. A positive result will confirm the presence of a hereditary cancer syndrome and a negative result will reduce, albeit not eliminate, the likelihood of an inherited cancer. As a rule, moderate-risk families should be offered genetic tests that are available clinically. If testing is only available on a research basis, then counselors will need to determine if the family meets eligibility criteria before raising it as an option with clients.

8.3.2.5. Monitoring Suggestions

There are no standard monitoring guidelines for moderate-risk families. Recommendations about monitoring are typically based on the specific pattern of cancer in the family, the types of cancer associated with the syndrome in question, and the availability, utility, and invasiveness of the monitoring options. Clients at moderate risk are often suggested to undergo some or all of the specialized and/or more frequent cancer monitoring appropriate for people with the syndrome. Management recommendations should come from the high-risk program's physician with input from the client's personal physician. However, it is appropriate for counselors to list the possible management options and facilitate the appropriate referrals. Over time, the results from the monitoring procedures may shift the client's probability of a hereditary cancer syndrome. As examples, the client depicted in Figure 8.3 will likely be advised to have a baseline colonoscopy and the counselor can set up a referral to a gastroenterologist. The client depicted in the less striking moderate-risk family (Fig. 8.4) can likely wait until age 50 to have a baseline colonoscopy, but based on the colon cancer in the family, may be advised to have colonoscopies every 5 years rather than every 10 years.

8.3.3. Cancer Risk Assessment: High Risk

In some ways, counseling clients at high risk for cancer is the most straightforward. Counselors can use published data on the cancer syndrome regarding the associated types of cancer, estimates of risk, genetic testing options, and appropriate monitoring.

8.3.3.1. Likelihood of Cancer Syndrome

Families at high risk either have patterns of cancer that meet criteria for a hereditary cancer syndrome or have patterns of cancer that are highly suggestive of a hereditary cancer syndrome. Counselors should describe the features of the specific hereditary cancer syndrome and compare it to the client's personal and family history. In the case of the family depicted in Figure 8.5, the client should be told that the pattern of cancer in her family is consistent with Hereditary Diffuse Gastric Cancer (HDGC) syndrome. The counselor can then describe the features of HDGC syndrome, including the 50% or one in two chance that she has HDGC as well. Clients may need time to adjust to the information and their reactions may vary from satisfaction that they have an answer regarding the cause of cancer to disbelief or fear. Some clients may want to know why such a diagnosis had never been made before; they may feel bitterness at past providers or hope that the counselor's assessment is wrong. It is important to provide written literature, including information about support groups and other resources. Counselors should also provide clients with fact sheets, brochures, Web-based resources, and information about support groups or organizations. Given the volume and complexity of information that needs to be conveyed to high-risk clients, it may be helpful for counselors to review the information at a later date through follow-up telephone calls or visits.

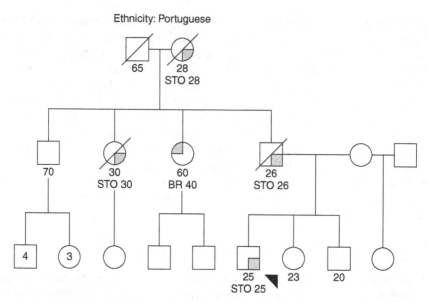

FIGURE 8.5. Pedigree depicting a client at high risk for having HDGC syndrome. BR = breast cancer, invasive; STO = stomach cancer, diffuse type.

8.3.3.2. Risk of Developing Cancer

In a few cancer syndromes, the presence of certain characteristics makes it obvious that a client has the genetic predisposition and the associated risks of cancer. Examples include Basal Cell Nevus syndrome, Familial Melanoma, and Neurofibromatosis. However, in most hereditary cancer syndromes, there is nothing about the client's physical appearance to distinguish carriers from noncarriers. Therefore, the cancer risks for high-risk clients are generally based on the cancer risks associated with the syndrome, the client's position in the pedigree, and the inheritance pattern of the syndrome. The client's age and gender may also affect the cancer risks depending on the syndrome in question. As an example, the client depicted in Figure 8.5 can be told that her risk of diffuse gastric cancer would be about 80% and her risk of breast cancer would be about 40% *if* she has HDGC. However, the counselor can also remind the client that she has a 50% chance of *not* having HDGC.

8.3.3.3. Risks for Other Family Members

The likelihood that other relatives have the inherited syndrome is largely based upon their placement in the pedigree. The age and gender of relatives may affect their risks of developing syndrome-related malignancies. In syndromes with less than 100% penetrance (which is the majority), it is not possible to rule out risks to offspring of unaffected individuals. However, given the size of the family, it may be possible to identify the branches of the family that are at highest risk. Genetic counselors should let clients know which other relatives are at increased risk and can also offer to help the client disseminate the information through the family. This can include writing a family letter for the client to send to relatives or by acting as a resource if other relatives have questions that the client cannot answer. The client in Figure 8.5 may be aware that her younger brother is at increased risk but should also be reminded that her paternal cousins (especially the offspring of her two paternal aunts) are also at increased risk for having HDGC. The counselor can also reassure the client that her younger half-sister would not be considered at high risk since she has a different father.

8.3.3.4. Option of Genetic Testing

Genetic testing is clinically available for most of the major hereditary cancer syndromes. High-risk clients should be offered genetic testing in order to determine the exact genetic mutation in the family. Identifying a positive genetic test result will confirm the diagnosis and also allows other family members to have the option of targeted genetic testing. In the family depicted in Figure 8.5, the client's brother who has been recently diagnosed with diffuse gastric cancer would be the best candidate for *CDH1* genetic testing. If a *CDH1* mutation is detected in the family, then the client—and other relatives—would have the option of predictive genetic testing. Genetic counselors also need to remind clients that genetic testing may not uncover the specific genetic mutation in the family. In addition, a negative result does not nullify a clinically based diagnosis in a family likely to have an inherited cancer; the lack of a positive result only means that the family's underlying genetic mutation is unidentifiable by current technologies.

8.3.3.5. Monitoring Suggestions

Clients who are at high risk for having a specific hereditary cancer syndrome will typically need to be monitored for the syndrome-related cancers (provided that such monitoring tests exist). Clients at high risk will typically be advised to undergo specialized screening tests beginning at earlier ages and at more frequent intervals as compared with clients at low or moderate risk. Genetic counselors can review the existing published data and guidelines for individuals at risk for a specific cancer syndrome. It may also be helpful for counselors to discuss the rationale for and the limitations of the suggested screening tests. The counselor should then refer the client to physician specialists who have experience in caring for individuals who are at risk for hereditary cancers. The client depicted in Figure 8.5 should be informed about the recommendations for frequent upper endoscopy procedures as well as the options of chromatin dye endoscopy, gastric biopsies and even prophylactic gastrectomy. If a specific CDH1 mutation is identified in the family, then it is reasonable to wait until the client undergoes targeted genetic testing to clarify her own risks of cancer. If the client has the familial CDH1 mutation, then she will need to follow the screening guidelines for individuals with HDGC syndrome (refer to Table 5.8). If the client tests negative for the familial CDH1 mutation, then she does not need to be screened for gastric cancer unless she has other risk factors.

8.4. CASE EXAMPLES

The following three cases illustrate counseling challenges that can arise during the discussions of risk.

Case 6: "Do we have to talk about this?"

When the genetic counselor first spoke the words "colon" and "rectum," Marcus, age 18, made a face and practically put his hands over his ears. The counselor substituted the words with "intestines" and "bowel," but each term seemed to make Marcus more uncomfortable. She finally stopped describing FAP and tried to regroup.

Marcus' family was well known to the High Risk GI Clinic. The family was clinically diagnosed with FAP about 10 years ago. At that time, Marcus' two older brothers had undergone baseline colonoscopy exams and were found to have multiple colorectal adenomas. Both of them have subsequently undergone total colectomies. The family had been offered genetic testing, but they were not interested. Marcus and his younger sister were too young to be screened at the initial family visit, but both of them had negative colonoscopy exams when they turned 13; no screening has been done since this time. (See Fig. 8.6 to see the family's pedigree.)

Marcus and his siblings have lived with their maternal grandmother since their mother died from cancer. Their biological father is also deceased. The family is originally from Bermuda.

About 6 months ago, one of Marcus' cousins agreed to have genetic testing and was found to carry a specific APC mutation. Suddenly it was possible to determine which relatives were at risk for developing polyposis instead of relying on colonoscopy exams (which most of the relatives were not doing). Marcus' grandmother received a family letter that discussed the positive APC result and encouraged at-risk relatives to be tested. The purpose of today's appointment was to arrange genetic testing for Marcus and, depending on the test results, to arrange appropriate screening procedures. Marcus' younger sister is scheduled to come in for a separate appointment.

The genetic counselor looked over at Marcus who was slumped down in his chair, a backwards baseball cap on his head. He looked miserable. The

Ethnicity: Bermudian

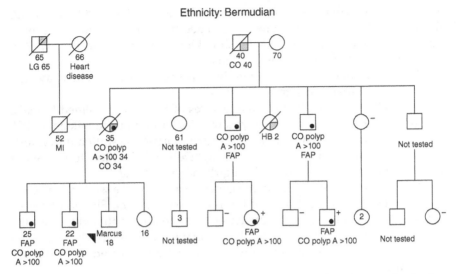

FIGURE 8.6. Marcus' family history. This family has FAP. (See the text for further discussion of this case.) LG = lung cancer; CO = colon cancer; CO polyp A = colorectal adenoma; HB = hepatoblastoma; MI = myocardial infarction.

counselor decided to try a direct approach. "Okay Marcus, this is no fun. I bet you'd rather be somewhere else right now, wouldn't you?"

"You got that right," said Marcus with a heavy sigh.

"I can certainly understand that. But your grandmother is worried about you staying healthy. You want that too, right?"

Marcus shrugged his shoulders. "I guess so."

"Well, we want that too, which means there are things I need to talk about with you. And there are things the doctor needs to talk about with you."

"I know," said Marcus with another big sigh.

The counselor sensed that Marcus was resigned to hearing the information but he certainly wasn't interested in participating in the discussion. She searched for a way to better connect with him. She had tried to chat with him earlier but it had gotten her lots of one-word answers and shrugged shoulders. She didn't recognize the symbol on his cap and didn't know if it was a sports team or a band logo. She decided that guessing might make things worse, so she decided on a different approach.

She put aside her chart and pen. "Okay here's the deal. The doctor and I each have things we need to talk about with you. Whenever I meet with someone, I have three topics that I need to talk about. First, I need to ask about the family history—which is already done thanks to your cousin and grandmother. So we can check that off the list. Second, I need to describe the features of FAP, which is what we've been doing. Third, I need to talk about the genetic blood test. The sooner we can get through each topic, the sooner you can get out of here. So let's finish talking about FAP and then we can move on to the last topic. How does that sound?"

Marcus shrugged his shoulders but also nodded and said okay. The counselor took that as a sign of progress.

"We talked a little bit about the features of FAP. But it seemed to make you uncomfortable. Does it make you worried or nervous to talk about it?"

"It's not that. It's just kind of. . . ." began Marcus. He shifted uncomfortably in the chair. Then he burst out with, "Do we really have to talk about this? It's hard to . . . I mean you're a girl and everything."

Comprehension dawned on the genetic counselor. He was embarrassed to talk about his GI tract and bodily functions with her. She had been so focused on possible cultural differences that she hadn't thought about the factors of gender and age. She had hoped that her own relatively young age would allow her to connect better with him; instead, it seemed to make him less comfortable.

"I think I see the problem. Would it be easier to talk about the features of FAP with a man? Like the doctor?" The counselor felt a little resentful that her gender made a difference but she did her best to put those feelings aside.

Marcus nodded.

"OK, how about this—I won't give you any more details about FAP and I won't ask you any more questions about your health if you agree to talk about these two things with the doctor. Deal?"

"Deal," said Marcus, and he even gave her a half smile.

"Good. Alright, then that brings us to the last topic. And that has to do with the genetic test. Is it something you want to have done?"

"Well, I don't *want* to have it," said Marcus. "But I will. It's important to my grandmother."

"Yeah that was a dumb thing for me to say, wasn't it? No one 'wants' to have the test," agreed the genetic counselor. "But it sounds like you are willing to have the test. It is your decision, you know."

"Yeah, I know," said Marcus.

The counselor asked him if he would like his grandmother to join them. Marcus agreed and he seemed more relaxed with his grandmother in the room. The genetic counselor discussed testing in a simplified way. She gently reminded Marcus that he could still have FAP even though he didn't have any polyps at age 13. She then said that a negative *APC* result meant no more colonoscopies until he was 50 years old, which brought a huge smile to his face. "That would be awesome," said Marcus. His grandmother agreed.

They wrapped up the session. The counselor told the gastroenterologist what she had—and had not—been able to cover during the session and he agreed to review the features of FAP and get the medical history. Afterwards, the physician commented on how difficult it was to get Marcus to talk to him, which made the counselor feel better about their interaction. Marcus' APC results are pending.

Case 6 wrap-up: This case suggests ways to counsel clients, who are embarrassed or uncooperative, regarding their cancer risks and testing options.

Case 7: "So you are saying I will get pancreatic cancer."

Siobhan was named after her maternal grandmother who died in her fifties from pancreatic cancer. Siobhan's mother had died last year from the same disease. Siobhan was understandably concerned about her own risks. She came to the session with medical records confirming that both women had primary adenocarcinoma of the pancreas.

The genetic counselor thanked her for bringing in the confirmatory records and continued collecting the client's personal and family history information. Siobhan related that she had recently had an early-stage melanoma removed from her upper arm. The counselor noted Siobhan's fair complexion and asked about her ethnicity. Siobhan told him that her mother was Irish and her father was English and Danish.

After gathering the rest of the family history information, the counselor showed the pedigree to Siobhan (Fig. 8.7). The family certainly appeared to have a cluster of pancreatic cancers. In addition to the affected mother and grandmother, a maternal cousin had also reportedly died from pancreatic cancer.

Using a flipchart of diagrams and illustrations, the counselor described the difference between sporadic and inherited forms of cancer. He then explained that hereditary pancreatic cancer may be caused by a mutation in a specific gene, but that so far researchers had found only a few genes associated with inherited pancreatic cancer. This meant that the currently available genetic tests were seldom able to identify the exact genetic cause in families with hereditary pancreatic cancer. Siobhan asked detailed questions about each diagram and took copious notes.

"So you are saying I will get pancreatic cancer," Siobhan said in a calm, matter-of-fact voice.

The counselor blinked in surprise since he did not think he had said anything of the kind.

"Umm, actually that is not what I am saying. You *may* have a higher chance of getting pancreatic cancer, but we don't know that for sure. First of all, we do not know if there is a cancer syndrome in your family. Even if there is a cancer syndrome in the family, you may not have it because you may not have inherited the altered gene that causes it. And even if you have inherited the altered gene, you may never get cancer. That is a lot of 'ifs.' Does that make sense?"

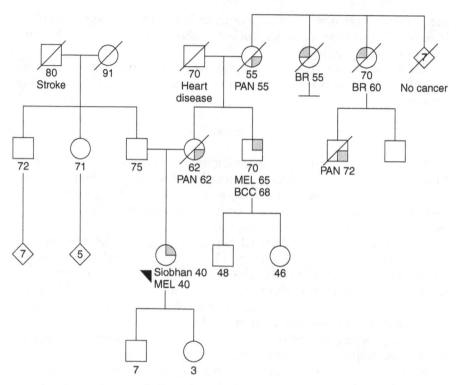

FIGURE 8.7. Siobhan's family history. The paternal side of the family is English and Danish; the maternal side of the family is Irish. (See the text for further discussion of this case.) BR = breast cancer, invasive; PAN = pancreatic cancer; BCC = basal cell carcinoma; MEL = melanoma.

"Absolutely," said Siobhan as she scribbled more notes. "But it sure looks genetic. And since I've had cancer myself, I must have the altered gene. I'm so worried about my children. Can they be tested?"

The genetic counselor realized that the client was taking what he was saying and leaping to her own conclusions. Given her fears about pancreatic cancer, he couldn't blame her for thinking that way. The counselor decided to be more concrete in his answer. Instead of reiterating that she and her children might not have an inherited risk for pancreatic cancer, he used her question to segue into discussing the possible cancer syndromes.

"Being able to test your children is one of the main benefits of genetic counseling and testing. Here are the steps we need to do before we can test them: We need to talk about the possible genetic conditions that your family might have. Then we need to test one person in the family to try and find the genetic cause of cancer in the family. After we find the genetic cause of cancer, then we can test your children as well as other relatives. However, in some families there is no obvious genetic cause of cancer. So, genetic testing was not helpful, but everyone would still be followed carefully for signs of cancer."

After Siobhan finished writing it all down, the counselor repeated the information to make sure that she had written it down correctly and also to stress the point that there were several steps that needed to happen before anyone could be tested.

Siobhan looked over what she had just written. Chewing nervously on her pen, she asked, "What kind of genetic condition do you think our family has?"

The counselor discussed the possibility that Siobhan's family could have either Familial Atypical Mole Melanoma (FAMM) syndrome or Hereditary Breast–Ovarian Cancer syndrome (HBOCS). He described the features of FAMM and HBOCS, but stressed that the family had only a small likelihood of having either syndrome.

Siobhan worried aloud about the possibility that she might have both conditions. The counselor explained that this was extremely unlikely and reiterated that most people with pancreatic cancer did not have either condition.

Reviewing her notes, Siobhan said, "Well, it seems pretty obvious that I have this FAMM syndrome since I've had melanoma. I must have it, right?"

The counselor patiently explained the difference between sporadic melanoma and FAMM-related melanomas. He said that it was difficult to determine whether her melanoma was due to her fair skin (and disappearing ozone layer) or whether it was evidence of a hereditary cancer syndrome. He then went on to explain that most people with FAMM have several dysplastic or abnormally shaped moles.

Siobhan immediately showed the counselor several small normal-appearing freckles (nevi) on her shoulders and neck. After making sure that the client was seeing a dermatologist regularly, the counselor indicated that these freckles did not look dysplastic to him. However, he stressed that this was not his area of expertise and he encouraged the client to ask her physician specifically about these nevi if she was concerned about them. He also reminded her that melanomas and other skin cancers were much more likely to occur in fair-skinned people who had gotten a lot of sun exposure. Siobhan admitted to spending a lot of time in the sun when she was younger and that she had gotten several bad sunburns as a child.

The genetic counselor steered the conversation back to testing. Siobhan eagerly agreed to undergo *TP16* and *BRCA* testing and Siobhan signed the appropriate consent forms. As they wrapped up the session, the counselor asked if she had any other questions.

"Oh, I have lots of questions. But I'll wait until I get the results back," said Siobhan. The counselor said that sounded like a good plan.

Case 7 wrap-up: This case suggests ways to counsel clients, who misinterpret or misunderstand the discussions of cancer risk.

Case 8: "I can't seem to focus on anything right now."

Nina, age 34, had recently completed her treatment for breast cancer, which was diagnosed 1 year ago. Nina related that she had noticed a lump in her breast 4 weeks before her due date. She says that the months following her diagnosis were a blur—she had undergone an emergency cesarean section to deliver her second child and was immediately started on a course of neo-adjuvant radiation therapy to shrink the tumor. She then had a lumpectomy, several courses of chemotherapy, and was currently taking tamoxifen.

The genetic counselor listened to the story of what Nina had gone through over the past year and asked how Nina was doing now.

"I'm fine," said Nina although her exhausted and disheveled appearance belied her words. "Tired all the time, but I guess that's normal with two children under age 5."

The genetic counselor made a mental note to further explore this issue later in the session, but continued with the collection of the family history intake. Once the pedigree was completed, she showed it to Nina. (See Fig. 8.8.) Given Nina's unusually young age of diagnosis, it was appropriate to discuss the option of BRCA testing, but the remainder of the family history made it less likely that she had an inherited form of breast cancer.

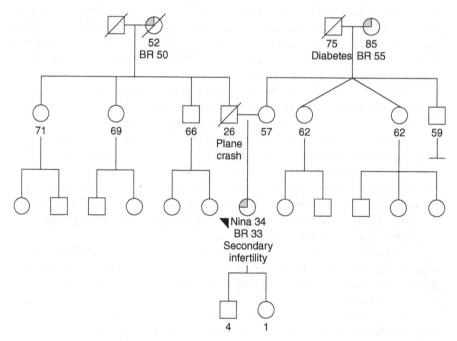

FIGURE 8.8. Nina's family history. (See the text for further discussion of this case.) BR = breast cancer, invasive.

The counselor used the client's pedigree to describe the features that were and were not suggestive of hereditary breast cancer. The counselor pulled out her set of diagrams and statistical tables, but before she launched into her basic description of genetics, the counselor noticed that Nina looked worried and asked her if something was wrong.

Nina said apologetically, "I have to warn you, I'm not very good with math and science."

"That's OK," assured the counselor. "I will take it slow. Please let me know if something doesn't make sense to you."

The counselor proceeded to describe the *BRCA1* and *BRCA2* genes, the associated risks of cancer, and the parameters of genetic testing. Nina asked several basic questions and kept apologizing that she "just didn't get it." When Nina asked the same question for the third time, the counselor realized that the client was simply not able to focus on the conversation. The counselor put down the diagrams and shifted the focus of the session.

"Let's take a break from talking about this stuff. You are right, it can be very complicated. And sometimes our brains are so full of other things; it is difficult to take in anything else." The counselor hesitated—how do you ask people if they are mentally and emotionally okay without offending them? She decided to start by asking a few general questions. "It sounds like you have had a really tough year."

"It was tough," agreed Nina. "I'm so glad it is over."

"Is it difficult to talk about this kind of stuff?" The counselor pointed to the family tree and the diagrams of the *BRCA* genes.

"Oh no," said Nina. "I need to get all the facts. I know how important it is for me to have this test."

The counselor got the sense that Nina was saying what she thought the counselor wanted to hear. The counselor realized that she would have to utilize a more direct approach. She took a deep breath and said as tactfully as she could, "I noticed that you seem to be having some problems concentrating on our conversation. I know that math and science aren't your thing, but it seems to be more than that. Have you noticed this before? Do you sense that this is a problem?"

It initially felt like Nina was going to deny that there was a problem, but then her eyes filled with tears. "Yes it's a problem. I can't seem to focus on anything right now. I can't even read the newspaper; my mind starts wandering. I don't know what's wrong with me. And I'm so emotional about everything. I don't get it. It's not me at all. I barely cried at all when I found out I had cancer; I just wanted to get started with my treatment. I stayed so positive the whole time. My husband fell apart, my mom fell apart; I'm the one who kept everyone going. And now look at me—I'm a mess. I can't sleep even though I'm tired all the time and it takes every ounce of energy to get through the day. The littlest thing will start me crying and I'll start reliving the whole experience and getting scared that the cancer will come back. It's crazy."

The genetic counselor made some empathetic responses, but otherwise simply listened to Nina talk. She then explained that Nina's inability to focus on things was actually quite normal given all that she had been through and assured her that it should get better over time. The counselor explained that it was partly chemically based, a side effect from her cancer treatments, and partly emotionally based—it was very natural for cancer patients to stay mentally focused so that they could get through the necessary treatment only to fall apart afterwards.

As Nina wiped away her tears, she said it was a relief to hear that she wasn't crazy. The counselor agreed that Nina "wasn't crazy" and reminded her that she had been through two huge life events over the past year—a baby and a cancer diagnosis. No wonder she was having difficulties with her sleep and her daily activities! The counselor then asked if Nina had ever talked to a therapist or psychologist.

"No, I never really thought about doing that," admitted Nina. "I just keep telling myself how grateful I should be for having two beautiful children and my cancer in remission."

"Well it is always good to feel grateful for what we have. But it is also important to allow ourselves the time and space to feel all the other emotions we might have like grief, fear, or anger. We have a wonderful psychologist who works here at the hospital. I would like to set up an appointment for you to meet with her. Would that be alright?"

Nina thought about it for a minute and then agreed to meet with the psychologist. The genetic counselor made an appointment for Nina to meet with the psychologist the following week. The counselor also paged Nina's oncologist, who called Nina that evening and ended up prescribing a low-dose sleeping medication for her.

Nina and the counselor agreed to shelve the discussions about genetic testing for at least the next 6 months. The counselor asked Nina to call her if she wanted to talk and promised to check in with her in a few days.

About 1 year later Nina came back in for genetic counseling and testing. Things went very smoothly the second time around.

Case 8 wrap-up: This case suggests ways to counsel clients who are having difficulties attending to or comprehending the risk discussions.

8.5. FURTHER READING

Baty, BJ. 2009. Risk communication and decision-making. In Uhlmann, W, Schuette, JL, and Yashar, BM (eds), A Guide to Genetic Counseling. Wiley-Blackwell, Hoboken, NJ, 207–250.

Dixon, SD, and Konheim-Kalkstein, YL. 2010. Risk Communication: a complex process. In LeRoy, BS, Veach, PM, and Bartels, DM (eds), Genetic Counseling

Practice: Advanced Concepts and Skills. Wiley-Blackwell, Hoboken, NJ, 65–94.

Eeles, RA, and Murday, VA. 2004. The cancer family clinic. In Eeles, RA, Easton, DR, Ponder, BAJ, and Eng, C (eds), Genetic Predisposition to Cancer, 2nd edition. Arnold Publishers, London, 391–403.

Hopwood, P, Howell, A, Lalloo, F, et al. 2003. Do women understand the odds? Risk perceptions and recall of risk information in women with a family history of breast cancer. Community Genet 6:214–223.

Uhlmann, WR. 2009. Thinking it all through: case preparation and management. In Uhlmann, W, Schuette, JL, and Yashar, BM (eds), A Guide to Genetic Counseling. Wiley-Blackwell, Hoboken, NJ, 93–131.

Veach, PM, LeRoy, BS, and Bartels, DM. 2003. Collaborating with clients: providing information and assisting in client decision making. In Facilitating the Counseling Process: A Practice Manual. Springer, New York, 122–149.

Weil, J. 2000. Nondirective counseling, risk perception, and decision-making. In Weil, J (ed), Psychosocial Genetic Counseling. Oxford University Press, New York, 117–152.

Yelland, JM. 2004. Genetic counseling for inherited cancer syndromes. In Ellis, CN (ed), Inherited Cancer Syndromes: Current Clinical Management. Springer, New York, 30–60.

GENETIC TESTING AND COUNSELING

I know there are women who fear testing, but. . . . At the moments when I'm feeling particularly down and pessimistic it helps to think that even if I don't survive my cancer, my getting tested has probably saved the lives of the next generation in my family.

(Marsha Posusney in Dizon and Abu-Rustum, 2006, p. 122)

Cancer genetic counseling visits typically involve discussions about genetic testing. In fact, clients often come to the genetic counseling sessions with an expectation of being tested. This chapter describes the major elements of the testing and counseling process, which includes the logistics involved in arranging a test and providing pretest and posttest genetic counseling. The chapter ends with three genetic counseling cases.

9.1. THE LOGISTICS OF ARRANGING TESTS

The logistics of testing involve determining the client's appropriateness for texting, selecting the right tests, choosing the right laboratory, explaining the testing process to clients, and assessing the client's interest in and readiness to be tested.

9.1.1. DETERMINING IF FAMILY IS APPROPRIATE TO TEST

Since only 5–10% of cancer cases have a strong hereditary component, genetic testing is not appropriate for every client. Determining eligibility for a

Counseling About Cancer, Third Edition. Katherine A. Schneider.
© 2012 Wiley-Blackwell. Published 2012 by John Wiley & Sons, Inc.

specific genetic test relies on a thorough assessment of the client's personal and family histories of cancer. Families who are offered genetic testing for a specific hereditary cancer syndrome should have at least a reasonable probability of obtaining positive test results.

Once it is deemed appropriate to offer cancer genetic testing to a specific family, the next issue is to decide which family member is the best candidate for testing. Ideally, testing should be initially performed on the person in the family who is most likely to carry the gene mutation. This might be a relative who has had one of the syndrome-related malignancies or a relative who is deemed an obligate carrier (i.e., the individual has a parent and a child who have had syndrome-associated cancers).

Testing a relative who is affected (i.e., has cancer or other clinical signs of the syndrome) provides the most informative results for the family. If the affected relative tests positive, then other relatives will have definable increased risks and will be able to have targeted genetic testing. If the affected relative tests negative, then there are two possible explanations: (1) The cancer in the family is not due to an inherited risk factor, or (2) the cancer in the family is due to a mutation in a region or gene for which a test was not performed. Testing unaffected individuals is also possible, but it is an indirect way of linking a specific genetic mutation with the cancers in the family and may yield less informative results. The rationale for testing an affected relative prior to testing at-risk relatives may seem obvious to genetics providers, but this concept can be puzzling to clients.

In families with no living (or available) affected relatives, testing should be offered to a first-degree relative of the affected family member. Again, from a genetics standpoint, the goal of testing is to identify the underlying cause of cancer for the family, that is, to obtain a positive test result. Therefore, it makes more sense to test someone at 50% *a priori* risk for having the gene mutation than a cousin who may only be at 12.5% risk. Part of the rationale for this approach is the financial burden on the family; an initial genetic analysis can cost thousands of dollars.

In determining a client's appropriateness for testing, counselors should also consider the factors presented in the succeeding sections.

9.1.1.1. The Client's Cancer Status

If there is no known mutation in the family then testing should begin with an individual who has had a syndrome-related cancer. If the client has not had cancer, then it is preferable to offer testing to one of the client's affected relatives.

If there is a known mutation in the family, then the client, regardless of cancer status, has the option of being tested. In syndromes with rare or unusual tumor types, such as Basal Cell Nevus syndrome or Neurofibromatosis, it may be possible to identify individuals with the syndrome without resorting to a genetic test. In syndromes with more common tumor types, such as colon or breast cancer, all relatives with cancer should be tested to distinguish between inherited and sporadic cases.

9.1.1.2. The Client's Age

The client's age at diagnosis may help sort out the likelihood that it is a hereditary or sporadic cancer. In general, the initial testing candidate should be the relative who developed cancer at the youngest age. For example, in a family with no known *BRCA* mutation and two sisters with breast cancer, one at age 60 and one at age 32, it makes more sense to initially test the sister diagnosed at the younger age. Counselors should be cautious when testing children, especially if there is no effective screening to offer to those with positive results. Children rarely derive any medical benefit from being tested for adult onset hereditary cancer syndromes.

9.1.1.3. The Client's *A Priori* Risks

If there is a known mutation in the family, then the risk of carrying the mutation is based on the client's placement in the pedigree. For example, if the syndrome follows a dominant inheritance pattern, clients with an affected first-degree relative will have a 50% risk of carrying the mutation and their children will be at 25% risk. In general, testing each branch of the family should begin with the oldest living at-risk family member. Thus, testing a grandparent will determine whether it is necessary to offer testing to his/her children and grandchildren. If certain relatives are not available or interested in testing, then testing should be offered to their children or siblings. This is especially true if there are specific medical interventions that can be offered to individuals with the hereditary cancer syndrome.

9.1.2. SELECTING THE RIGHT TESTS

> It is important to keep in mind that the availability of genetic testing does not obligate its use.
>
> *(Uhlmann, 2009, p. 114)*

One goal of the pedigree assessment is to determine whether the client should be offered testing for one or more of the known cancer susceptibility genes. Clinical genetic testing is now available for many of the major hereditary cancer syndromes. (See Table 9.1.)

The types of genetic tests that cancer genetic counselors can order are presented in the succeeding sections.

TABLE 9.1. CLINICALLY AVAILABLE CANCER GENETIC TESTS

Gene	Syndrome
ALK/PHOX2B	Familial neuroblastoma
APC	FAP
ATM	Ataxia telangiectasia
BLM^{ASH}	Bloom syndrome (Ashkenazi Jewish founder mutation)
BMPR1A/SMAD4	Juvenile polyposis syndrome
BRCA1/BRCA2	Breast–ovarian cancer syndrome, hereditary
BWS	Beckwith–Wiedemann
CASP10	Autoimmune lymphoproliferative syndrome
CDH1	Gastric cancer, hereditary diffuse
CDK4/CDKN2A	Melanoma, cutaneous malignant
FANCA–FANCN	Fanconi anemia
FH	Leiomyomatosis and renal cell cancer, hereditary
FLCN	Birt–Hoge–Dubé syndrome
MEN1	MEN1
MET	Renal cell carcinoma, hereditary papillary
MLH1/MSH2/MSH6/PMS2/ TACSTD1	Lynch syndrome
MYH	MYH-associated polyposis
NF1	Neurofibromatosis, type 1
NF2	Neurofibromatosis, type 2
PRKAR1A	Carney complex
PTCH	Nevoid basal cell carcinoma syndrome
PTEN	PTEN hamartoma syndrome
RB1	Retinoblastoma, hereditary
RECQL4	Rothmund–Thomson syndrome
RET	MEN2
RPL5/RPL11/RPL35A/RPS7/ RPS10/RPS17/RPS19/ RPS24/RPS26	Diamond–Blackfan anemia
SDHB/SDHC/SDHD	Paraganglioma–pheochromocytoma, hereditary
STK11	Peutz–Jeghers syndrome
TP53	LFS
TSC1/TSC2	Tuberous sclerosis complex
VHL	Von Hippel–Lindau syndrome
WT1	Wilms' tumor, familial
XPA/XPC	Xeroderma pigmentosa

Sources: Lindor et al. 2008. Natl Cancer Inst Monogr 38: 1–93; Gene Tests (http://www.genetests.org).

9.1.2.1. Diagnostic Test

The purpose of a diagnostic test is to confirm or exclude a genetic disorder in an individual who has a malignancy or other features associated with a specific hereditary cancer syndrome. Prenatal or preimplantation genetic tests are also examples of diagnostic tests. Examples of diagnostic tests in cancer genetics include tests for Beckwith–Weidemann syndrome, Bloom syndrome, Fanconi anemia, Neurofibromatosis, and Werner syndrome.

9.1.2.2. Presymptomatic Test

The purpose of a presymptomatic test is to determine if an asymptomatic individual carries a gene mutation that is associated with an absolute (100%) likelihood of cancer or other syndromic features. One example is the analysis of the *APC* gene, which is associated with Familial Adenomatous Polyposis (FAP). Genetic tests for other syndromes that confer 90% or higher risks of malignancy (and are sometimes considered presymptomatic) include the following: *TP53* (Li-Fraumeni syndmore), *RB1* (retinoblastoma), *RET* (Multiple Endocrine Neoplasia, type 2), and *XP* (Xeroderma Pigmentosa).

9.1.2.3. Predictive Test

The purpose of a predictive test is to determine if an asymptomatic individual carries a gene mutation that is associated with an increased but not absolute risk of cancer or other syndromic features. The likelihood of the syndrome is reduced but not eliminated if the individual tests negative unless agenemutation has previously been identified in the family. Most of the clinical cancer genetic tests fall into this category, including tests for Hereditary Breast–Ovarian Cancer syndrome, and Lynch syndrome.

9.1.2.4. Carrier Test

The purpose of a carrier test is to determine if an asymptomatic individual has a gene mutation for a specific autosomal recessive or X-linked genetic disorder. Examples include testing the unaffected parents, siblings, or children of an individual diagnosed with Bloom syndrome, Fanconi anemia, or MYH-associated polyposis.

9.1.2.5. Screening Test

The purpose of a screening test is to determine if a certain population group has an increased likelihood of carrying a specific gene mutation. These types of tests may be useful in determining the need for DNA studies, especially in people with low probabilities of having inherited cancer. At the present time, one of the best examples of screening tests used in cancer genetics is the tumor block analysis for individuals with colorectal or uterine cancers. Individuals with high microsatellite instability (MSI) or absent immuno-histochemistry (IHC) of one or more of the mismatch repair genes will be advised to undergo additional DNA testing.

9.1.3. TEST SELECTION CHALLENGES

In the selection of the appropriate genetic tests for a specific client, genetic counselors need to consider the prior likelihood of a positive result, the logistics involved in ordering the test, and any other relevant factors (e.g., time sensitive requests; potential risks and benefits).

Genetic counselors can face a variety of challenges when determining which genetic tests are most appropriate to offer to clients. These challenges include the following presented in the succeeding sections.

9.1.3.1. The Pedigree May Suggest More Than One Cancer Syndrome

The client's personal and family history may be suggestive of two or more different cancer syndromes for which testing are available. For example a client diagnosed with adenomatous colorectal polyps may have Lynch syndrome, attenuated FAP, or MYH-associated polyposis. In some cases, the client's personal history may suggest one syndrome while the family history suggests another. For example, a female client with clear cell renal cell carcinoma may have been referred to the genetic counselor to arrange *VHL* testing, but the counselor may also need to address the fact that the client is Ashkenazi Jewish with a family history of breast cancer. In these types of situations, counselors must decide whether the genetic tests for different syndromes should be performed simultaneously or sequentially.

9.1.3.2. The Cancer Syndrome May Be Caused by Alterations in More Than One Gene

Certain hereditary cancer syndromes are caused by mutations in two or more genes. For example, Lynch syndrome can be caused by mutations or deletions in at least five different mismatch repair genes. Counselors may want to arrange testing in a sequential fashion, beginning with the analyses of the genes that are most likely to contain alterations based on the prevalence data and/or the client's IHC tumor block results.

9.1.3.3. Testing Is Useful for a Small Percentage of Cases

Even in families with clusters of cancer, there is a good likelihood that the genetic test results will come back negative (i.e., uninformative). The currently available genetic tests pick up only a small fraction of hereditary cases. Perhaps the genetic defects cannot be detected by current technologies or there may be other as-yet undiscovered genes involved in the syndrome. This includes clients who have significant histories of melanoma, lymphoma, or prostate cancer.

9.1.3.4. Client's Insurance May Not Cover All Genetic Tests

Decisions about which genetic tests to order may be at least partially based on the client's level of insurance coverage. Genetic counselors may want to arrange testing for the genes that are covered by the client's insurance before moving on to tests that will incur significant out-of-pocket expenses. Of course, the ordered tests need to be appropriate for the specific client; it is not necessary for a client to undergo comprehensive testing if a specific gene mutation has been identified in the family (even if insurance would pay for the comprehensive test). If the client has to self-pay for testing, then counselors should order sequential tests, beginning with the test that is most likely to yield a positive result.

9.1.4. CHOOSING THE RIGHT LABORATORY

It often falls to the genetic counselor to select the genetic testing laboratory. With the exception of BRCA testing in North America, which is performed by a single laboratory due to current patent restrictions, counselors typically have a choice of which laboratory to use. Hereditary cancer syndromes are similar to other orphan genetic diseases in that certain laboratories specialize in performing the analysis for select cancer syndromes. Therefore, certain laboratories provide RET analysis, while other laboratories offer MET or RBI testing. Testing a client for a single disorder may necessitate that specimens are sent to more than one laboratory. A good example of this is Lynch syndrome testing—ordering the tumor block analysis and DNA sequencing and deletion testing for the MSH2, MSH6, MLH1, PMS2, and EP-CAM (TACSTD1) genes may require sending specimens to two or more different laboratories!

Cancer genetic counselors typically deal with several different laboratories, so one of the first tasks of the genetic testing process is to determine which molecular genetics laboratory to use. Here are some strategies for finding an appropriate testing laboratory:

- Go to the Gene Tests website (http://www.genetests.org), which lists both clinical and research laboratories for many of the genetic syndromes.
- Query other cancer genetics colleagues who may have arranged similar testing in the past. One excellent resource is the National

Society of Genetic Counselors Cancer Special Interest Group discussion forum.

• Conduct a literature search and contact the researchers who have published work on the gene(s) in question.

Genetic testing can be performed in a clinical or research laboratory. The major differences between clinical and research laboratories are described below.

9.1.4.1. Clinical Laboratory

Clinical laboratories are service laboratories that offer molecular analysis of specific genes for a fee. Genetic testing for hereditary cancer syndromes is quite specialized. Each clinical laboratory has their own requisition forms, billing systems, specimen requirements, and shipping instructions. Certain laboratories have consent forms that need to accompany the specimens. The test results are typically available in 2–6 weeks, depending on the gene that is being analyzed.

9.1.4.2. Research Laboratory

The interests of research laboratories include locating and characterizing the disease gene, perfecting the methods of analysis, and determining the gene frequency within specific populations. These efforts are important in furthering our understanding of inherited forms of cancer and often lead to the development of a clinical genetic test. Participation in a research study may require extensive documentation of the cancer diagnoses in the family, completion of questionnaires, and collection of blood and/or tissue specimens. There is typically no charge for DNA testing performed in research laboratories; however, it may take several weeks or months for results to be forthcoming. In some cases, only aggregate test results will be released, not individual test results. Prior to study enrollment, clients need to know whether they can expect to receive any test results. If the research laboratory does agree to disclose preliminary research results, clients need to be aware that any positive result would need to be confirmed in a clinical laboratory. Clients should not make any medical decisions based on the test result nor any other relatives be offered testing, until the result is confirmed.

In the past, cancer genetic tests were kept in the research sector for several years before becoming clinically available; nowadays, it seems as though tests for hereditary cancer syndromes become clinically available soon after the gene's discovery, sometimes simultaneously with the research studies. This rapidity presents new challenges to genetic counselors to stay abreast of the newly available tests but also to make sure that clients are aware of the limited knowledge base regarding newly discovered gene mutations and their relationship to cancer development.

9.1.5. Laboratory Features to Consider

In deciding which genetic testing laboratory to use, counselors can consider the features which are presented below.

9.1.5.1. Clinical Certification

All laboratories in the United States performing clinical tests are required to have certification. There are two levels of certification for DNA-based tests: The Clinical Laboratory Improvement Amendments (CLIA) of 1988 or the voluntary proficiency program through the College of American Pathologists (CAP) and the American College of Medical Genetics (ACMG). The CAP certification is more rigorous, but either is acceptable. It is important to be aware that test results generated from nonclinically certified laboratories should not be disclosed to clients except as preliminary research results (which require clinical confirmation).

9.1.5.2. Technique and Accuracy

Laboratory techniques vary and include linkage analysis, multiplex ligation-dependent probe amplification (MLPA), single-strand conformational polymorphism (SSCP), Southern blotting, and DNA sequencing. The type of analysis that is used depends on the gene in question and whether there is a known mutation in the family. Accuracy rates also vary depending upon the techniques used. Ideally, the genetic test should have close to 100% sensitivity, meaning that a positive result is truly a positive result. The specificity of a test (whether a negative result is truly negative) is usually lower than the sensitivity. Ascertaining the specificity rate is more difficult, since it means estimating the number of mutations that were missed. Members of families with known mutations can be reassured that single-site analysis has close to 100% sensitivity and specificity.

9.1.5.3. Billing Policies

The cost of genetic testing for hereditary cancer syndromes can range from about 500 to 4000 U.S. dollars and billing practices differ from lab to lab. Some labs require referring providers to set-up institutional accounts so that the referring hospital is responsible for paying the laboratory and collecting the money from the client. Other laboratories require up-front payment from clients (by check or credit card) regardless of whether they have insurance preapproval.

9.1.5.4. Customer Service

Genetic counselors may also look for a laboratory that is "user friendly." Genetic counselors can determine whether the laboratory offers online forms and specimen kits, readily available prices, assistance with insurance approval or billing problems, reliable turnaround time for results, and staff members (often genetic counseling colleagues) who are available to resolve any issues that arise during the testing process.

9.1.6. EXPLAIN THE LOGISTICS OF THE TESTING PROCESS

The logistics of the testing process should be clearly outlined to clients. (Also refer back to Table 8.1.) This discussion can include the following simple yet important details presented below.

9.1.6.1. Number of Visits

Clients should be aware—upfront—whether the testing program requires a certain number of counseling visits. Most cancer programs require (or encourage) two genetic testing visits: a pretest visit (which can be combined with the risk assessment visit) and a results disclosure or follow-up visit. Although many programs have shifted to telephone disclosures, some programs still require that results be given during in-person visits.

9.1.6.2. Team of Providers

Clients should be aware of the names and roles of each provider they will be meeting with at each of their testing appointments. The team of providers may consist of a genetic counselor, nurse practitioner, and a physician (usually an oncologist). Testing programs should also have a clinical psychologist or other mental health provider on staff to meet with clients and provide mental health backup with challenging cases. A few programs encourage all clients to meet with a social worker or psychologist during the testing process; again, it is important for clients to be aware of this beforehand.

9.1.6.3. Informed Consent Procedure

All clients who undergo genetic testing should sign appropriate written consent. The consent form can originate from the testing laboratory or from the testing program. The consent form should describe the possible test results, implications of the results to the client and family, accuracy and limitations of testing, and potential risks and benefits of testing (see Table 9.2). It is also important that clients have ample opportunity to ask questions about the test and have taken the time to consider all the possible

TABLE 9.2. Topics to Discuss during the Informed Consent Process for Cancer Genetic Tests

- Description of the condition for which testing is being done
- Logistics of the testing procedure
- Possible test results
- Accuracy and limitations of testing
- Risks and benefits of learning the test results
- Alternatives to testing
- Options to defer, decline, or cancel the test
- Options to defer or decline learning the result
- Privacy and confidentiality policies regarding the genetic test result
- Contact information for program staff

Sources: Geller et al., 1997.

ramifications of testing. Thus, there should be an informed consent *process*; handing clients a form to sign is not sufficient.

9.1.6.4. Test Logistics

Clients count on genetic counselors to make the appropriate arrangements for each genetic test. This includes the correct test requisition forms, required signatures from the client and referring provider, completed billing information, correctly labeled tubes, sufficient amount of specimen collected, and shipping instructions.

9.1.6.5. Results Timing/Disclosure

One question that clients invariably ask is when results will be available. For clinical genetic tests, the answer usually lies somewhere between 2 and 6 weeks. Obtaining results from research laboratories can take much longer. Since DNA testing often takes longer than anticipated, it is prudent to provide a range of time rather than specifying an exact date. Clients should also be informed that second blood samples are sometimes necessary and that this is seldom indicative of a deleterious mutation. The method of disclosure should also be discussed beforehand. Some cancer testing programs routinely disclose results by telephone while other programs require that results be disclosed in person unless there are extenuating circumstances (e.g., client is too ill to travel).

9.1.6.6. Cost of Testing

Clients have sometimes complained that they receive information about every aspect of genetic testing—except how much it will cost. The total cost of testing typically includes the provider visits, the blood draw, and the DNA analysis. Clients need to be aware of all major testing-related charges because they may need to contact their insurer beforehand to determine the extent of coverage or to obtain the appropriate referrals. It is always better to figure out the client's potential costs *before* the blood specimen has been shipped to the laboratory.

Medicare, as well as many of the group health insurance plans, will pay for *BRCA*, *APC*, and *MSH2/MLH1/MSH6* genetic testing if the client meets the plan's testing criteria. For example, a client's insurance plan may cover the cost of *BRCA* testing if any of the following criteria are met:

- The client has a personal history of breast cancer plus two relatives with breast or ovarian cancer
- The client has a personal history of breast cancer under age 40 plus one relative with breast or ovarian cancer
- The client has a personal history of ovarian cancer plus one relative with breast or ovarian cancer
- The client has a personal history of male breast cancer plus one relative with breast or ovarian cancer
- The client has a personal history of breast cancer and ovarian cancer (no other cancer family history required)
- The client has a personal history of breast or ovarian cancer plus Ashkenazi Jewish heritage
- The client has a known gene mutation in a first- or second-degree relative

When ordering other cancer genetic tests, counselors may need to write letters of medical necessity, call the insurance company to explain the rationale for the test, and/or help the client to appeal a denial of coverage. All clients undergoing genetic testing should be warned about potential charges even if they have prior approval from their insurance company. Clients may be responsible for certain charges if they have insurance policies that:

- Require clients to pay a set portion of the fee. For example, in an 80/20 policy, the client would be responsible for 20% of the bill.
- Require clients to pay a certain deductible each year. If the deductible has not already been met, then clients will have to pay for at least part of the genetic test even if the test has been preapproved.
- Require clients to pay the remainder of the bill (balanced billing) after the insurer pays the laboratory what they consider to be the "usual and customary" price, which may be considerably less than the actual bill.

For some clients, the cost of cancer genetic testing is prohibitively expensive. Some hospitals and laboratories have set up philanthropic funds to help defer the costs of testing for people who do not have adequate funds. In addition, a few genetic testing laboratories are willing to arrange individual payment plans with clients so that the bill can be paid over a number of months.

9.1.6.7. Confidentiality Practices

Counselors will want to reassure clients that the genetic test results and other information shared during the testing process will remain confidential in a manner similar to other protected medical information. Clients who receive positive results should be asked for verbal or written permission prior to releasing results to anyone, including other family members. When testing a cancer patient with advanced disease, counselors should obtain the names and contact information of one or two individuals (preferably blood relatives) to whom the result can be disclosed in the event of the patient's demise. Since most cancer genetic tests are now offered on a clinical basis, it has become the standard of care in most programs to place a copy of the test result in the client's permanent medical record. Testing programs can decide whether there will be any exceptions to this policy for clients who are especially worried about their privacy.

9.1.7. ASSESSING THE CLIENT'S INTEREST AND READINESS

Clients request cancer genetic tests for a variety of reasons, ranging from "I don't want to keep having colonoscopies if I don't need them" to "I just need to know." Counselors should ask clients if they are undergoing testing in order to make specific medical decisions, for the sake of other family members, or for another reason. Ascertaining why clients are interested in testing can provide valuable insight into their concerns as well as their overall understanding of the test. Clients may need to be reminded that DNA testing looks for the presence of a cancer susceptibility gene, not evidence of cancer. Clients who undergo genetic testing may need to be reminded that they should continue being monitored for signs of cancer. For example, a woman with a suspicious breast lump needs to have imaging studies and a possible biopsy regardless of negative *BRCA* results.

Genetic counselors should describe the option of genetic testing in a nondirective and impartial manner and then help clients to reach their own decisions about it. During this process it may be helpful to review the possible test results (see Section 9.2.1) and the potential risks and benefits of testing (see Section 9.2.3).

A client's interest in genetic testing is in part influenced by the hereditary cancer syndrome itself. Although there are exceptions, interest in genetic testing tends to be lower in the following situations:

- The cancer syndrome can be reliably detected by physical exam (e.g., Basal Cell Nevus syndrome)
- The client has a form of cancer that is rarely familial (e.g., leukemias and lymphomas)
- There are few effective detection or prevention strategies available for people with the syndrome (e.g., Li–Fraumeni syndrome [LFS])

Interest in genetic testing tends to be higher for syndromes in which:

- It is rarely possible to identify people with the syndrome by other means (e.g., Hereditary Breast–Ovarian Cancer syndrome)
- There are potentially effective early-detection or risk-reduction strategies for people with the cancer syndrome (e.g., Multiple Endocrine Neoplasia, type 2 [MEN2])
- The recommended surveillance for people with the cancer syndrome is burdensome, invasive, or expensive (e.g., FAP)

Interest in testing varies among families and even within families. Some clients greet the availability of testing as an opportunity while others see it as more of a threat. Factors that may influence a client's interest in testing are presented in the succeeding sections.

9.1.7.1. Personality Type

Individuals may be more likely to pursue genetic testing if:

- They have a direct locus of control; that is, they feel that they are in control over whether they develop cancer
- They believe that the more information they have, the better they can protect or prepare themselves
- They have greater faith in available monitoring or prevention strategies
- They deal better with certainty than uncertainty, even if the news is bad
- They cope better with risk with actions or obtaining more information

9.1.7.2. Galvanizing Events

The decision to be tested may be triggered by a precipitating event. These galvanizing events are often cancer-related incidents, such as an abnormal cancer screening result or a new cancer diagnosis in the client or family.

However, noncancer-related events can also trigger decisions to be tested. Examples include a planned move to another state or country, the birth of a baby, or the imminent loss of health insurance.

9.1.7.3. Emotional Reactions/Well-Being

Clients who are overly anxious or apathetic may be less likely to pursue genetic testing. Clients who are anxious may be fearful about learning their results and clients who are apathetic may not see the value in learning the information. Clients may experience a spectrum of emotional responses to their risk status and the option of genetic testing. Any type of strong reactions may influence the client's decision to be tested, although not always in uniform ways. For example, some clients who are grieving the cancer-related death of a relative may decide they are not emotionally ready to be tested while others may decide that being tested is what their relative would have wanted them to do. Any underlying mental health disorder in clients can add a layer of complexity to their decisions about being tested. In addition, clients who have personal histories of anxiety, depression, eating disorders, or substance abuse problems may be less equipped to deal with all the emotions engendered by the testing discussions. Clients who are emotionally vulnerable who do decide to proceed with testing may need extra programmatic support. (See Section 9.2.5 for more information.)

9.1.7.4. Readiness to Learn Result

Clients who elect to be tested need to be emotionally and intellectually prepared to hear their results. It is important for genetic counselors to explore with clients the possible reactions to a positive or negative test result. Clients who "don't want to think about it until they have to" may be less willing to discuss potential reactions to results ahead of time, and thus, may require additional posttest counseling and support. Clients who indicate that they would be devastated by a positive test result should strongly consider deferring the test until they have processed some of these feelings or they have additional mental health supports in place.

9.1.7.5. Timing Issues

It is important for counselors to let clients know that genetic testing is optional and that the timing of testing is up to the clients themselves. In most cases, there is no urgency to making the decision of being tested. (Exceptions include situations in which the client's surgical or medical decisions are on hold until the test results are back, but these are uncommon events.) In most cases, clients can take time to consider whether they are ready to learn their genetic test results. Even in situations of testing a terminally ill client, the family can decide to store a specimen of blood or saliva until the family is ready to pursue genetic testing.

It is also helpful for counselors to explore what else is going on in clients' lives that might impact their reactions to the test results. Examples include a new diagnosis, a seriously ill relative, or a major life event such as a new baby, divorce, or loss of job. Clients who are already sad or stressed may have even more acute reactions to positive genetic test results and it may be useful to remind clients that they can defer testing until a later time. Counselors should also recognize that certain anniversary dates can affect a client's decisions about testing. For example, there may be a specific time of year that the client is more focused on cancer-related issues (or feels more vulnerable) due to a prior cancer diagnosis or a cancer-related death in the family. Certain birthdates may also trigger decisions about testing; clients may suddenly "need" to be tested when they approach the age of their affected relative who was diagnosed with or died of cancer. Clients who lost a parent to cancer may also seek genetic counseling and testing when their own children reach the ages they were at when their own parent died.

9.1.7.6. Religious/Cultural Beliefs

Clients who hold strong religious beliefs that their destiny is in "God's hands" may be less interested in pursuing genetic testing options. They may feel that genetic testing is contradictory to their beliefs or they may feel as though their families would not support a decision to be tested. It is important for counselors to be respectful of their clients' belief systems and to recognize that some people will be less interested in genetic testing because of these beliefs. At times a client may express a viewpoint that makes the counselor uncomfortable (e.g., the client objects to screening guidelines or believes the cancer is retribution for a past misdeed). In these cases, it might be useful for the counselor to seek guidance from someone who is knowledgeable about the client's religious or ethnic culture in order to help the counselor know how best to proceed.

9.1.7.7. Understanding of the Test

Clients who are interested in being tested should have a clear understanding of what the genetic test results can and cannot tell them. Alerting clients of all possible implications and consequences of being tested should be considered part of the informed consent process. For example, clients may want to learn their genetic test results to help clarify the need for extra imaging procedures, but they may not have considered all the ramifications of a positive result, such as the fact that other close relatives would also be at increased risk.

9.2. Pretest Counseling

The purpose of pretest counseling is to give people sufficient information to make an informed decision about whether or not to proceed with testing. The pretest session should include discussions about the following topics: the possible test results, the accuracy and limitations of testing, the implications of testing for the client and relatives, the potential risks and benefits of learning this information, and making the decision about testing. The amount of time spent discussing each topic may vary depending upon the client's prior knowledge about testing, number of questions asked, and any special issues that are of concern to the client or counselor. Most pretest counseling sessions are between 30 and 60 minutes.

9.2.1. Possible Genetic Test Results

Clients should be aware of the different answers they might receive from genetic testing. The range of possible test results depends on the type of genetic test that has been ordered. This section describes the possible test results for five types of genetic tests.

9.2.1.1. Comprehensive DNA Analysis

Comprehensive DNA testing typically refers to sequencing tests. This type of test involves an analysis of the entire coding sequence of the gene plus a certain number of DNA nucleotides at each splicing junction. Comprehensive analysis is generally recommended for a client who is either the first person in the family to be tested or the member of a family for which testing, so far, has revealed only negative results.

The possible test results for comprehensive DNA analyses are:

- *Positive*—A positive result is one in which a specific germline mutation has been identified in one copy of the gene. The germline mutation will either be a frameshift mutation (which is always deleterious) or a missense mutation that has been shown to affect the function of the gene. A positive result will likely explain the pattern of cancer in the family and means that the client has increased risks of specific malignancies. Other relatives will also be at increased risk for carrying the mutation, but now have the option of undergoing a targeted genetic test.
- *Indeterminate negative*—An indeterminate negative result is one in which no mutation or variant has been identified in either of the two gene alleles. This result may decrease the likelihood that the client has an inherited predisposition to cancer, but does not eliminate the possibility. The family could have a mutation in the analyzed gene

that cannot be detected by current technologies or could have a mutation in another gene that has not yet been identified. In families at high risk for a hereditary cancer syndrome, an indeterminate negative test result should not be viewed as reassuring news. The client may have increased cancer risks and it may still be appropriate to discuss additional monitoring options. Sometimes it is helpful to offer testing to other relatives to try and identify a positive result in the family.

- *Variant of uncertain significance* (VUS)—Clients need to be aware that not all genetic test results will yield definitive results. Whenever comprehensive DNA analyses are performed, there is a chance that a novel DNA change will be identified. This type of result is termed a VUS. Typically, a VUS is a missense mutation (i.e., change in a single DNA nucleotide) that cannot be definitely characterized as either a functional, deleterious mutation (i.e., positive result) or a polymorphism of no clinical significance (i.e., negative result). Receiving a VUS result should not alter estimates of risk or recommendations about screening, although clients may want to delay decisions about prevention strategies until the VUS has been clarified. At the current time, it can take months or years for a VUS to be formally reclassified. Other family members should not be offered predisposition testing until the VUS has been determined to be a deleterious mutation. However, the testing laboratory may request blood samples from additional family members as part of their efforts to clarify the VUS. Family members asked to donate samples for such a study need to be aware that these efforts may still not yield a definitive answer. The testing laboratory will reclassify the result when they have sufficient information. Answering the following questions maybe useful in reclassifying a VUS:

  - Is there a known deleterious mutation on the opposite allele? Most dominant cancer syndromes are caused by a mutation in one of the two alleles. The presence of two mutated alleles is either not compatible with life (e.g., the *TP53* or *BRCA1* gene) or causes a different genetic condition (e.g., the *BRCA2* or *PMS2* gene). Thus, if the mutation and VUS are on opposite alleles (in *trans* not *cis*), then it is much less likely that the VUS is deleterious.

  - Does the variant result track with the cases of cancer in the family? Family studies (i.e., cosegregation studies) involve testing other affected relatives for the VUS to help determine whether it is deleterious. For example, if the client with a VUS has a strong maternal history of cancer, then identifying the VUS in the client's father would be reassuring, because it is clearly not tracking with the cancer in the family. Alternatively, if the client's mother carries the VUS, then the variant is still not necessarily deleterious, but the possibility cannot be ruled out.

- Does the variant result occur in a section of the gene that is conserved across species? The laboratory can also assess whether the VUS has occurred in an evolutionarily conserved region of the gene, by looking at the gene sequences that have remained constant across various species. VUS results that occur in conservatively conserved regions of the gene are more likely to be deleterious.

- Does the new amino acid change the formation or properties of the molecule? Variants that cause major (nonconservative) changes in the amino acid or molecule are more likely to be deleterious. Counselors can consult with other laboratories or review available data on the VUS via publications or database resources, such as PolyPhen or SIFT genome.

9.2.1.2. Single-Site Analysis

Clients can be offered single-site analysis when a specific gene mutation has previously been identified in their family. As the name suggests, this type of genetic testing focuses on a few specific nucleotides of DNA. If single-site genetic testing is ordered, then two results are possible:

- *Positive*—A positive result is one in which the familial mutation has been identified. This result means that the client has the cancer syndrome in the family and that the client has increased risks of the syndrome-related malignancies. In addition, the client's offspring are now at increased risk (usually 50%) for carrying the mutation. A positive result does not alter the likelihood that the client's siblings carry the mutation unless this is the first positive result in their branch of the family.

- *True negative*—A true negative result is the absence of the familial mutation in either copy of the gene. The client's descendents are no longer at risk for carrying the familial mutation and will not ever need to be tested. A true negative result does not alter the likelihood that the client's siblings could carry the mutation.

9.2.1.3. Founder Mutation Testing

In this type of testing, an individual is tested for one or more specific mutations that are more prevalent in the individual's ethnic group or geographic region. For example, people of Ashkenazi Jewish heritage who undergo *BRCA1* and *BRCA2* testing are usually tested for three specific founder mutations: the 187delAG and 5385insC mutations in the *BRCA1* gene and the 6174delT mutation in the *BRCA2* gene. It is estimated that people of Ashkenazi Jewish heritage have a 2% probability of carrying one of the three *BRCA* founder mutations. For this reason, all Ashkenazi Jewish clients who are tested for a familial *BRCA* mutation should be tested for all three founder mutations rather than single-site analysis because of the small chance they could have inherited a mutation from the other parent.

Founder mutation testing may yield the following results:

- *Positive*—The client carries one of the founder mutations that are more prevalent in the ethnic group and are known to cause a specific cancer syndrome. This type of mutation is more likely to have been inherited from a parent than to be a *de novo* event. In some instances, a client will test negative for the familial mutation but will be found to have a different founder mutation. In this situation, other relatives may need to be notified and retested for the new positive result in the family.

- *Indeterminate negative*—The client does not carry one of the founder mutations for a specific disorder. This type of negative result may be more reassuring than an indeterminate negative result in the general population. For example, Ashkenazi Jewish clients who test negative for the *BRCA* founder mutations have reduced their likelihood of an inherited predisposition by about 90%. Clients who test negative for the founder mutations can be offered more comprehensive DNA analyses of the genes if their *a priori* risk of having the syndrome is high enough to warrant it (perhaps a 10% risk or higher).

- *True negative*—The client does not carry the founder mutation that is known to be in his or her family. Thus, the client does not have the hereditary cancer syndrome that has been identified in the family. In addition, the client has tested negative for the other founder mutations.

9.2.1.4. Genomic Rearrangement Testing

A subset of individuals with hereditary cancer syndromes will have large deletions rather than nucleotide errors. In rare cases, the entire gene may be deleted. Standard DNA sequencing will not detect these genomic rearrangements. For example, in the Dutch population, there are two *BRCA1* founder deletions that can only be detected by MLPA or Southern blot analysis. In some cases, the molecular laboratory will perform the deletion studies together with the DNA sequencing analysis, but most of the time, the deletion studies must be ordered separately. The possible results from genomic rearrangement studies are described below:

- *Positive*—A positive result means that at least one exon of the gene is absent. This result means that the person has the hereditary cancer syndrome. In a few syndromes, having a large deletion rather than a mutation might alter the cancer risks.

- *Indeterminate negative*—An indeterminate negative result means that each region of the gene is intact. Thus, a large rearrangement of the gene is not the underlying explanation of cancer for the client. Alternative genetic and nongenetic explanations can be explored.

- *True negative*—The client does not carry the large deletion that is known to be in his or her family. Thus, the client does not have the hereditary cancer syndrome that has been identified in the family.

9.2.2. ACCURACY AND LIMITATIONS

Genetic tests are never 100% accurate due to the parameters of testing and the potential for human error. Counselors should inform clients of the test's accuracy rate and describe mechanisms in place to prevent or minimize errors, such as careful labeling of the specimen tubes and meticulous record keeping. Single-site DNA analysis should be close to 100% accurate while comprehensive DNA sequencing has a lower rate of accuracy, due to the high number of indeterminate negative results (a portion of which may be false negatives).

It is also important that clients understand the inherent limitations of cancer genetic test results. For a positive result, these include the concepts that:

- *A positive result is not synonymous with cancer*—Penetrance is high for many of the hereditary cancer syndromes, but is rarely 100%. Clients need to understand that positive results are not a guarantee that cancer will develop, especially with currently available detection and prevention strategies. In addition, the absence of cancer does not mean the test results are wrong (which is a separate issue!).

- *Uncertainties about cancer remain*—Clients may overestimate the power of DNA testing, so they need to be cautioned that results will still leave many unanswered questions. A positive result confers an increased risk of cancer, but does not resolve which type of cancer will develop, at what age the cancer will be diagnosed, or how amenable the cancer will be to treatment.

Negative test results carry the following limitations:

- *Does not rule out an inherited susceptibility*—Families need to be counseled that the absence of a gene mutation does not exclude an inherited predisposition to cancer. For example, about 25% of classic LFS families do not carry a detectable germline *TP53* mutation or large deletion. In these cases, the likelihood of a hereditary cancer syndrome should also consider the client's clinical features and the pattern of cancer in the family. Some clients with indeterminate negative results may have gene mutations that are undetectable by current technologies or they may have mutations in a different gene for which they were not tested.

- *Does not guarantee that cancer will not occur*—Individuals with indeterminate negative results should be made aware that they may still have increased risks of cancer. Individuals with true negative results can be reassured that their risks of developing cancer are the same as the average person—which are not insignificant risks. This is quite different from other types of genetic conditions in which noncarriers have disease risks approaching zero.

9.2.3. POTENTIAL RISKS AND BENEFITS OF TESTING

When there are proven strategies to prevent or cure inherited forms of cancer, there will be less emphasis on the risks versus benefits of genetic testing. This has been the case for the *RET* and *APC* genetic tests, both of which are routinely offered to affected probands and their at-risk relatives. However, for most genetic tests, detailing the pros and cons of testing is a key part of the pretest session. (See Table 9.3.)

The potential risks of learning one's genetic test results are as follows:

- *May increase cancer worry and sadness*—For clients, the most anxiety-producing aspect of genetic testing may be facing the possibility that they have an inherited susceptibility to cancer. Clients should be told that they may experience increased sadness and/or cancer worry if they test positive, although these emotions tend to be of

TABLE 9.3. POTENTIAL RISKS AND BENEFITS OF CANCER GENETIC TESTING

Risks
- May increase cancer worry and sadness
- May be of questionable medical benefit
- May lead to genetic discrimination
- May strain family relationships

Benefits
- May end uncertainty about one's gene status
- May be a negative (normal) result
- May impact medical management decisions
- May clarify cancer risks for other relatives

short duration. More serious emotional sequelae appear to be rare among people being tested for hereditary cancer syndromes.

- *May be of questionable medical benefit*—For many of the inherited cancer syndromes, there are no proven strategies to reliably detect the cancers at an early stage. Even in syndromes that do offer some strategies for reducing one's risks of cancer through prophylactic surgery, lifestyle changes, or chemoprevention, the prevention of cancer is not possible. Some clients become less interested in genetic testing when they are told that there is no way to guarantee the prevention of the associated cancers.

- *May lead to genetic discrimination*—Some people decide against having genetic testing because they are concerned about possible genetic discrimination. Despite the protective legislation and the lack of documented cases, clients continue to express concerns about insurability if they receive positive results. Genetic counselors can reassure clients that they are unlikely to experience any adverse effects in terms of health insurance or employment because of a cancer genetic test. It may be helpful to describe the Genetic Insurance Nondiscrimination Act (GINA), which was signed into law in 2008. (See Table 9.4.) Clients may also be concerned about the impact of a positive genetic test result on other types of insurance policies for which there are no legislative protections, including life, short-term disability, and long-term care insurance policies. Military service eligibility may also be impacted.

TABLE 9.4. GENETIC INFORMATION NONDISCRIMINATION ACT (GINA) OF 2008

GINA provides protections to people who seek genetic counseling and testing.[a] Specifically, this legislation:
- Prohibits health insurers from requesting or requiring genetic information of an individual or the individual's family members
- Prohibits health insurers from using genetic information of an individual or the individual's family members for decisions regarding coverage, rates, or preexisting conditions[b]
- Prohibits employers from using genetic information for hiring, firing, or promotion decisions
- Prohibits employers from using genetic information for any decisions regarding terms of employment

Source: National Human Genome Research Institute (2009), http://www.genome.gov/pages/policyethics/geneticdiscrimination/GINAinfodoc.pdf.

[a]The insurance provisions do not apply to life, disability, and long-term care insurance plans. The employment provisions do not apply to employers with fewer than 15 employees.

[b]The Health Information Portability Amendment of 1998 also disallows health insurers from using pre-existing conditions for decisions regarding coverage or rates.

- *May strain family relationships*—Some clients shy away from testing because they do not want to deal with the familial ramifications of a positive result. A positive genetic test result can send a ripple effect through the family and may strain familial relationships. While some people enter testing with the sole intent of sharing the results with their relatives, others see the task of informing their at-risk relatives as an unwelcome burden. Whether clients decide to share their results with all relatives or to keep the results secret, there are potential ramifications to familial relationships.

The potential benefits of learning one's genetic test results are as follows:

- *May end uncertainty about one's gene status*—Clients who undergo testing have often lived with their cancer worries for a long time. The burden of not knowing whether one is at increased risk may add to the difficulties of the situation, especially within a family in which cancer is so prevalent. Learning one's gene status may provide a sense of control over the cancer syndrome—and one's destiny. There has also been some research to suggest that family members who elect not to be tested actually have higher anxiety scores than those who were tested and found to carry the genetic predisposition. For some people, it is the "not knowing" that is hardest to live with.

- *May be a negative (normal) result*—Clients undergoing testing usually have a 50% or better chance of *not* being found to have a mutation. Clients with true negative results are not at increased risk for developing a syndrome-related cancer and their offspring cannot inherit the familial mutation. Thus, learning a true negative result may have both a psychological and a medical benefit. Clients who receive indeterminate negative results may also be relieved by their results, although they need to be cautioned that the test has not ruled out the possibility of an inherited predisposition to cancer.

- *May impact medical management decisions*—One of the purposes of genetic testing is to identify individuals who are at high risk for developing cancer. Individuals who do have an inherited susceptibility to cancer will often be advised to undergo specialized surveillance tests or to undergo monitoring at earlier ages and/or more frequent intervals than is customary. There may also be risk-reduction strategies available, such as chemoprevention or prophylactic surgery.

- *May clarify risks for other family members*—A positive result can directly impact the cancer risks of other relatives, especially the client's children. Inherited gene mutations (as opposed to *de novo* mutations) confer increased risks to the client's siblings and parents as well as other more distant relatives including aunts, uncles, and cousins.

A positive result also allows other at-risk relatives the opportunity to have a targeted genetic test. For some clients with cancer, the main motivation for testing may be to clarify the risks for their relatives. A true negative result also clarifies the (lack of) risk for the client's current or future children.

9.2.4. Making Decisions About Testing

One important aspect of cancer genetic counseling is to assist clients in making decisions about genetic testing. Although some clients come to the genetic counseling sessions with their minds made up to either proceed or decline testing, a number of clients will be undecided about whether or not they wish to be tested.

According to genetic counselor and psychotherapist, Jon Weil, the main goals of the client's decision-making process are as follows:

- The client's decision should be based on an adequate assessment of options and consequences and be consistent with his or her values.
- The client should feel that he or she made the best decision possible at the time.
- The genetic counseling process should support and facilitate implementation of the client's decision (Weil, 2000a; Baty, 2009).

Genetic counselors can employ the strategies presented in the succeeding sections to assist clients in making decisions about cancer genetic testing (also see Table 9.5).

TABLE 9.5. Strategies to Assist Clients in Making Decisions About Cancer Genetic Testing

- Present all the relevant facts
- Offer assistance, not advice
- Provide encouragement and support
- Help clients to structure the discussion in a way that is useful and value neutral
- Consider brainstorming or using best-case/worst-case scenarios
- Explore how clients have dealt with other health-related decisions
- Identify other people (partner, relative, friend, physician) whose input might be helpful to the client
- Encourage the client to reflect and deliberate before reaching a decision

Sources: Weil (2000b); Baty (2009).

9.2.4.1. Present All the Relevant Facts

It is important for counselors to provide all of the pertinent information about the genetic test and the hereditary cancer syndrome for which testing is being done. This discussion should include information about the possible genetic test results as well as the impact of these results on the client's risk status and monitoring recommendations.

9.2.4.2. Offer Assistance, Not Advice

The genetic counselor's role in the decision-making process is to assist clients as they make their own decisions about testing. This follows the tenet of nondirective counseling, which places the emphasis on providing information and support rather than on advice or personal opinions. Some genetic counselors worry that they will influence client decisions about testing. This does not seem to be the case. Even clients who pointedly ask for advice seem to weigh the answers against their personal filter of preferences and experiences.

9.2.4.3. Provide Encouragement and Support

Some clients may need to work through their emotional reactions to the situation. This may include feelings of grief and fear. Counselors can help empower clients to make appropriate decisions about testing and can then support them in these decisions. For example, if the client defers testing to a later time, the counselor can inform the referring physician and other program staff and explain the reasons why the client has made this decision.

9.2.4.4. Help Clients to Structure the Discussion in a Way That Is Useful and Value-Neutral

Some clients struggle with even knowing how to think about making this type of decision and are not sure what questions to ask. It may be helpful for counselors to frame or structure the discussion by helping clients to focus on the factors that are most important to their heath, families, and value systems.

9.2.4.5. Consider Brainstorming or Using Best-Case/Worst-Case Scenarios

It might be helpful for clients to brainstorm all of the different alternatives or outcomes associated with a specific course of action. Counselors can also consider exploring different hypothetical situations with clients. For example, counselors can ask clients to imagine the best-case or worst-case scenario relating to a certain decision.

9.2.4.6. Explore How Clients Have Dealt with Making Other Health-Related Decisions

Some clients have difficulty making the decision about testing because it is such a novel situation. It may be helpful for counselors to ask clients how they have made other types of health-related decisions. Perhaps the clients will be able to use similar strategies to make the decision about testing.

9.2.4.7. Identify Other People Whose Input Might Be Helpful to the Client

Clients may want to talk over the option of testing with certain people in their lives before making a final decision. Many clients will seek input from their spouse/partner, relatives, close friends, or personal physicians. These conversations may take place before or after the genetic counseling session. Counselors can also encourage clients to speak to specific relatives, such as their parents, siblings, and adult children whose cancer risks may be impacted by the genetic test result.

9.2.4.8. Encourage the Client to Reflect and Deliberate before Reaching a Decision

Clients may feel pressured to make a decision about testing during the initial counseling visit. Counselors can remind clients that this type of testing is rarely a matter of urgency and that they should take as much time as they need to make the decision that is right for them.

9.2.5. Psychological Assessment

Genetic testing for cancer susceptibility is often a major event in a person's life. Learning the results of a genetic test—regardless of whether it is positive or negative—can have a significant impact on one's emotional well-being. For this reason, it is important for genetic counselors to discuss the potential emotional ramifications of testing and to assess the client's emotional vulnerability. Although research has shown that most people undergoing *BRCA* testing cope well with their results, less information has been published regarding genetic testing for other cancer conditions. It is important for testing programs to have safeguards in place to assess and support the subset of clients who experience some type of serious emotional distress.

Topics to ask clients undergoing cancer genetic testing are presented in the succeeding sections.

9.2.5.1. Current Emotional Well-Being

Because the testing process can exacerbate psychological problems, counselors should assess the client's current emotional well-being. This line of questioning can include queries about the client's mood and any changes in eating or sleeping habits. (See Section 10.2.1 for more information.)

9.2.5.2. Anticipated Impact of Results

It may be helpful for clients to verbalize what it might be like to learn they have positive or negative genetic test results. This exercise may be a way of assessing the potential of a severe adverse reaction. It may also help initiate discussions about possible medical management decisions and communicating the result to other family members. It may also be useful to ask clients if they expect to receive a particular result. Some clients will be convinced that they carry a gene mutation, while others will be convinced that the result will be negative. For some clients, there is a certain rationale to their expectations (the client with adenomatous polyposis should expect a positive *APC* result), but in other cases, it may be due to intuition or wishful thinking. Learning whether clients anticipate certain results and why they expect these results may be helpful in providing support when the result is disclosed.

9.2.5.3. Coping Resources

Everyone develops their own ways of coping with difficult situations, although some strategies are healthier than others. Counselors can explore with clients how they plan to cope with their results. It may also be helpful to learn how they have handled other stressful events in their lives. While some people cope with stressful events by reaching out to friends or going to the gym, others may isolate themselves or numb their feelings through the use of alcohol or drugs.

9.2.5.4. Support Network

Clients who do not seem to have any close friends or family members may need some extra psychological support. This may also be the case when the client's choice of support seems questionable (such as a clinically depressed sister or a 13-year-old son). Some people may have other more introspective ways of coping with worry or sadness rather than turning to other people. It is also possible that clients do have support people in their lives, but prefer not to discuss them during the counseling session.

9.2.5.5. Other Major Life Stressors

Any number of stressful life events could be present at the time a client decides to be tested. These events may be cancer related (terminally ill relative) or may be completely unrelated (job stress, family problems). Cancer-related stressors should be considered carefully as they might cause a more intense reaction to the genetic test result. Noncancer-related stressors should not be ignored, because a positive test result could add a second, potentially overwhelming, stressor. This is because clients who are in the midst of some type of upheaval are unlikely to have the same reservoir of emotional resources as clients who are not dealing with this type of situation. Counselors can explore with clients about whether this is the right time for them to be tested in light of the other events going on in their lives.

It is also important for testing programs to have a protocol in place to deal with clients who require additional psychological support. A client should be referred to a mental health professional if there is any concern about the person's ability to cope with the results due to previous cancer experiences, lack of support, or other major life stressors.

A program's decision to defer or deny genetic testing should only be considered if providers have evidence that disclosing a test result could lead to suicidal ideation or could cause incapacitating depression or anxiety.

9.3. RESULTS DISCLOSURE AND FOLLOW-UP

The goals of the results disclosure and follow-up interactions are to disclose and discuss the genetic test results with clients. This section describes the preparation and logistics involved with results disclosure, strategies for disclosing results successfully, possible client reactions, and topics to discuss in follow-up. The section ends with three case examples.

9.3.1. PREPARATION AND LOGISTICS

This section discusses the logistics involved in the disclosure of cancer genetic test results.

9.3.1.1. Mode of Results Disclosure

Cancer genetic test results can be disclosed by telephone or at an in-person visit. Results should not be given via email, fax, or letter, in part due to confidentiality concerns with these modes of communication. Counselors should consider the following issues in terms of the disclosure:

- *In-person disclosures*—Before the results visit, the genetic counselor should confirm the appointment time with the client and ensure that a meeting room has been arranged. It is also important to consider the setting in which the results will be disclosed. Counselors should pay attention to the layout of the room by making sure there are sufficient chairs and that the seating arrangement will allow everyone to feel included in the conversation. If possible, avoid having the client seated on an exam table or the counselor seated behind a desk. The room should have a door that can be completely shut to ensure privacy. Clients are also encouraged to bring a support person with them, such as their spouse/partner, family member, or close friend. Some clients bring an entire entourage with them; others prefer to come alone.

- *Telephone disclosures*—Prior to disclosing the results by phone, the genetic counselor should confirm that the client has the privacy and ability to speak freely. Genetic counselors are encouraged to schedule the disclosure phone calls in advance or at least to determine the best time of day to contact clients. This is the best way of avoiding disclosure to clients who are in the midst of a traffic jam, busy office, or their child's day care—none of which are conducive to a meaningful discussion. Unless prior arrangements have been made, all results should be given directly to the client. If the client is not available, then the counselor should leave a message for the client to call back. Counselors should provide clients with both their telephone and pager numbers so as to minimize the likelihood of playing phone tag with anxious clients.

- *What the counselor needs to know*—Genetic counselors should have a list of topics that they plan to cover at the disclosure, although they need to be flexible in case the client has alternative questions or concerns (or needs time to process the news before holding an in-depth discussion). Prior to any disclosure of results, genetic counselors should:

  - know how the result will be disclosed and make the appropriate arrangements (e.g., set-up an appointment or conference call; alert other providers if appropriate)

  - review the lab report, resolve any questions about the result, and confirm that it is the client's result

  - compose a set list of topics to cover during the results disclosure, focusing on items of immediate importance to clients

  - anticipate any possible counseling challenges (unexpected result, complex family dynamics, vulnerable client)

  - prepare materials to give to the client (lab report, summary letter, fact sheet, support group information)

- *What the client needs to know*—Clients need to know what to expect from the results disclosure interaction, by knowing in advance:

- how the result will be disclosed
- the type of result that will be disclosed
- who will be present at the results disclosure phone call/session
- approximately when they can expect to receive results

9.3.2. THE RESULTS DISCLOSURE

I'm not the news, just its messenger. I'm almost scared as you are. I'm not sure how to say it. I hope you will forgive me. I don't want to tell you. I don't want to tell you. I don't want to tell you. And you don't want to know.

(Resta, 2009, p. 12)

The results disclosure can be the most difficult aspect of the testing process for the client—and the counselor. This section discusses useful strategies for disclosing a cancer genetic test result in a professional yet empathetic manner.

9.3.2.1. Disclose the Result Early in Conversation

The few minutes prior to the results disclosure may be among the most anxiety-provoking for clients. Thus, it is best to disclose the result early in the conversation, unless the client had requested otherwise. It is also important that the disclosure visit or phone call occur at the time it has been scheduled; delays will only enhance client worry.

9.3.2.2. Use Direct and Clear Language

When disclosing the result, counselors should state the result in simple, straightforward language. Counselors should choose an approach with which they are comfortable and that seems to be appropriate for this client. For example, the counselor can say, "The Lab found that you *do* have the *FH* alteration that is in your family." Counselors may wish to alert clients that they are about to learn their result and/or offer some expression of empathy: "Are you ready to learn your result? OK. The test showed that you have an alteration in the *PTEN* gene. I wish I had better news for you." Other counselors may prefer to give the result in a bit more formal manner: "The Genetics Laboratory looked for mutations in three genes associated with Lynch syndrome. The DNA analysis did identify a mutation in the *MSH2* gene. This result explains why you developed colon cancer."

9.3.2.3. Allow Clients Time to React

After disclosing the result, pause. This gives clients a chance to consider the news and react to it. Don't launch into detailed explanations or even encouragement that a positive result is not that bad. At that moment, the news may be emotionally jarring, and clients might need time to react and regroup. Counselors should hold off from providing information or offering statements of encouragement until the initial reactions subside.

9.3.2.4. Be Empathetic but Professional

Counselors will want to acknowledge the client's disappointment and sadness by being appropriately empathetic. For some clients, especially those who have never had cancer, a positive genetic test result may be the worst news they have ever received. It is natural for counselors to be affected by a client's distress, but they need to retain a professional manner. Counselors will not be effective providers if they become emotionally distraught themselves. Some clients will accept and even seek demonstrations of comfort from the counselor (such as a gentle touch on the arm), but others will become uncomfortable by these gestures. Counselors need to learn to read client signals and respect the counselor–client boundaries.

9.3.2.5. Let Clients Set the Remaining Agenda

The remainder of the results disclosure discussion should be tailored to the clients' needs. Upon hearing their results, some clients will have dozens of questions, while others may need more time to process the news. In the event of a positive, variant, or unexpected result, it may be best to schedule a follow-up phone call or appointment to review the information rather than expecting to cover all the topics during the initial disclosure conversation. Counselors may also wish to remind clients with positive results that the most important thing for them to do is simply adjust to the news. They do not need to rush out and inform all their relatives nor do they need to schedule immediate appointments especially if they are feeling overwhelmed by the news.

9.3.2.6. What Happens Next

It is important for clients to have a good understanding about what happens next. This might include providing the answers to the following questions:

- Does the client need a follow-up genetic counseling appointment? How will it be scheduled?
- How will referrals to other specialists be made? Does the client need to call them or will the counselor facilitate these appointments?
- Will a copy of the genetic test result go in the medical record?
- Will the client be sent a copy of the result along with a summary letter? When can they expect to receive it?

- Who will inform the referring physician of the result—the counselor or the client?
- If the client's relatives have questions or want testing appointments, whom should they contact?

9.3.3. POSSIBLE CLIENT REACTIONS

This section describes the types of emotions and reactions that may occur among individuals who receive different types of cancer genetic test results. The majority of reactions are minor or transient; however, counselors should be prepared for the rare client who has a more intense reaction.

- *Positive result*—Clients who are told they have a gene mutation that predisposes them to cancer may experience a variety of emotions, including sadness, disappointment, shock, fear, anger, and disbelief. For the most part, clients with positive results adjust well to the news; only rarely are therapeutic or medicinal interventions necessary for clients with positive cancer genetic test results. However, a positive test result can trigger delayed grief reactions, feelings of isolation or vulnerability, or strained family relationships. Alternatively, clients with positive results may experience feelings of relief or closure that they have an explanation for the cancer in their family or because they finally know their gene status. Positive results can also lead to increased feelings of control, greater motivation to pursue cancer monitoring, and closer ties to some of their relatives.

- *Learning an indeterminate negative result*—Clients are typically relieved to hear that they do not have a genetic mutation. The degree of reassurance afforded by an indeterminate negative result depends on the prior likelihood that the family has a cancer syndrome. Clients who are at low risk for having a certain cancer syndrome may be told that the negative result lowers the likelihood that they have the syndrome. Clients who are at high risk for having a certain cancer syndrome need to be carefully counseled that it is still likely that they have the syndrome despite the negative results.

- *Learning a true negative result*—Clients who receive true negative results generally react with relief, joy, and decreased cancer worry. Clients may also experience survivor guilt regarding other affected relatives and may have regrets about major life decisions they have made. (For example, choosing a spouse based on their care-taking abilities rather than other factors.) Clients with true negative results may also feel excluded when relatives with positive results get together and share their concerns or plans. Clients who have lived with their cancer fears for a long time may find it disconcerting to

adjust to their altered risk status and may find it difficult to completely believe the news or to let go of their monitoring practices.

- *Learning a VUS*—Clients who receive VUS results may be confused
  more than anything else by this inconclusive finding. Clients may
  also express feelings of frustration, anger, or disappointment that the
  genetic test did not provide them with an unequivocal answer. Being
  in genetic limbo for months or years can be difficult for clients and
  it may be as stressful as being in a family that has tested positive. In
  fact, clients may need to be reminded (on more than one occasion)
  that a VUS result is *not* a positive genetic test result.

The majority of clients who receive positive test results cope satisfactorily
with the news. In fact, one of the consistent findings of clinical research
studies has been the lack of people who "fall apart" upon learning their
results. Yet having said this, most cancer genetic counselors have dealt with
one or more clients who have experienced a more intense reaction or required
greater programmatic support.

It is rarely possible to predict the clients who will experience greater
levels of distress. However, general factors that might contribute to greater
distress among clients with positive results are described in the succeeding
sections.

9.3.3.1. The Client Has Significant Baseline Depression or Anxiety

Clients who have underlying depressive or anxiety disorders may find their
symptoms exacerbated by the news of a positive result. This is especially
true if the mental health condition is not being adequately managed.

9.3.3.2. The Client Has Other Major Stressors in His or Her Life

Clients who are dealing with other stressful situations may have fewer emotional reserves to cope with the impact of a positive genetic test result.
Clients may be surprised by the intensity of their reactions, but it is more
likely to be a function of the cumulative stresses in their lives.

9.3.3.3. The Client Has Never Had Cancer

For clients who have never had cancer, receiving a positive test result may
be the most difficult (or frightening) news they have ever experienced and
may cause intense feelings of sadness, vulnerability, or cancer worry.

9.3.3.4. The Client Has a First-Degree Relative Who Died of Cancer

Having one or more close relatives who have died of cancer may intensify
the meaning of a positive genetic test result. Upon hearing their results,

clients may identify more strongly with their affected relatives or may experience delayed grief reactions, both of which may magnify the clients' reactions to their test results.

9.3.3.5. The Client Did Not Expect the Result

Clients may have a more difficult time adjusting to their gene status if the result they received was unexpected. This includes clients who unexpectedly receive positive results as well as those who are surprised by negative results. The unexpected results may be disorienting to clients and may make it more difficult to believe the news or to adjust their practices accordingly.

9.3.3.6. The Client Has Children

For clients who have children, one of the most distressing aspects of a positive result is the realization that their children could also be at risk. Even individuals who are sanguine about their own risks of cancer may have a difficult time sharing the news with their offspring or watching them undergo genetic testing or cancer screening. Positive test results may lead to intense feelings of parental sadness and guilt.

9.3.4. Post-Results Discussions and Follow-Up

Following the disclosure of a cancer genetic test result, there are several topics that genetic counselors will want to discuss with clients. These discussions may take place directly after the result has been given or during later follow-up visits or telephone calls. The nature of these interactions will vary from client to client, depending on the test result, the client's cancer status, and the relevance of each topic to the client's situation. Clients should always be encouraged to recontact the genetic counselor at a later date if they have any further questions about their results.

Topics to discuss with clients following results disclosure are presented in the succeeding sections.

9.3.4.1. Implication of the Result to the Client

Counselors may want to open the discussion by asking clients what their understanding is of the results. Clients have already been told, probably more than once, what the results mean in terms of their cancer risks. Despite this, clients often ask for clarification once they learn their own results. It is important for counselors to remind clients of the uncertainty and variability inherent in the test results. Counselors should also focus on the information that is most relevant to the client's specific situation. For example, discussions about a positive *BRCA2* result will vary depending on the client's gender, age, and cancer status.

9.3.4.2. Medical Management Options

Clients with positive test results are usually provided with syndrome-specific monitoring guidelines and referred to the appropriate medical specialists. Clients should also be encouraged to seek advice from their primary care physicians. In addition, there may be other options, such as chemoprevention or prophylactic surgery, for clients with positive results to consider. Clients may feel urgency to make certain medical management decisions (such as prophylactic surgery) but should be reminded that they have time in which to carefully consider these options. Some clients find it difficult or overwhelming to be faced with making decisions about their medical management. Yet in some ways they are the lucky ones. Clients at risk for sarcomas or pancreatic cancer have few effective monitoring or risk-reduction options available to them.

For clients with positive results, the recommendations and options for medical management are the major focus of the post-disclosure discussions. Clients with indeterminate negative or VUS results can consider screening options based on their uncertain or potentially increased cancer risks. Although clients with true negative results are often able to reduce their monitoring practices, they may benefit from a general discussion of cancer monitoring and living a healthy lifestyle.

9.3.4.3. Implication of the Result to the Client's Family

A cancer genetic test result has potential implications for the client's biological relatives. Clients with positive test results should be encouraged to share the information with their close relatives. Disseminating this information to the family can prove to be emotionally difficult, especially if the relationships are already strained or if the news is unexpected. Most clients with a positive result do end up sharing the information with at least some of their relatives. It may be helpful for counselors to identify the existing communication patterns within the family and also to remind clients about the confidentiality practices of the testing program. Some families operate in secrecy regarding who is being tested; others are much more open. The counselor may also want to explore possible barriers for communicating the results to at-risk relatives. As examples, clients may be reluctant to share the results with relatives who are estranged from the family or with relatives who are likely to become unduly upset by the news. The client should be the one to decide how to disclose the result to other family members, but counselors can help clients figure out how best to disseminate the information through the family. Counselors can also provide assistance in other ways such as writing a family letter, fielding questions from other family members, or making referrals to local genetic counseling services. In the case of clients who test positive for *APC* mutations (FAP) or *RET* mutations (MEN2), health-care providers may have a legal obligation to ensure that first-degree relatives are aware of their risks. However, this is the exception, not the rule. (See Section 11.3.11 for more information about this topic.)

9.3.4.4. Follow-Up Interactions

Genetic counseling services do not usually end with the disclosure of the genetic test result. Counselors may want to provide one or more follow-up telephone calls and to send summary letters to clients. It may also be appropriate to offer clients additional follow-up appointments to further discuss the information. Clients with positive test results may find it useful to have a follow-up appointment to review the information once the initial reaction to the news has subsided. For some clients with indeterminate negative or VUS results, it might be appropriate to discuss further genetic testing options. Testing programs can make follow-up telephone calls or visits a standard part of the testing process or can offer such services to the subset of clients who request or seem to need additional information or support.

9.3.4.5. Adjustment to the Result

It is important to continue assessing how well (or how poorly) clients are coping during the weeks and months following the results disclosure. Some clients may benefit from meeting with a mental health professional. The emotional response to testing seems to be the most intense in the first few weeks or months after learning the results, but tends to dissipate over time. However, specific issues and concerns may arise in the future, as the client's children become older or when another relative is diagnosed with cancer. It is important for clients to be aware of resources that are available to them if and when they need additional information or support in the future.

9.3.4.6. Review of Genetics

Clients may be confused about the risks of cancer or passing the gene mutation to offspring, especially as time passes. Clients who remain cancer free may begin to question their positive results. Or clients with true negative results may request predictive testing for their not-at-risk children. Thus, counselors may find themselves reviewing basic information about genetics, inheritance, and variable expressivity. Even clients who seem to have a good grasp of these concepts may not remember the information over time or may not be able to relate the information to their own situation.

9.3.4.7. Referrals to Specialists

Genetic counselors can also help make sure that clients are referred to the appropriate medical specialists. Clients with positive results will need to meet with various medical specialists to arrange the appropriate monitoring tests and follow-up. Clients with indeterminate negative or VUS results may also benefit from referrals to medical or mental health specialists. Genetic counselors to have a network of physicians, surgeons, and mental health providers for whom to refer clients.

9.4. CASE EXAMPLES

This section contains three case examples regarding clients who are offered genetic testing.

Case 9: "Why can't anything be simple?"

Maya cradled her 6-week-old daughter in her lap while her husband sat nearby. The genetic counselor congratulated the couple on the birth of their beautiful baby—after years of secondary infertility—and for recently attaining a prestigious research grant.

Maya, age 36, and her husband were both scientists working in a joint laboratory at the medical center.

The genetic counselor went on to collect the family history information. Maya's mother had undergone a simple mastectomy for invasive ductal carcinoma of the left breast at age 51 and was doing well at age 62. Over the past year, two of Maya's first cousins have been diagnosed with breast cancer—one at age 38 and one at age 35. The family originally came from India and most of the relatives (including the two affected first cousins) still reside there. (See Fig. 9.1 for Maya's pedigree.)

This couple expressed concern about Maya's risk of breast cancer because of the family history of breast cancer and all of the hormones she has taken in order to conceive and carry a pregnancy to term.

The genetic counselor explained that she could not readily quantify the risks of breast cancer based on the use of hormones, but offered to conduct a literature search. She reminded the couple that most breast cancer cases are due to a combination of risk factors. Thus, the risk of breast cancer associated with hormones might differ depending on the presence of other breast cancer risk factors, such as a germline *BRCA* mutation.

The counselor began to describe the *BRCA* genes but realized that as scientists working in cancer research they probably knew more about these genes than she did! Therefore, she switched to discussing the logistics of testing and explained that the relatives who had had breast cancer were the best candidates for genetic testing.

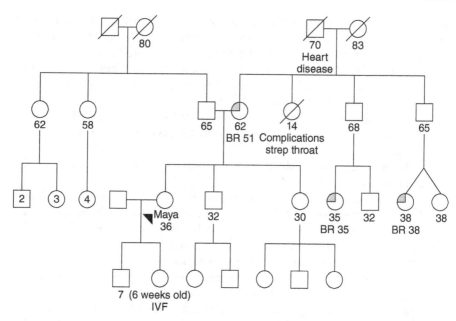

FIGURE 9.1. Maya's pedigree. This client was offered genetic testing to look for mutations in the *BRCA1* and *BRCA2* genes, which are associated with hereditary breast–ovarian cancer syndrome. (See the text for further discussion of this case.) BR = breast cancer, invasive; IVF = *in vitro* fertilization.

"I understand this reasoning," said Maya in a soft but assured voice. "However, my relatives live a fair distance away from any of the major cities in India. I know they would agree to be tested but arranging it would be difficult for them. My mother is coming to visit us this summer, but that's not for several months. I think I'd rather go forward with the tests myself." The husband nodded in agreement and said that he thought it was important for them to learn this information.

The genetic counselor described the genetic testing process. The couple understood the possible test results as well as the inherent limitations of testing an unaffected individual. The counselor also reminded the couple that they could delay testing and explored whether the recent birth of their baby might make it more difficult to receive a positive test result.

"No, I see it differently. I am doing this for my daughter. Knowledge is power." Maya held up her sleeping daughter and gave her a kiss. Her husband nodded in agreement.

The genetic counselor went through the informed consent form, ascertained the patient's insurance coverage, and made arrangements for a blood specimen to be drawn that day. She explained that she would call Maya with the results. She also offered to set up an appointment for Maya to meet with the program breast oncologist to discuss the hormonal risk factors, but Maya preferred to wait until the *BRCA* results were back.

Eighteen days later, the counselor contacted Maya at her work number. Maya greeted her hurriedly and said, "OK, what are the results, I'm ready to hear—is it positive or negative?"

"Well, actually it is a little more complicated than that. The *BRCA1* gene came back negative. But you were found to have a DNA variant in the *BRCA2* gene."

After a short pause, Maya said, "A variant result; that is one of the inconclusive results, correct?"

"That is correct," affirmed the counselor. "It is a missense change that the laboratory has not seen before. It may turn out to be a normal DNA variation or it may turn out to be a deleterious mutation. Most *BRCA* variants turn out to have no clinical significance."

"But some of them turn out to be deleterious?" persisted Maya.

"That is also correct," agreed the counselor. "Some *BRCA* variants are eventually reclassified as deleterious mutations."

The counselor brought a copy of the test result to Maya's lab and agreed to meet with the couple that afternoon. At that visit, they discussed the *BRCA2* variant result at length and compared published articles regarding similar variant results. The counselor reminded them that it was not unusual for variants to be found in less commonly tested ethnic groups.

The counselor broached the option of testing other relatives. "It would be helpful to determine whether this variant is tracking with the cases of breast cancer in the family. Do you think that your mother would be willing to be tested?"

"Yes I'm sure she would be willing," said Maya.

"You said the lab would test her for the variant at no charge, is that correct?" queried the husband.

"Yes, that is true. But I actually think it would be helpful for your mother to have comprehensive *BRCA* testing. If she were to have a different *BRCA* mutation, then that would be useful information for the family—and it might lower the likelihood that this *BRCA2* variant result is deleterious," explained the counselor.

Several months later, Maya's mother came in to meet with the genetic counselor, accompanied by her son-in-law who also acted as the interpreter. The patient's mother seemed to have a good understanding of why she was being tested and she granted permission for the results to be disclosed to her daughter or son-in-law.

A few weeks later, the genetic counselor called Maya with her mother's test results. The mother was also found to carry the *BRCA2* variant result. Maya and her husband came in for another discussion about the genetic test results. The counselor stressed that the Lab still did not have sufficient information to reclassify the variant result. While the husband expounded on possible ways to study the BRCA variant, the counselor noticed that Maya seemed to be quieter and less attentive to the conversation compared with prior visits.

The counselor turned the conversation toward the emotional implications of the inconclusive variant result. She remarked that this type of uncertain result could be more stressful than a positive result and asked how Maya was feeling about it.

At first Maya said she was fine but then she admitted that she was feeling upset and frustrated by the whole situation. Her husband put his arm around her as she spoke about her years of infertility treatments—the agonizing roller coaster of emotions and all the ambiguous test results along the way. "This brings it all back. The worry, the uncertainty, the waiting. Why can't anything be simple?"

Maya also said that her reluctance to meet with the breast oncologist stemmed from her fear that she was at increased risk for developing breast cancer. "Meeting with the oncologist would make it real—it would say that I truly am at increased risk and my daughter is also at increased risk. It may not be logical, but that is how I feel."

The genetic counselor listened attentively. Afterwards they explored ways to help reduce Maya's distress regarding the inconclusive result. The counselor offered to talk to the breast oncologist and obtain medical recommendations on Maya's behalf. Maya seemed relieved by this plan and promised to meet with the breast oncologist at some point.

Maya and her husband also agreed to temporarily shelve discussions of the variant result. The counselor encouraged them to contact her if they had any questions and promised to contact them if she learned any updates about the variant result.

"I hope we get more information soon," said the husband with a sigh. "Otherwise, it is tempting to see about doing the lab work ourselves."

"One grant at a time, dear," said Maya dryly.

Case 9 wrap-up: This case describes a counselor disclosing a variant result and helping the client deal with its medical and emotional impact.

Case 10: "How can I have a syndrome if I don't have the gene?"

Elizabeth was in the midst of getting her sixth chemotherapy treatment when she met with the genetic counselor.

"Call me Liz," said the patient as she set aside her book and removed her reading glasses. The counselor recognized the book as one that she had recently read and they spent the first few minutes chatting about the entertaining plotline and quirky characters. They then shifted to discussing the family history and the option of genetic testing.

Liz had been diagnosed with Stage II right-sided colon cancer at age 52—2 years after a normal screening colonoscopy. She had undergone a complete hysterectomy at age 35 due to severe endometriosis. Her mother had been diagnosed with uterine cancer at age 40 but was doing well in her eighties. The maternal grandfather and a maternal uncle had both died from colon cancer in their fifties. Liz's diagnosis of cancer was the first in her generation but her brother, age 48, was found to have a large adenoma in his right colon. The completed pedigree certainly looked like a textbook example of Lynch syndrome! (See Fig. 9.2.)

The genetic counselor described the features of Lynch syndrome and explained that Liz's family met clinical criteria for the condition. Liz expressed concern about her niece and nephews. She said that she would probably not tell her mother about it. "My mother would be sad to learn she might have passed it on to us," said Liz. "But I will share the news with everyone else."

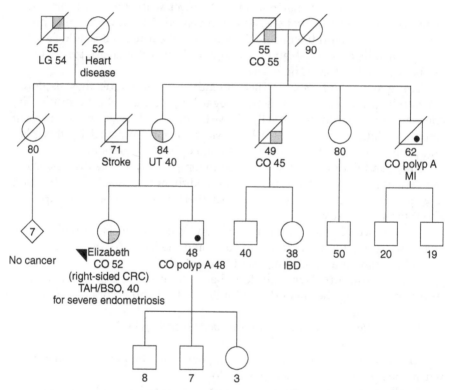

FIGURE 9.2. Elizabeth's pedigree. This client was offered tumor block and blood DNA studies to look for mutations in one of the mismatch repair genes associated with Lynch syndrome. (See the text for further discussion of this case.) CRC = colorectal cancer; IBD = inflammatory bowel disease; LG = lung cancer; CO = colon cancer; CO polyp A = colorectal adenoma; UT = uterine cancer; TAH/BSO = total abolominal hysterectomy with bilateral salpingo-oopherectomy.

The counselor arranged for Liz to be tested for the *MLH1*, *MSH2*, and *MSH6* genes. They arranged to meet again in 3 weeks at Liz' next chemotherapy visit to discuss the results.

The DNA test results did not detect a deleterious mutation in the *MLH1*, *MSH2*, and *MSH6* genes. Liz beamed with relief at the news. The counselor stressed that Liz (and her family) still had Lynch syndrome despite the negative test results. She also discussed the option of doing additional genetic tests.

Liz seemed to understand the limitations of the indeterminate negative results and gave permission for the counselor to obtain a tumor block specimen for the purposes of performing microsatellite (MSI) and IHC analyses.

As the counselor rose to leave, Liz said happily, "I can't wait to tell my brother that we don't have that gene problem! He will be so relieved that he doesn't have to worry about his kids."

The counselor sat back down again. Again she endeavored to explain that in all likelihood the family did have some kind of "gene problem" but that these tests were not able to find it. The counselor told Liz that there were additional genes that could cause Lynch syndrome and that the tumor block analyses might be able to help pinpoint where the genetic error might be. In the meantime, everyone in the family should probably follow the guidelines for people with Lynch syndrome.

Over the next few months, the counselor had several conversations with Liz. The tumor block analysis revealed an MSI-high result, which is highly suggestive of an inherited tumor, and the IHC result showed an absence of the *MSH2* and *PMS2* genes. The patient underwent *PMS2* testing, which also came back negative. Once again, the patient expressed great joy about the negative result and once again the counselor tried hard to explain why the negative result was not really "good news."

Liz's oncologist and surgeon both recommended that Liz have a total colectomy. Liz was initially resistant to this plan but a follow-up colonoscopy identified two small flat adenomas in the cecum and these findings convinced her to have a complete colectomy.

The program gastroenterologist also stressed the importance of annual colonoscopies for adult members of the family and uterine cancer screening for all at-risk female relatives. The genetic counselor and gastroenterologist wrote a summary letter to Liz as well as a family letter that urged all at-risk family members to follow the monitoring guidelines for people with Lynch syndrome.

About a year later the counselor met with Liz to discuss *EPCAM* (*TACSTD1*) gene testing. She began to discuss the test in more detail but Liz interrupted her and said that by now she knew the process. What she really wanted to know was whether the counselor had read a historical biography that had recently hit the bestseller list. The counselor admitted that she had not read it yet and asked if Liz would recommend it. Liz had lots of complaints about the book but ultimately recommended it. The counselor recognized that Liz enjoyed the break from all the medical conversations and promised to read the book and let Liz know what she thought about it. She then went through a curtailed conversation about the *TACSTD1* gene and arranged for Liz to have blood drawn and sent to a different genetics laboratory. As they wrapped up the brief session, the counselor asked if Liz had any other questions.

"My oncologist still seems to think I have that Lynch syndrome. So does my surgeon. Can you talk to them?" said Liz.

In a gentle but firm tone of voice, the counselor replied, "Your doctors believe that you *do* have Lynch syndrome. I do too. There are five members of your family over three generations who have had colon cancer or uterine cancer. That tells us that you and your family do have Lynch syndrome."

"How can I have a syndrome if I don't have the gene?" asked Liz in a puzzled tone of voice.

The counselor realized that her natural tendency to use qualifying words like "probably" and "seems to" was contributing to the patient's confusion. "You do have an error in one of your genes. The Lab hasn't found it yet but there is a genetic error in your family."

"But you've looked at all those genes and they came back fine," Liz argued.

"That's true," agreed the counselor, "and that does make it confusing. Here is what your results mean: either the problem is in one of the genes we have already looked at but it cannot be detected by current technologies *or* the error is in a different gene that we haven't looked at yet. That is why we keep inviting you to have more genetic tests. The tests keep getting better and the researchers keep finding more genes, like the *TACSTD1* gene that we are testing you for today. Does that make sense?"

"I guess it makes sense," said Liz slowly. "In other words, it is just like one of those books in a series." 'To be continued. . . . '

"That is exactly right," said the counselor as she booked Liz's next visit. "Plus, we can talk about the next book on your list. Maybe you can give me a hint as to what you've chosen..."

Liz said with a laugh, "Not a chance. This way we are both waiting for news."

Case 10 wrap-up: This case describes the disclosure of negative results and finding ways to convey what it means (and doesn't mean).

Case 11: "I wanted an answer—but did it have to be this one?"

The genetic counselor met with Jon's parents, Ellen and Greg. The first thing the counselor noticed was that the parents had the bewildered "deer in the headlights" look of individuals whose children are newly diagnosed with cancer. She opened the session by asking how their son was doing.

"Better than we are," said Ellen with a wan smile.

"He seems to be doing alright," said Greg in a guarded tone of voice. "But we are still waiting for the results of the latest computed tomography (CT) scan."

About 4 weeks ago, their 9-year-old son, Jon, had been diagnosed with an osteosarcoma of the femur. The parents initially thought that their son had bruised his leg during a soccer match. However, when the pain worsened, they took their son to the emergency room of a local hospital, which found the tumor and transferred Jon to the pediatric unit of the cancer center. When the pediatric oncologist learned that there was a family history of cancer, she referred the family for genetic counseling.

The genetic counselor took the family history information. Greg and Ellen were both cancer free in their thirties. Ellen reported no history of cancer on his side of the family, but Greg reported that a paternal uncle had died at age 2 from a brain tumor and a paternal aunt had died from breast cancer in her thirties. This aunt's daughter had also developed breast cancer in her thirties and had recently tested negative for BRCA mutations. Greg's father had died from throat cancer at age 40. The father had smoked cigarettes, but the counselor noted the earlier-than-usual age of diagnosis.

Once the family history information was complete (see Fig. 9.3), the counselor explained that Jon's cancer might be due to an inherited susceptibility. She talked about the features of the family tree that suggested a genetic link—the ages of onset, the types of cancer, and the cancers over three generations.

The genetic counselor mentioned that Greg's family—and Jon—might have a rare hereditary cancer syndrome termed LFS. The counselor described the option of genetic testing and reviewed the pros and cons of TP53 testing. She stressed that this test could be done at a later time or not at all; but the parents were eager to proceed with the test.

The counselor asked what the couple hoped to gain from the genetic test results. The parents spoke of the oncologist's concern about radiation therapy but mainly spoke of wanting an explanation for why this happened.

"I want to do whatever I can to help Jon. And I am looking for an answer. So if the answer is an altered gene, I want to know that. I've also been scouring the Internet for possible environmental causes. I mean, how can we protect our family if we don't know what caused the cancer in the first place?" said Greg.

The counselor began to say that most cases of cancer were not linked to a single cause but was interrupted by Ellen who said, "Oh we know that. Still, if there *is* an answer, we want to find it out. We need to know how best to take care of our son—and our daughter."

The counselor informed the parents about the limitations of genetic testing and that uncertainties would remain regardless of the results. After

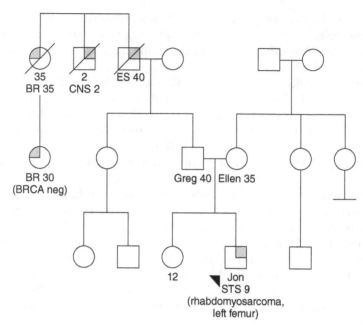

FIGURE 9.3. Jon's pedigree. This family was offered genetic testing to look for germline mutations in the *TP53* gene, which is associated with LFS. (See the text for further discussion of this case.) BR = breast cancer, invasive; CNS = brain tumor, unspecified type; ES = esophogeal cancer; STS = soft tissue sarcoma.

a detailed discussion, the parents signed consent for their son to undergo *TP53* testing and a blood specimen was drawn and sent to the genetics laboratory.

Four weeks later, the genetic counselor disclosed the positive *TP53* results to Jon's parents. Ellen and Greg expressed disappointment at the news but their reactions seemed somewhat muted. The counselor conjectured that the couple might still be emotionally drained from their son's cancer diagnosis. As the counselor considered ways to discuss the impact of the news, Greg abruptly changed the subject by asking if he and Ellen could be tested for the *TP53* mutation that day. It seemed to be easier for the couple to deal with tangible actions rather than feelings at this point, especially if they thought it might be useful for their children. The counselor suggested that Greg be tested first for the *TP53* mutation (since he had a higher chance of testing positive). However, Ellen and Greg were adamant about being tested that day, so the counselor made the appropriate arrangements. The counselor asked them what their reactions would be if one of them (likely Greg) tested positive.

Greg shrugged his shoulders. "We will deal with the news whatever it is. The important thing is that we gather as much information as we can."

Ellen added, "That's right—we need to get as many answers as we can. I feel like it is the responsible thing to do."

The counselor asked Greg about his possible emotional reactions to a positive result but he responded with, "Oh, it will be fine." The counselor paused to see if Greg would expand on that statement, but he did not. Given all that the couple was dealing with at the moment, it was possible that they were unable to articulate their emotional reactions.

As predicted, Greg was found to carry the *TP53* mutation. The parents accepted the news stoically at first but Ellen became teary at the thought that her daughter might also be at high risk. "I wanted an answer—but did it have to be this one?" "I know," said Greg. "I thought it would help to know why Jon got cancer. But now I'm not sure."

Greg put his arm around Ellen as they discussed the result—and its implications—with the counselor. The couple still seemed uncomfortable (with unable) to articulating their emotional reactions. Rather, they were interested in figuring out how to share the news with their children and other relatives. The counselor offered some potential strategies for disclosing the results to the family, but encouraged the couple to first take some time to process the information themselves.

Jon's clinical course was not easy, but he tolerated the chemotherapy reasonably well and his tumor was resected successfully. The genetic counselor left a few telephone messages for the family, but she did not hear from them. A few months later, the counselor met up with Greg at one of Jon's follow-up appointments. Greg was in much better spirits at this visit. Jon was doing well and was back in school. He was even talking about rejoining the soccer team in the spring.

The counselor was happy to hear that things were "returning back to normal" for the family. She knew that the parents were vigilant about Jon's health and had informed all of his physicians about the positive *TP53* result. However, Greg had yet to follow up on any of the recommended appointments or screening tests.

During a lull in the conversation, the genetic counselor said, "One of my jobs is to review the information so it doesn't get forgotten. I am very glad to hear that your son is doing so well—that is excellent news." She then looked at Greg. "Now I'd like to spend a few minutes focusing on . . . "

"My daughter," interjected Greg. "I guess it is time to consider the option of testing her. To be honest I haven't thought about it at all since our last conversation."

The counselor said, "Well, we can certainly talk about the option of testing your daughter for the familial *TP53* mutation, but first, I would like to talk about *your* health."

Greg admitted that he had been too busy to set up any appointments for himself and launched into a description of his hectic schedule.

"I understand that—but now that things are starting to settle down a little it seems like a good time for you to focus on your own health. We talked about so many things when we last spoke, it may have been a bit overwhelming. How about we make an appointment for you to meet with one of the oncologists in our High-Risk Program? She has lots of experience taking care of people with LFS. You could also discuss the other screening recommendations with her. And you and I could talk again as well."

"That sounds like a good plan. I keep telling my son how important these doctor's appointments are. Guess I'd better follow my own advice," said Greg with a sigh.

Case 11 wrap-up: This case describes a counselor disclosing a positive test result and helping the family deal with its ramifications.

9.5. FURTHER READING

American Cancer Society. Genetic testing: what you need to know. http://www.cancer.org.

Baty, BJ. 2009. Risk communication and decision-making. In Uhlmann, WR, Schuette, JL, and Yashar, BM (eds), A Guide to Genetic Counseling, 2nd edition. Wiley-Blackwell, Hoboken NJ, 207–250.

Dizon, DS, and Abu-Rustum, NR. 2006. Prevention, screening and advocacy. In 100 Questions & Answers about Ovarian Cancer, 2nd edition. Jones & Bartlett, Sudbury, MA, 122.

Faucett, WA, and Ward, PA. 2009. Understanding genetic testing. In Uhlmann, WR, Schuette, JL, and Yashar, BM (eds), A Guide to Genetic Counseling, 2nd edition. Wiley-Blackwell, Hoboken, NJ, 207–250.

Geller, G, Botkin, JR, Green, MJ, et al. 1997. Genetic testing for susceptibility to adult-onset cancer: the process and content of informed consent. JAMA 277: 1467–1474.

GeneTests: Medical Genetics Information Resource (online database). University of Washington, Seattle. 1993–2011. Available at http://www.genetests.org.

Lindor, NM, McMaster, ML, Lindor, CJ, et al. 2008. Concise Handbook of Familial Cancer Susceptibility Syndromes—second edition. J Natl Cancer Inst Monogr 38:1–93.

Resta, R. 2009. Before the call. J Genet Counsel 18:12.

Uhlmann, W. 2009. Thinking it all through: case preparation and management. In Uhlmann, WR, Schuette, JL, and Yashar, BM (eds), A Guide to Genetic Counseling, 2nd edition. Wiley-Blackwell, Hoboken, NJ, 93–132.

United States Department of Health and Human Services. Genetic information non-discrimination act (GINA). http://www.genome.gov.

Veach, PM, LeRoy, BS, and Bartels, DM. 2003. Collaborating with clients: providing information and assisting in client decision making. In Facilitating the Genetic Counseling Process: A Practice Manual. Springer, New York, 122–149.

Weil, J. 2000a. Cancer risk counseling. In Psychosocial Genetic Counseling. Oxford University Press, New York, 168–181.

Weil, J. 2000b. Decision making. In Psychosocial Genetic Counseling. Oxford University Press, New York, 137–152.

PSYCHOSOCIAL ASPECTS OF CANCER COUNSELING

> A number of words such as "joining," "mutuality," "attunement" and "empathy" have been used to describe the effective [genetic counselor–patient] relationship. To illustrate further it can be likened to a dance where the task of the professional is to be "in step" with the patient and not vice versa.
>
> *(Evans, 2006, p. 75)*

To be effective, cancer risk counselors need to focus on the informational aspects *and* the psychosocial aspects of counseling sessions. This chapter describes the types of psychosocial issues that clients may have, presents genetic counseling strategies for effectively dealing with these issues, and discusses when and how to make psychosocial referrals. The chapter ends with three case examples.

10.1. THE PSYCHOSOCIAL FEATURES OF CLIENTS

This section considers the psychosocial impact of cancer risk from the client's point of view, focusing on emotional responses, coping strategies, and family issues. This section also discusses how these factors might affect various aspects of the client's life, as well as the genetic counseling interactions.

10.1.1. COMMON EMOTIONAL RESPONSES

Clients may exhibit a range of emotional reactions as they grapple with learning their heightened cancer risks and options for genetic testing or

Counseling About Cancer, Third Edition. Katherine A. Schneider.
© 2012 Wiley-Blackwell. Published 2012 by John Wiley & Sons, Inc.

cancer surveillance. These emotional responses can be broadly categorized as either pleasant (e.g., relief, joy) or unpleasant (e.g., fear, anger). Given the topics being discussed, it is not surprising that cancer genetic counseling sessions elicit far more unpleasant than pleasant reactions in clients.

It is important to recognize that clients can display multiple (even conflicting) emotions throughout the genetic counseling and testing process. The extent to which these emotional responses impact the counseling interactions depends upon several factors, including:

- the intensity of the client's emotions
- the extent to which the client feels threatened
- the types of coping strategies that are triggered by the emotional reactions (See Section 10.1.2 for more information about coping strategies.)

Cancer risk clients may exhibit the emotional responses presented in the succeeding sections (also see Table 10.1).

10.1.1.1. Anger

Clients may feel angry about their increased cancer risks or the uncertainties, with which they live. This anger may present as nonspecific hostility or may be displaced onto a specific target, such as the "messenger" (e.g., counselor) or a trivial annoyance (e.g., scheduling problems). Clients may express their anger through the use of sarcastic comments or barbed humor. Expressions of anger are often an attempt to relieve anxiety or stave off depression.

TABLE 10.1. COMMON EMOTIONAL REACTIONS OF CANCER GENETIC COUNSELING CLIENTS

- Anger
- Anxiety
- Fear of disfigurement and disability
- Fear of dying
- Grief
- Guilt and shame
- Loss of control
- Resiliency and other pleasant emotions
- Sadness
- Sense of identity
- Sense of isolation
- Stress and trauma

Clients who feel as though anger is not a socially acceptable emotion may try to disguise or ignore their feelings. Over time, clients who inadequately deal with their feelings of anger may end up turning these emotions inwards toward themselves, thus engendering feelings of guilt and shame.

10.1.1.2. Anxiety

All high-risk individuals experience some degree of anxiety about developing cancer. A certain amount of anxiety is appropriate and even expected in clients as they face their cancer fears during doctor's appointments, screening tests, and genetic counseling appointments. In fact, it may be beneficial to have a certain level of anxiety, since it can motivate people to undergo appropriate cancer surveillance. However, some clients have anxieties about cancer that are pervasive and constant. Excessive anxiety can have a paralyzing effect on clients, leading to an avoidance of screening practices or a denial of symptoms. Severe anxiety may be manifested in a number of ways, including insomnia, hypochondria, phobias, eating disorders, or a general withdrawal from daily activities. In extreme cases, clients have made their high-risk status the focal point of all that is wrong in their lives. Thus, they may blame their unhappiness on their fears of cancer rather than the actual source of anxiety (e.g., job stress, unhappy marriage). This is termed displacement anxiety.

10.1.1.3. Fear of Disfigurement and Disability

A client's fear of cancer may be focused on the physical effects of the cancer disease and/or treatment. These concerns include fears about hair loss, scars, excised organs, loss of energy, or diminished mental capacity. Clients may worry about being a burden to their families, because they would no longer be able to work or would have decreased strength or mobility. These fears may be heightened in clients who have taken care of one or more relatives with cancer. Clients may or may not be able to articulate their fears about disfigurement and disability, but the intensity of these fears will almost certainly impact their decisions about cancer screening and genetic testing.

10.1.1.4. Fear of Dying

A fear of death is a universal emotion, but the level of one's fear can vary widely in terms of intensity and intrusiveness, which is the degree to which a particular fear intrudes on one's thoughts during daily activities. A person's fear of death may be intensified by being at increased risk for cancer or by his or her past experiences with cancer (e.g., having watched relatives die of cancer). Clients who are parents may also express fears about dying while their children are still too young to take care of themselves. Having a certain level of fear about dying of cancer may motivate people to be extra vigilant about their health. However, too much fear can lead to hypochondria, risk-taking behaviors, or a never-ending search for something to protect them from developing cancer.

10.1.1.5. Grief

Successful grieving follows a continuum, with the most painful memories occurring near the time of the loss followed by a gradual distancing from the loss over time. Clients frequently display feelings of grief for relatives who have died of cancer even if the losses occurred long ago. These clients may have experienced several cancer-related deaths, which may have led to incomplete cycles of grieving. Incomplete grieving is more likely to occur in certain situations, such as when a loss has occurred suddenly or unexpectedly. (See Table 10.2.) Unresolved grief reactions can, over time, lead to a veneer of a chronic sadness that overshadows all other activities. This phenomenon is termed chronic sorrow.

10.1.1.6. Guilt and Shame

Experiencing one or more adverse events can trigger feelings of guilt and shame. Examples of adverse events include abusive situations, serious car accidents, or chronic illnesses. People typically have little or no control over an adverse event; however, they may feel as though they could or should have done something different to try and change the outcome. This type of guilt is frequently present in people with family histories of cancer. Clients may feel that they could have done more for their affected relatives by taking them to different physicians or visiting them more often. These internal feelings of guilt may lessen as time goes by or may intensify into shame, which is the feeling that others would harshly judge one's actions or thoughts.

TABLE 10.2. Types of Losses That Are More Likely to Cause Incomplete Grieving Among Clients

---

- The client's loss was sudden or unexpected
- The client's loss occurred in a significant relative (e.g., parent, sibling, or child)
- The client's loss occurred when he or she was too young to process it
- The client's loss has been compounded by other losses, which cause the grief process to begin again
- The client's loss occurred in an individual with whom the client had emotional difficulties or some type of unfinished business
- The client's loss was not discussed in the family either during or after the experience

---

Source: Gettig (2010, p. 112).

People who experience this type of guilt and shame often rehash past events via internal dialogues or repetitive thoughts, which can ultimately lead to lowered self-esteem and even self-loathing. Cancer counseling clients who feel guilt and shame may be reluctant to share certain aspects of their family history information or they may be unusually sensitive to any implied criticisms of their prior actions. Clients who are free from cancer or the familial gene mutation may also feel guilty when contrasting their own good fortune with other relatives who have cancer or the gene mutation. This phenomenon is termed survivor guilt.

10.1.1.7. Loss of Control

People at increased risk for cancer have little to no control over whether or when a malignancy will occur. Living with this type of uncertainty can cause intense feelings of distress and vulnerability. This in turn may cause lowered self-esteem and an inability to cope with day-to-day activities. In an effort to feel less helpless or vulnerable, some high-risk individuals seek as much information as possible about ways to prevent cancer while others spend as little time as possible thinking about their risks of cancer. In the counseling discussions, clients who are struggling with control issues may either lash out at counselors or emotionally withdraw from the discussions. Clients may also seek alternative ways to manage their feelings of vulnerability by turning to holistic remedies, spiritual practices, or addictive substances.

10.1.1.8. Resiliency and Pleasant Emotions

Clients with significant histories of cancer may have developed of resiliency. Clients may feel that they have the inner strength and fortitude to face their risks of cancer because they have survived previous adverse events. These clients may feel empowered by learning information about their cancer risks and medical management options. Cancer counseling clients may also display one or more pleasant emotions, including:

- *Relief*—that someone is finally listening to them
- *Hope*—that their risks are not as high as they think
- *Comfort*—that they will be cared for by excellent providers
- *Encouragement*—that they have developed a plan of action

10.1.1.9. Sadness

High-risk individuals often live with underlying feelings of sadness regarding the past illnesses or deaths in their family as well as their own risks of cancer. A client's sadness might be due to feelings of fear, grief, and vulnerability. Clients may also experience bitterness or resentment that their family must face such trials and tribulations while other families do not. The knowledge that one is at increased risk for developing cancer can negatively affect many types of life experiences (See Section 10.1.4). Over time, these persistent feelings of sadness may manifest as clinical depression or feelings of hopelessness.

10.1.1.10. Sense of Identity

Individuals with genetic disorders, including hereditary cancer syndromes, may feel defined by their aberrant genes. This might inspire some high-risk individuals to join the fight against cancer by becoming advocates, researchers, or health-care providers. However, more frequently, a cancer-focused sense of self engenders feelings of helplessness and isolation that over time can lead to lowered self-esteem and self-worth. While a positive genetic test result can exacerbate a person's cancer-focused identity, a person with a true negative test result may feel lost or unsettled as their sense of identity (i.e., one who will develop an inherited cancer) is proven false.

10.1.1.11. Sense of Isolation

People with high cancer risks have to face concerns that may be distinctly unique from their partner, friends, or coworkers. This is especially true for young people. Even their physicians may be unfamiliar with a family's rare hereditary cancer syndrome. This can cause clients to feel as though no one can truly understand their fears and concerns. These feelings of isolation can cause clients to feel unsupported, anxious, or vulnerable.

10.1.1.12. Stress and Trauma

Clients with personal or family experiences with cancer may continue to rehash (and even relive) their ordeals. Over time, the grief caused by the multiple illnesses and losses in families can be traumatizing. Clients may report depression, anxiety disorders, sleep disturbances, or physical ailments. In fact, some clients in families with hereditary cancer syndromes may show signs of posttraumatic stress disorder (PTSD). Clients with PTSD may display agitation at the recall of certain events or they may withdraw completely from the discussions.

10.1.2. POSSIBLE COPING STRATEGIES

Individuals rely on coping strategies to help them deal with adverse (anxiety-provoking) situations. Adverse situations will trigger a specific emotional response in a person, which he or she handles by use of a learned coping strategy. Thus, client responses that seem to occur out of the blue or make little sense may indicate that the client is invoking the use of a coping strategy to manage his or her intense emotional reactions.

Christine Evans, a psychotherapist, writes that people invoke their personal coping strategies to answer the three following questions (2006, p. 28):

- How do I see this problem?
- How do I deal with the feelings that are triggered by this problem?
- What can I do to resolve this problem?

Coping strategies, therefore, contain both an emotional aspect and a cognitive aspect. The emotional aspect of coping is responsible for assessing, containing, and reducing the distress caused by an anxiety-provoking situation. Examples of emotion-focused strategies include commiserating with friends, listening to music, or going to the gym. The cognitive aspect of coping is responsible for analyzing the situation, sorting through possible solutions, and deciding how best to resolve the situation. These cognitive-focused strategies will only kick in once the person's emotional distress is at a manageable level. Examples of cognitive-focused strategies include seeking advice, making plans, or reading "self-help" books.

Individuals develop their cadre of coping strategies based on past experiences and the success (or failure) of previously tried coping strategies. Coping strategies are continually evolving and are an important part of normal functioning. It is worth noting that the success of a coping strategy may be based on its ability to provide immediate emotional relief rather than its ability to resolve problems, successfully.

Coping strategies can be either adaptive (healthy responses to a stressful situation) or maladaptive (inappropriate and potentially harmful responses). Almost all coping strategies can be either adaptive or maladaptive depending on their context and degree of use. For example, the use of magical thinking can range from the harmless practice of wearing a lucky shirt to a feared medical appointment to delusions that one's cancer can only be cured by aliens from space.

Cancer risk clients may demonstrate a variety of coping strategies during the cancer genetic counseling and testing discussions. These coping strategies are described below. (Also see Table 10.3.)

10.1.2.1. Accepting Responsibility

Individuals who seek appointments in high-risk clinics may feel as though this is the responsible thing for them to do. Taking responsibility for one's own health allows people to feel somewhat in control in terms of whether they develop cancer. Thus, they faithfully maintain their surveillance

TABLE 10.3. TYPES OF COPING STRATEGIES THAT MAY BE EMPLOYED BY CANCER COUNSELING CLIENTS

- Accepting responsibility
- Anxious preoccupation
- Cognitive avoidance
- Confrontational approach
- Denial (includes distraction, disbelief, deferral, and dismissal)
- Displacement
- Distancing
- Escape–avoidance
- Fatalism
- Fighting spirit
- Humor
- Intellectualism
- Magical thinking
- Obsessions and compulsions
- Planning
- Positive reappraisal
- Projection
- Rationalization
- Regression
- Relying on social support
- Relying on spiritual or holistic practices
- Seeking approval from caregivers
- Self-controlling
- Stoic acceptance

Source: Weil (2000); Djurdjinovic (2009).

schedules and pursue options that reduce their risks of cancer. However, this strategy can also cause people to be less empathetic toward relatives who develop or die from cancer. This so-called blame the victim mentality allows clients to psychologically distance themselves from their own concerns about developing cancer. Alternatively, individuals may feel responsible for adverse events (e.g., cancer-related illnesses or deaths) that are out of their control, which can ultimately lead to self-criticism, guilt, or shame.

10.1.2.2. Anxious Preoccupation

Some clients seem to be consumed by their worries about cancer. These clients spend an enormous amount of time and energy worrying about the possibility that they will develop cancer someday. This type of obsessive brooding can lead to somaticizing thoughts, phobias, hypochondriachial behaviors, insomnia, panic attacks, or full-blown anxiety disorders.

10.1.2.3. Cognitive Avoidance

Cognitive avoidance is the suppression of thoughts about adverse situations that are frightening or overwhelming. This is a useful strategy that gives individuals the space to avoid thinking about a perceived threat until they are emotionally ready to handle it. Note that cognitive avoidance differs from denial in that the individual acknowledges the existence of the adverse situation, but consciously chooses not to think about it. Cognitive avoidance can be used as a temporary measure that allows people to control their emotions before employing cognitive-focused strategies to resolve the issue. Cognitive avoidance can also be used when there is nothing more one can do at that time (such as the people who quell their cancer worries while in-between their regular screening appointments.)

10.1.2.4. Confrontational Approach

Some individuals seem to think that the only way for them to get appropriate care is to "fight" their way through the medical system. Such clients may berate staff members scheduling appointments, make frequent (or unrealistic) demands on health-care providers, and argue about the accuracy of the information presented to them. Genetic counselors should keep in mind that clients who are confrontational or combative typically use these strategies to lessen feelings of anxiety, helplessness, or vulnerability.

10.1.2.5. Denial

Denial is the repression of something that is unpleasant or unwanted. Clients who are acutely frightened about developing cancer may try to ignore or refute any statements suggesting that they are at risk. Manifestations of denial can include the nondisclosure of information (such as forgetting to mention certain relatives with cancer) or brushing aside the genetic counselor's interpretation of risk. For example, a client may say: "Yes, my two uncles had gastrointestinal stromal tumors, but I'm sure it was because they ate lots of spicy food, not because of a gene mutation." Counselors need to recognize that a certain level of denial can be a helpful coping strategy. Some people who state that they will "never get cancer" are simply expressing their optimism and hope. On the other hand, clients who declare that they will never get cancer—and also refuse to seek medical care for appropriate screening or evaluation—may be operating under denial.

There are several distinctive versions of denial, including the following four types:

- *Distraction*—In this coping strategy, the client attempts to shift the conversation to avoid a topic that is anxiety provoking. For example, a client might say, "I know we are talking about my risk of colon cancer, but what did you think about the news that scientists have found an antiaging gene?"

- *Disbelief*—In this coping strategy, the client hears but does not accept the information because it is too emotionally distressing to process. This coping strategy allows clients to maintain a shred of hope that the information is wrong, while at the same time preparing themselves to accept the "bad news." As an example, a small number of clients who receive positive genetic test results will insist on being retested. Even though the second test will invariably confirm the initial result, it has given the client some extra time to come to terms with the news.

- *Deferral*—This strategy implies that clients accept the information at face value but do not seem to absorb all of its implications. This strategy keeps people from becoming emotionally and mentally overwhelmed. For example, upon disclosure of a positive *MSH2* genetic test result, a client might say, "Wow, I sure have a high risk of colon cancer. Thank goodness my last colonoscopy was clear so I'm all set for the next 10 years."

- *Dismissal*—In this strategy, the client directly—and often angrily—challenges the credibility of the information or even the competence of the provider. This strategy gives clients an excuse to end interactions that have become too uncomfortable or intense. For example, a client who is distressed by the idea of *BRCA* testing might fume that "I came here to find out about my risk of pancreatic cancer and now you tell me I should be tested for a breast cancer gene. What is this—some kind of scam?"

10.1.2.6. Displacement

In this coping strategy, feelings toward one person (or situation) are directed toward another person. This is a situation commonly experienced in genetic counseling. Clients who are angry or distressed by their increased cancer risks may redirect these emotions toward a health-care provider or an aspect of the testing process. For example, a client may express anger that his genetic test result is not available when initially promised, but his anger likely stems from the anxiety that he might have a gene mutation. In addition, some clients may find it easier to gather information on behalf of other relatives rather than to acknowledge that it pertains to them as well. For example, a client with children might say, "My two sisters are really concerned about their children. Are my nieces and nephews at increased risk for getting cancer?"

10.1.2.7. Distancing

Clients who have experienced significant losses in their lives may utilize a strategy termed distancing. This strategy allows individuals to remain emotionally detached from their past experiences or from other people. Distancing may make it difficult for people to maintain close relationships with partners, family members, or even health-care providers. Clients who seem unfriendly or unwilling to share any personal stories may be employing this strategy.

10.1.2.8. Escape–Avoidance

Individuals who utilize escape–avoidance strategies are trying to protect themselves from adverse situations that invoke strong emotional responses. They may be hoping that the situation goes away or may be hoping for a miracle solution, anything so that they do not have to deal with the situation themselves. Clients who utilize escape–avoidance tactics may continually defer genetic counseling or testing appointments or they may interrupt the cancer risk discussions with unrelated questions or stories. These types of clients are hoping not to hear the information about their cancer risks.

10.1.2.9. Fatalism

High-risk individuals may hold fatalistic views about their chances of developing (and dying from) cancer. In a sense, clients who are fatalistic have accepted their high risks of cancer; however, they have taken it to an extreme and may believe that they are destined to develop cancer regardless of what they do. Thus, they may be less interested in pursuing genetic testing or risk-reduction options than clients who believe it is possible to reduce their cancer risks.

10.1.2.10. Fighting Spirit

Watching close relatives die of cancer can act as a powerful motivator to avoid a similar fate. Utilizing this strategy may cause people to be especially vigilant about their cancer monitoring practices and eager to participate in clinical trials. In some cases, the individuals might choose to become cancer clinicians, researchers, or advocates. A fighting spirit is a useful coping strategy as long as clients feel as though the medical providers are working with them, not against them. In certain cases, clients may feel that they need to battle the health-care system for the services they need or they may focus on nonmedical ways to reduce their cancer risks (e.g., holistic or spiritual practices).

10.1.2.11. Humor

Individuals may utilize dark humor to help them cope with their series of adverse experiences. One client joked, "We don't call them funerals anymore, we call them family reunions." The ability to speak humorously about one's cancer experiences or high-risk status can be a valuable coping strategy. Clients may also interject jokes or sarcasm into the genetic counseling session to relieve their rising tension or to deflect attention from serious topics. Taken to an extreme, clients may use humor in ways that are inappropriate or disruptive.

10.1.2.12. Intellectualism

Some clients feel that the key to controlling their cancer fears is to learn all the information they can, i.e., knowledge is power. The process of gathering information gives people a greater sense of control over, being at increased risk for cancer. For clients utilizing an intellectual coping strategy, the standard discussion of risk estimates is inadequate; they will want to know how these figures were derived and may insist on seeing the original journal citations. This thirst for data may be helpful in that it allows people to feel more in control in regard to their cancer risks. This strategy may also lead to close bonds between clients and the health-care providers who satisfy their need for more information. However, clients can become overwhelmed—and more anxious—by the many facts and figures or they can become frustrated if there is limited information available (which is the case for many of the rare cancer syndromes). Clients who utilize intellectualism may also be trying to avoid how they *feel* about their cancer risks.

10.1.2.13. Magical Thinking

Magical thinking refers to any ideation that is based on fantasy, superstition, or illogical thinking. Magical thinking is often employed to make sense out of a series of frightening experiences. Clients may utilize a type of fallacious reasoning to explain why their cancer risks are increased. For example, a female client might say, "I know I'll get breast cancer like my mother, because I look just like her." Clients may also utilize magical thinking to help them cope with new anxiety-provoking situations, for example, "I want to schedule my mammogram on a Thursday, because that is my lucky day." Bargaining, which can be considered a type of magical thinking, refers to the promises one makes to oneself in the event that a potential threat turns out to be alright. For example, a client might say, "If this genetic test result turns out OK, then I will re-join the gym and take much better care of myself from now on." In most cases, this coping strategy is a temporary way to reduce one's fears, while not interfering with daily functioning or adherence to screening protocols. Taken to an extreme, a person may be delusional or psychotic and are therefore no longer able to distinguish between fantasy and reality.

10.1.2.14. Obsessions and Compulsions

These types of coping strategies are considered maladaptive because they tend to make things worse rather than better. Obsessions and compulsions mask a person's emotional distress and do not foster any cognitive-focused strategies. Thus, the person never actually handles or resolves any type of adverse situation. Examples of obsessions and compulsions include alcohol addictions, anorexia, bulimia, cutting, hair pulling, and obsessive hand washing. These behaviors often have their roots in past traumas and low-self esteem. Obsessive–compulsive disorder (OCD) can also take the form of excessive neatness, cleanliness, or other rituals that help clients to create a sense of order and control.

10.1.2.15. Planning

Some individuals are comforted by creating plans of action for what they would do if they were ever diagnosed with cancer. This might involve seeking consultations with oncologists or discussing "what-if" scenarios with friends. This strategy can help people cope better with their high-risk status, even if they never follow through with the plans they have made. Clients who utilize this strategy may need to be reined in if they continually focus on unlikely or distant events. For example, counselors may need to remind clients who want to discuss experimental therapy options for metastatic disease that they have a cancer predisposition gene, not cancer.

10.1.2.16. Positive Reappraisal

Some individuals have the ability to focus on the positive aspects of past tragic or traumatic experiences. They may feel that these experiences have given them greater self-resilience, a heightened appreciation for life, or closer bonds with family members. These clients may see a positive cancer gene test result as a wake-up call to take better care of their health. Clients who utilize positive reappraisal techniques may be able to adapt to adverse situations better than those who utilize other types of coping strategies.

10.1.2.17. Projection

Projection occurs when people ascribe one of their own undesirable traits to another person. Individuals may utilize this coping strategy when they feel it is too distressing or shameful to admit having similar attitudes or behaviors. For example, a client who has not seen a physician for several years may bemoan the foolishness of a relative who refuses to be screened for cancer. Another example is the client who frets that the genetic counselor does not like him or her when in reality it is the client who dislikes the counselor, because of his or her distressing questions.

10.1.2.18. Rationalization

Rationalization describes the process of giving plausible explanations for a specific action, while the real reason for the behavior is to avoid a distressing situation. Clients may use various excuses to explain why they did not show up for appointments that are emotionally difficult or screening tests that are physically uncomfortable. For example, "I meant to come to the appointment but I got really busy at work that day. Plus I couldn't find the packet of information you sent me about the appointment and I figured I should not come in without it."

10.1.2.19. Regression

Individuals who deal with chronic high-stress situations may revert to the helpless, dependent behavior typical of childhood. This coping strategy allows the individual to feel taken care of and safe during stressful situations. Clients who regress to younger ages may rely on others to schedule the appointments, drive to the medical center, and ask relevant questions of providers. During the counseling session, a client may say "I am not sure what to do. What do you think—should I have the genetic test?" Another client may say "I can't possibly drive into the city by myself. I will have to check and see if my friend can drive me to the appointment."

10.1.2.20. Relying on Social Support

Some high-risk individuals surround themselves with a strong network of relatives and friends. This support network may provide clients with emotional support or other types of support such as child care, meals, or financial assistance. Clients might speak of being especially close to their relatives and friends and they may express their gratitude for the many supportive people in their lives. However, taken to an extreme, clients may develop extra needy personalities, and an overreliance on others, causing friends and relatives to feel burdened or used.

10.1.2.21. Relying on Spiritual or Holistic Practices

Some high-risk individuals rely on their religious or spiritual practices as their main coping strategy. This may involve going to a church, temple, or mosque or may involve personal practices such as meditation, prayer, or yoga. These activities can help individuals to calm their emotions and quiet their minds so that they can begin to deal with the anxiety-provoking situation. Clients may also seek holistic practices to reduce their levels of stress (acupuncture, Reiki, or hypnosis), to boost their immune system (vitamins or green tea), or to help treat cancer (natural remedies). In rare cases, a search for spiritual or holistic practices may lead clients toward fringe cults or harmful practices.

10.1.2.22. Seeking Approval from Caregivers

High-risk individuals may be "model patients," carefully following all suggestions set forth by their health-care providers. This attitude may be viewed as prudent given their cancer risks, but might also reflect a need to obtain approval from their caregivers. This type of coping strategy may increase compliance to screening guidelines, but can exacerbate feelings of dependence and vulnerability if carried to an extreme.

10.1.2.23. Self-Controlling

Individuals who practice this coping strategy seek to control themselves *and* their environment, which includes anyone with whom they come in contact. These controlling clients can provoke a variety of difficult interactions from scheduling appointments on their timetable to providing information to their satisfaction. Individuals who are controlling are often trying to reduce their feelings of vulnerability or helplessness. Self-controlling individuals may also have trouble expressing their emotions or maintaining relationships.

10.1.2.24. Stoic Acceptance

Individuals who experience recurring anxiety-producing situations may adapt to their high-risk status over time. Cancer counseling clients who display stoic acceptance have successfully dealt with the emotional reactions invoked by their high-risk status and they have assimilated the information while not allowing it to monopolize their lives.

10.1.3. The Impact of Clients' Cancer Fears on the Counseling Session

Adverse situations can invoke mild, moderate, or severe levels of anxiety. For example, misplacing one's car in a shopping mall parking lot is mildly anxiety provoking while being in a major motor vehicle accident is extremely anxiety provoking. The level of anxiety invoked by a specific situation helps determine which of the person's coping strategies will be utilized. Mild anxiety levels may actually enhance a person's ability to handle adverse situations while severe anxiety levels tend to trigger feelings of overwhelming fear and stress (which are not conducive to thinking logically or clearly).

Cancer genetic counseling sessions cause some level of anxiety for all clients. Anxiety can be caused by several aspects of the counseling process, including decisions to undergo genetic testing and learning one's genetic test results. (See Table 10.4.) Cancer counseling clients who become highly anxious about the cancer risk discussion (or the idea of such a discussion) may behave in ways that are unproductive, such as:

- Canceling or coming late to appointments
- "Acting out" during the counseling session
- Misinterpreting or disregarding the information given to them
- Utilizing the information in inappropriate ways (e.g., rejecting the screening recommendations or demanding unnecessary screening procedures)

The following factors presented in the succeeding sections may impact a client's level of anxiety during the cancer genetic counseling session.

10.1.3.1. Baseline Anxiety

A client may have cancer-specific fears or a more generalized anxiety disorder; either type of anxiety can contribute to a client's emotional reactions during the counseling discussions. Not surprisingly, clients with high levels of baseline anxiety are more likely to be distressed by the cancer risk discussions compared to nonanxious clients. The counseling session may also trigger other unpleasant emotions such as grief, agitation, or frustration in clients with heightened baseline anxiety.

TABLE 10.4. ANXIETY-PRODUCING ASPECTS OF CANCER GENETIC COUNSELING

- Being referred to a cancer genetic counselor
- Setting up the cancer genetic counseling appointment
- Rehashing all the cancer diagnoses in the family
- Hearing about the increased risks of cancer
- Making decisions about genetic testing
- Awaiting the genetic test results
- Learning the genetic test results
- Considering how to tell relatives about the genetic test results
- Undergoing the cancer screening tests and awaiting the results

---

10.1.3.2. Prior Experiences with Cancer

A client's prior cancer experiences often influence his/her reactions to the risk discussions. Clients who have relatives who were diagnosed with cancer may have heightened fears about their own risks of cancer. The extent of impact of these prior cancer experiences depends on the client's level of attachment to the affected relative, the client's involvement with the relative's care, and whether the relative survived the cancer or succumbed to the disease. Clients who have personal histories of cancer may also find that the counseling discussions bring back painful memories of their own diagnoses.

10.1.3.3. Age and Gender

There are several ways in which the age of clients may influence their levels of anxiety during the counseling session. Clients may have increased fears about cancer if they are nearing the age at which other relatives were diagnosed or if they are in the "high-risk" age group for the syndrome being discussed. For example, the risk of eye malignancies in a child with an *RB1* gene mutation is highest between the ages of birth and 5 years. Therefore, a discussion of hereditary retinoblastoma with parents of an infant is bound to be more anxiety provoking than a similar discussion with parents of a 10-year-old child. The age of clients may also play a role in how well or poorly they handle adverse situations or process distressing risk information. Thus, teenagers may feel invulnerable despite their high estimated risks of cancer while older people may fail to be reassured by their low cancer risks because they have relatives and friends who have developed cancer. In addition, certain cancer syndromes confer gender-specific cancer risks. For example, a female client is likely to have higher anxiety about the personal implications of a positive *BRCA* genetic test than a male client. It is also important for counselors to recognize that male and female clients might differ in how they process or express anxiety.

10.1.3.4. Type of Cancer

Being at increased risk of cancer—any type of cancer—is anxiety producing; however, certain cancers inspire greater fear than others. The prospect of developing a malignancy that is uniformly fatal is undoubtedly more frightening than the possibility of developing a cancer that is treatable. Thus, clients who are at risk for hereditary pancreatic or stomach cancer (which generally have poor prognoses) are more likely to be anxious than those at risk for papillary thyroid cancer or nonmelanoma skin cancer (which are both typically curable diseases).

10.1.3.5. Prior Perception of Risk

It is the client's perception of risk—not the actual numerical risk—that often has the greatest impact on his or her responses and actions. For example, individuals who are convinced that they are going to get cancer someday may demand all the screening practices of those at highest risk even if their actual estimates of cancer risk do not support these practices.

10.1.3.6. Ethnic and Cultural Factors

Ethnocultural factors may influence the client's level of cancer-related fears and subsequent reactions and behaviors. Clients of different cultures may perceive the risk information differently than the counselor intended or they may be concerned about aspects of the risk information that the counselor has not addressed. In addition, clients whose primary language differs from that of the counselor may have difficulty understanding all the nuances of the information.

10.1.4. IMPACT OF THE CLIENTS' CANCER FEARS ON OTHER ASPECTS OF THEIR LIVES

Clients' fears about cancer can impact other aspects of their lives, including the following presented in the succeeding sections.

10.1.4.1. Daily Activities

Clients may express the opinion that it is not a matter of *if* they will develop cancer, but *when* they will develop it. These clients are performing their day-to-day activities with an undercurrent of fear about developing cancer. Sometimes specific events will trigger anxieties about cancer, such as hearing about an old friend diagnosed with cancer or reading about a new cancer drug. Clients who can discuss their anxieties openly with family members or friends tend to be less affected by their high-risk status.

10.1.4.2. Lifestyle Behaviors

Clients are generally eager to reduce their cancer risks in any way they can. One way people can reduce their overall risks of cancer is through lifestyle changes, such as exercising more regularly and avoiding risky behaviors such as smoking cigarettes or excessive tanning. Making lifestyle changes may give clients a greater sense of control despite little evidence that hereditary cancer risks will be substantially reduced. Conversely, clients may blame themselves if they are not making these lifestyle changes (which could lead to lowered self-esteem). A small number of clients may even be engaging in daring or risky behaviors since they feel as though their future is overshadowed by the risk of cancer.

10.1.4.3. Medical Care Practices

Recommendations about surveillance range from routine clinical examinations to more specialized procedures, such as colonoscopy or magnetic resonance imaging (MRI) exams. Some individuals at high risk will pursue all recommended screening tests, while others stay away from doctors completely. A fear of cancer is certainly a strong motivator for people to be regularly screened for cancer although excessive fear can be counterproductive. A person's cancer fears may be influenced by their family's experiences with cancer, especially whether the recommended detection strategies worked in other family members and whether the relatives ultimately survived their cancers. The adherence to monitoring practices depends upon other factors as well, including the individual's level of concern about developing cancer and faith in the monitoring procedure as well as logistical issues, and the discomfort (or expense) of the procedure.

10.1.4.4. Major Life Decisions

High-risk individuals may make major life decisions based on their fears that they will someday develop cancer. Examples of major life decisions include educational goals, choice of career, selection of marital partner, and decisions about having children. In making these major life decisions, some clients are minimally influenced by their high-risk status. However, for others, the fear of developing cancer is a central concern, making it difficult to aspire to long-term career goals or sustain long-term relationships.

10.1.5. Clients and Their Families

Genetic information affects clients *and* their families. A family can be defined as a social system consisting of a group of individuals who are bound together by blood, marital contract, social obligation, or sharing a household. Families typically include individuals who are of different generations and who interact with each other over time. A family may include people of different ethnic backgrounds, religious beliefs, financial means, sexual orientations, or political views. Broadening the definition of family even further, individuals and couples can currently become parents through the use of sperm donors, egg donors, frozen embryos, surrogate mothers, or adoption.

A diagnosis of cancer can impact the family unit in a number of ways, from straining family resources to fracturing relationships. (See Table 10.5.)

TABLE 10.5. POTENTIAL WAYS IN WHICH A CANCER DIAGNOSIS CAN
IMPACT OTHER FAMILY MEMBERS

- Restricted social interactions
- Heightened tensions
- Fractured relationships
- Strained finances
- Emotional conflicts or awkwardness
- Unresolved grief
- Family pressure to accept or reject medical practices

Source: Patenaude (2005).

In a similar fashion, the identification of a hereditary cancer syndrome or specific gene mutation can impact the client's relatives, especially those who are also at risk.

Certain family characteristics may help shape a client's attitudes and fears and might also impact how (or whether) a genetic test result will be disseminated through the family. These family characteristics include the following in the succeeding sections.

10.1.5.1. Family Flexibility

This refers to a family's ability to cope and adapt to an adverse event, such as a cancer diagnosis. Families that are flexible are able to handle stressful events that arise and adapt to the altered needs of family members. For example, in the Smith family, the youngest sister, Betsy, was the person that everyone in the family depended on in times of need. When Betsy was diagnosed with cancer, her siblings realized that they needed to reverse the usual family roles and rallied together to provide her with extra care and support (which Betsy gratefully accepted). In contrast, families that are inflexible have a more difficult time changing their perceptions of a person's roles and needs, which can lead to hurt feelings, unmet needs, and strained relationships. For example, when Ned Jones was diagnosed with cancer, members of his family had a difficult time knowing what to do or how to help him. After all, Ned was the one who usually made the decisions and took care of everyone else. Ned's adult children felt so awkward about their father's atypical frailness and vulnerability that they began to avoid encounters with him. Ned's siblings tried to help him out, but they gave him so much unwanted advice and attention that Ned became resentful and eventually they all quarreled.

10.1.5.2. Family Attachment

All family relationships are not created equal; certain relationships may be especially close and loving, while others may be fraught with discord or drama. Adversity seems to bring some families closer together yet causes other families to fall apart. This can be explained, in large part, by the level of attachment that exists in the family prior to the adverse event. Families may be described as having either secure or insecure attachments. Attachment refers to how well or poorly a family handles emotions, supportiveness, conflict, and autonomy. Taking another look at the two examples listed above, we can see that Betsy Smith feels well supported by her siblings in part because they are respectful of her treatment decisions and her need for privacy at times. This is in contrast to how Ned Jones' relatives have reacted to his illness; his children have virtually abandoned him and his siblings have become overly involved in a way that feels intrusive.

10.1.5.3. Family Roles

A person may have set roles within the family system: he or she may be the designated responsible one, the adventurous one, the peacemaker, or the clown. These roles may be entrenched in their relatives' minds regardless of how the individuals have changed over the years. For example, to her relatives, the successful chief executive officer (CEO) of a marketing firm may still be viewed as the bratty little sister or the rebellious teenager. These roles (or the family perceptions of roles) may affect family relationships and communication patterns. For example, individuals who are the gatherers of genealogical or medical information in the family may be considered more reliable sources of information than the relatives who are viewed as attention seekers or hypochondriacs.

10.1.5.4. Family Obligations

Most people feel some type of moral responsibility toward members of their family. The amount of obligation a person feels regarding his/her relatives depends on multiple factors, including

- The degree of the relationship (e.g., one's child vs. cousins)
- The extent of the favor (e.g., visiting a relative in the hospital vs. donating a kidney)
- The emotional closeness of the relationship (e.g., beloved sister vs. estranged uncle)

10.1.5.5. Family Stories

Clients often relate stories about past events within the family. These family stories may recount a specific tragedy or triumph and may focus on a certain event or individual in the family. Even if the family stories are not helpful from a diagnostic standpoint, they may provide information about a client's motivations and attitudes. The family stories may also shed light on the family's level of attachment, flexibility, and pattern of communication.

10.1.5.6. Family Communication

In some families, cancer is an openly discussed topic, whereas in others it is seldom mentioned. Clients in families with an open communication style appear to be better at coping with their cancer risks than those in families that do not routinely discuss cancer. Some people may seek to distance themselves from their relatives or may avoid discussions of cancer. A family's communication style may also be influenced by other factors, including ethnicity, culture, religion, geographical region, and span of generations. Some clients willingly share newly learned information with their relatives, while other clients prefer to keep the information private. The client may have difficulty in tracking down certain relatives or the difficulty may have to do with how to tell specific relatives who are perceived as vulnerable or challenging. There may also be some type of "chain of communication" in the family that needs to be followed. For example, a client may share the news about his positive genetic test result with the maternal grandmother knowing that she will take care of disseminating it through the remainder of the family. Clients are more likely to share genetic information with their relatives in the following scenarios:

- *The client and relative are closely related.* A client is more likely to share genetic information with first-degree relatives than second- or third-degree relatives.
- *The client feels emotionally close to the relative.* A client is less likely to share the news with family members with whom there is little or no emotional attachment.
- *The client and relative live in the same geographic region.* A client is more likely to share the news with relatives who live in the same city than the out-of-state relatives whom he or she has not seen in years.
- *The client is in frequent contact with the relative.* A client may feel reluctant to share the news if the only point of contact with the relative is at large family gatherings or the once-a-year holiday cards.
- *The client feels morally obligated to tell the relative.* A client whose child is diagnosed with Fanconi anemia may feel more compelled to tell cousins of child-bearing age than elderly great-aunts or uncles.

10.2. Making a Psychosocial Assessment

10.2.1. Psychosocial Features to Assess

In a genetic counseling session, the psychosocial assessment begins with the collection of family history information. As a client relates stories about the family's cancer experiences, genetic counselors can begin to get a sense of the client's fears, hopes, and motivations.

Psychosocial questions can be incorporated into a routine series of questions asked of everyone or asked only when concerns are raised about a specific client's emotional well-being. The counselor's psychosocial intake should also include an assessment of the client features presented in the succeeding sections.

10.2.1.1. Current Emotional Well-Being

Counselors can assess possible symptoms of depression and anxiety by asking clients about any recent changes in their eating and sleeping habits. The counselor can also ascertain whether the clients are experiencing any unusual or intense sadness, anxiety, or stress. (See Table 10.6.) In addition, counselors can take note of:

- *The client's general appearance*—Two aspects of appearance to consider are grooming and motor activity (i.e., whether clients appear quiet or agitated). Clients who are poorly groomed may be clinically depressed, while constant fidgeting may signal a high level of anxiety.
- *The client's attention and concentration*—Throughout the session, counselors should pay attention to the client's level of attentiveness and

TABLE 10.6. Sample Questions for Cancer Genetic Counselors to Ask About the Client's Current Emotional Well-Being

- Over the past few weeks:
  - Have you had any problems sleeping?
  - Have you had any change of appetite?
  - Have you felt unusually anxious about anything?
  - Have you felt sad or depressed?
  - Are you crying more easily or more often?
  - Are you having a harder time getting things done at home or at work?
- Do you feel that your worries about cancer affect how well you are able to concentrate?
- Do you feel that your worries about cancer affect your relationships with your partner or family?
- Do you ever feel hopeless when thinking about your life or future?

concentration. Poor attentiveness and concentration may be indicators of high anxiety or distress.

- *The client's mood*—In psychology, mood refers to a pervasive, sustained behavior. A client's mood may be described as depressed, euphoric, or neutral.

- *The client's affect*—Affect refers to a person's emotional responses to a specific situation. (See Section 10.1.1 for examples of emotional responses.) In addition to registering the client's response, the counselor can note its appropriateness given the circumstances. For example, it is natural for clients to become emotional as they relate stories about relatives who have died from cancer. It is less typical for clients to burst into tears while counselors are arranging for them to have blood draws or obtain parking vouchers. (And this type of response would certainly warrant further exploration!)

10.2.1.2. Mental Health History

It may be helpful for genetic counselors to ask general questions about the client's mental health history and to ascertain whether the client is currently meeting with a mental health professional, such as a therapist, psychologist, social worker, or psychiatrist. (See Table 10.7.) This line of questioning allows clients to share information about their mental health history as well as their attitudes toward psychological counseling. All questions about clients' mental health histories should be asked with great sensitivity and tact. The client's answers may alert the counselor as to whether the risk discussion or genetic test results might trigger any adverse emotional sequelae. In addition, the counselor can begin to assess whether the client might benefit from meeting with a mental health professional (and whether the client might be

TABLE 10.7. SAMPLE QUESTIONS FOR CANCER GENETIC COUNSELORS TO ASK ABOUT THE CLIENT'S MENTAL HEALTH HISTORY

- Are you currently seeing a psychologist or therapist? If yes, how often?
- Have you ever met with a psychologist or therapist? If yes, how recently was this?
- What led you to meet with a therapist?
- Have you ever been told you have clinical depression or anxiety?
- Are you currently taking or have you ever taken any medications for psychological reasons?
- Have you ever tried to commit suicide? Have you ever seriously thought about committing suicide?
- Is there anything stressful going on in your life right now?

amenable to such a suggestion). Counselors might also find it reassuring to learn that clients who appear depressed or anxious are already in ongoing therapeutic relationships.

10.2.1.3. Emotional Reactions

High-risk clients have often witnessed one or more close family members who have been diagnosed with (and perhaps died of) cancer. The clients themselves may be short-term or long-term cancer survivors. Clients need to understand the significance of their family history from a genetic standpoint, but the psychological impact of the cancer history is also important. When collecting family history information, counselors can begin to ascertain how the client has been impacted by the diagnoses in the family and how their experiences might be impacting their current attitudes toward genetic testing or cancer screening. (See Table 10.8.) Clients can also be asked to describe their own fears and to explore the aspects of their situations that concern them the most.

10.2.1.4. Timing Issues

It is important for counselors to ask whether clients are currently dealing with any unduly stressful or anxiety-provoking issues (even if these issues have nothing to do with cancer). For example, learning about other potential stressors in the client's life can help counselors determine whether this is an optimal time for the client to undergo genetic testing, and if he or she proceeds with testing, whether the client may need any additional support services. Counselors can also try to ascertain whether a client's distress or motivations are due to a specific cancer-related anniversary date. Some clients will be aware of the emotional impact of certain dates or times of the year while others will be much less conscious of it.

TABLE 10.8. SAMPLE QUESTIONS FOR CANCER GENETIC COUNSELORS TO ASK ABOUT THE CLIENT'S EMOTIONAL RESPONSES TO THE INCREASED CANCER RISK

- How often do you think about your cancer risks?
  - Do you worry about getting cancer?
  - What worries you the most?
- Are there specific times when you are more worried?
- What do you usually do when you are worried (or upset, angry, etc.)?
- How close were you to your relative(s) who had cancer?
- Whose cancer experience affected you the most? In what way?
- How do you think these experiences have affected you?

10.2.1.5. Coping Strategies

Clients will have developed a variety of ways to cope with the possibility that they might someday develop cancer. (Refer back to Section 10.1.2.) It may be helpful to ask clients what they have done in the past when faced with a stressful situation (e.g., illness or hospitalization) and how well these strategies worked for them. (See Table 10.9.) A client's coping strategies may become evident during the counseling session depending on how much anxiety is triggered by the discussion. For example, a minor fear reaction might cause clients to perseverate over a specific point or to make a joke to ease the tension while more extreme fear might cause clients to lash out at the counselor or to shut down completely. Counselors should continually monitor their clients' emotional responses to the information presented and take note of how the client's level of fear might be impacting the counseling interaction. (See Table 10.10.) This will help counselors to determine whether they should halt the discussion of a specific topic or to delve further into the issue that triggered the client's reaction.

TABLE 10.9. SAMPLE QUESTIONS FOR CANCER GENETIC COUNSELORS TO ASK ABOUT THE CLIENT'S COPING STRATEGIES

- Is it difficult or easy for you to have a positive attitude?
- It's not unusual to feel overwhelmed and helpless about being at risk for cancer. Does this describe how you feel at times?
- Some people feel they want to leave everything to their physician. Is that how you feel?
- It sounds like you have been seeking a lot of information about your cancer risks. Has this helped you or do you think it makes you worry more?
- Are you the sort of person who tends to accept things as they are or do you question what goes on?
- Some people find it helps to avoid thinking about their risks of cancer. Are you that sort of person?
- When you are feeling worried, what do you usually do to feel better?
- What strategies seem to work the best for you? Why do you think that is?
- Do these strategies make you feel better right away? How about over time?
- Who can you talk to about these worries?

TABLE 10.10. SAMPLE QUESTIONS FOR CANCER GENETIC COUNSELORS TO ASK ABOUT THE CLIENT'S REACTIONS DURING THE COUNSELING SESSION

- How are you feeling about the information we have covered so far?
- Is any of the information confusing or upsetting to you?
- Is the information I am telling you what you expected to hear?
- Is it difficult discussing these issues? Which aspects are hardest to talk about? Do you feel comfortable sharing the reasons for this?
- You seem to be worried about something. Did I say something that upset you?

10.2.2. STRATEGIES FOR EFFECTIVE PSYCHOSOCIAL GENETIC COUNSELING

Cancer genetic counselors need to be able to balance the session's informational goals with the counseling needs of their clients. In the succeeding sections are some specific strategies for providing effective psychosocial cancer genetic counseling (see Table 10.11).

10.2.2.1. Convey Empathy

Empathy is a central tenet of genetic counseling. The importance of empathy is highlighted in Table 10.12. In order to convey empathy, the counselor must pay close attention to the client's verbal and nonverbal responses and must acknowledge these responses in a way that builds trust and rapport.

TABLE 10.11. STRATEGIES FOR PROVIDING EFFECTIVE PSYCHOSOCIAL CANCER GENETIC COUNSELING

- Convey empathy
- Stay attuned to verbal and nonverbal cues
- Employ active listening
- Ask rather than assume
- Ascertain the rationale behind questions and reactions
- Allow clients to express emotions
- Respect client boundaries
- Monitor client reactions
- Have strategies to deal with resistant clients
- Remain professional
- Help client with decisions and actions

Sources: Djurdjinovic (2009); Weil (2000).

TABLE 10.12. THE IMPORTANCE OF EMPATHY DURING A GENETIC COUNSELING SESSION

- Reinforcing the client to continue talking
- Providing clarification for both the counselor and the client
- Making the counselor seem similar to the client, thus increasing social attractiveness (the counselor is viewed as warm and likable)
- Providing a model for the client of how to be empathetic
- Facilitating the establishment of rapport and trust
- Helping clients feel understood by the counselor
- Helping clients manage their feelings
- Facilitating client risk-taking

Source: Veach (2003, pp. 52–53).

In other words, empathy can be defined as a process that involves answering the following three questions:

- Can I sense what you experience?
- Can I communicate this sense to you?
- Can you perceive this communication as my understanding you/ your experience? (Veach et al., 2003, p. 51).

It is important to recognize the difference between responding to a client with sympathy versus responding with empathy. Sympathetic responses are based on the counselor's perspective of the issue while empathic responses are based on listening to the client's perspective of the issue. A sympathetic genetic counselor might think, "I know this client must be really scared about her upcoming surgery, because that is how I would feel." In contrast, an empathetic genetic counselor might think, "This client seems really scared about her upcoming surgery because whenever she mentions it her voice trembles and then she quickly changes the subject."

A client's rejection of a counselor's empathetic response can cause strain or awkwardness (hopefully temporarily) during the counseling interaction. This is also termed an empathic break. If a client does not welcome a particular empathetic response from the counselor, it could be because:

- The counselor is off-target in reading the client
- The counselor is on-target in reading the client, but has not chosen the right empathetic response
- The counselor is on-target but the client does not want the emotion acknowledged
- It is too early in the counseling session for the client to acknowledge or discuss his or her feelings with the counselor

Counselors also need to learn to assess the client's emotional reactions without experiencing empathic distress, that is, the phenomenon of taking on another person's pain. Counselors who overly identify with a client's story may find themselves caught up in the emotions of the experience. This makes it difficult to see the client as a separate individual and may cause counselors to provide the client with false reassurances that everything will be OK so as to reduce their own levels of distress.

10.2.2.2. Stay Attuned to Verbal and Nonverbal Cues

Throughout the session, the counselor should pay close attention to the client's linguistic, paralinguistic, and nonverbal cues. Linguistic cues include the client's vocabulary and specific questions asked. One counseling technique suggests that counselors adopt the client's language choices and internally monitor the discussion's level of sophistication. For example, describing the carcinogenic process in detail will confuse the average client as much as simplistic analogies will annoy clients who have strong backgrounds in science. Paralinguistic cues refer to the volume, tone, and timing of the client's responses. To help promote empathy, counselors can subtly model the client's body position and can modulate the volume, tone, and timing of their responses. It is also important for counselors to pay attention to the nonverbal aspects of conversation, including the client's facial expressions, gestures, body position, and eye contact.

10.2.2.3. Employ Active Listening

This technique lets clients know that the counselor is listening to them and understands what they are is saying (or trying to say). Active listening techniques (listed in Table 10.13) can be as simple as nodding one's head or making brief vocalizations (such as "uh huh") to encourage the client to continue talking. Counselor responses should be sincere and honest; counselors should not pretend to understand a client's answer. Rather, counselors should ask clients to clarify their statements. One option is to say, "Help me to understand that last statement you made." (Also see Section 10.2.1.4.)

10.2.2.4. Ask Rather Than Assume

Clients will come to the genetic counseling session with different cancer experiences, backgrounds, and coping strategies. Asking questions about psychosocial issues should be a routine part of cancer counseling sessions (refer to Tables 10.6–10.10). The extent to which these issues need to be explored will vary from client to client. Counselors need to be careful not to questions that are emotionally laden, value laden, or could be viewed as confrontational. For example, asking a client, "So why aren't you being

TABLE 10.13. Ways to Let a Client Know That the Counselor Is Actively and Empathically Listening

- Use minimal encouragers—head nods, "uh huhs"
- Repeat key words
- Summarize what the client has said
- Use own words to repeat what client said
- React to nonverbal cues
- Listen for words that indicate the client's emotions
- Adopt client's word choices
- Mirror client's tone and manner of speech

Source: Djurdjinovic (2009, pp. 53–55).

screened for colon cancer?" is likely to lead to defensive responses. A better strategy is to say, "It looks like it is time to schedule your next colonoscopy. Let's spend a few minutes talking about this." This tactic paves the way for clients to discuss any potential barriers to screening so that the counselor and client can work together to resolve these concerns.

10.2.2.5. Ascertain the Rationale Behind Questions and Reactions

Some clients ask questions that seem trivial or irrelevant to the discussion at hand. In these situations, determining the rationale behind the questions might be more useful than continuing the discussion. Asking questions can be a way for clients to express their feelings, indicate what is important to them, or redirect the conversation away from an emotionally painful topic. In order to know how best to respond, counselors may find it useful to determine what kind of answer the client hopes to receive and how the client feels the information would be relevant to his/her situation.

10.2.2.6. Allow Clients to Express Emotions

Counselors should encourage clients to express their emotions freely, whether it is grief, fear, frustration, or anger. For some clients, the simple act of walking into a cancer clinic will invoke strong emotional reactions. Allowing clients to verbalize their emotions may help them to reduce their fears. It may also help the counselor to better understand the client's concerns and motivations. Some clients are reluctant to share their emotions and counselors may need to listen carefully for clues about the client's emotions during the session. For example, a client who denies any cancer-related anxiety might end up sharing information about his/her feelings when recounting a recent screening test: "I sure was scared when my doctor told me I might need a biopsy." In other cases, clients may end up pouring out feelings that have been bottled up for a long time. Counselors may be tempted to change the subject if the conversation becomes too emotionally charged but a few moments of empathetic silence may be more effective. Counselors can also reassure clients that it is normal to experience a range of emotions during this process. However, counselors do need to be careful not to open up intense emotional issues that are beyond their scope or the allotted time frame.

10.2.2.7. Respect Client Boundaries

Respecting and maintaining appropriate boundaries with clients is an important part of a counselor–client relationship. Some clients will freely discuss their fears and anxieties, while others will be much less forthcoming. Some clients may feel that a certain topic is too distressing or personal for them to discuss. By use of verbal or nonverbal cues, clients will generally indicate when their boundaries have been reached and it is important for counselors to respect these boundaries. Although the counselor may feel that it would be helpful for a client to "talk it out," a wiser course of action is to shelve the discussion; genetic counselors can use their judgment to decide whether or not to gently reintroduce the topic at a later time.

10.2.2.8. Monitor Client Reactions

Counselors should continually assess whether clients are feeling overwhelmed, confused, or distressed by the discussion. For example, during the cancer risk assessment, clients may ignore or refute the risk estimates given to them or they may concentrate on the facts and figures as a way of avoiding the emotional implications of risk. In addition, some clients will pretend to understand (because it is easier than admitting confusion) or will focus on the cancer risks of other relatives (because it is less daunting than focusing on their own risks). Counselors should always try to ascertain the probable emotion driving the client's response or question and determine how best to proceed. Sometimes simply acknowledging the client's reaction is helpful in starting a productive dialogue about these issues.

10.2.2.9. Have Strategies to Deal with Resistant Clients

So-called resistant clients behave in ways that prevent meaningful client–counselor connections and can also derail the genetic counseling interaction. Resistant clients manifest a variety of coping strategies to deal with their triggered feelings of distress (usually fear) and may appear apathetic, guarded, or openly hostile. Unless their high levels of distress are adequately dealt with, these clients will not be able to attend to the informational part of the genetic counseling session. Genetic counselors will need to find ways to actively engage clients who are withdrawn as well as to find ways to calm clients who are agitated. It may be helpful to make a general statement that many clients find the genetic counseling process to be anxiety producing or difficult. Gently acknowledging "the elephant in the room" (i.e., the true underlying trigger) may be the first step toward a more meaningful connection or discussion. Another approach is for counselors to try and resolve (or at least acknowledge) the surface issue that has triggered the client's resistance. Although it is not always easy, counselors should do their best to remain empathetic and professional even with clients who have unfriendly or hostile demeanors.

10.2.2.10. Remain Professional

Counselors should maintain an empathetic yet professional demeanor throughout the counseling interactions. Welling up with tears in response to a sad story is a human emotion—and cancer counseling is chock-full of sad stories. However, crying in front of clients may make it difficult for counselors to regain the focus of the discussion and is not generally helpful to clients who already know how tragic their circumstances are. (But debriefing afterwards with caring colleagues is a must!) When dealing with angry clients, the first impulse of the counselor might be to defend the source of the anger, whether it is aimed at program logistics, certain staff members, or the medical profession in general. However, this tactic will only further entangle the counselor in the conflict and could result in escalating anger on the part of the client. A better counseling strategy is to allow the client to vent for a short time, acknowledge his/her anger (which is different from agreeing with it), and then shift the discussion back to the genetic counseling discussion. By adopting this approach, the client is more likely to view the counselor as an ally rather than an adversary. When the client has become calmer, the counselor may be able to explore the underlying emotions that might have triggered the outburst.

Counselors who notice that a particular client interaction has become intense or strained (especially if it is not clear why this has occurred) might want to consider the possibility that the session has been impacted by one of the psychological phenomena described below:

- *Transference*—Transference is a set of expectations and emotional responses that a client brings to a provider–client relationship, which are based not on the provider's traits, but rather on the client's experiences with prior authority figures. Clients who display positive transference may be overly affectionate or idolizing, while clients who display negative transference may be mistrustful or hostile. Transference reactions often reveal unresolved conflicts from childhood due to abuse or trauma. However, some psychologists believe that all of us display transference reactions of sorts when entering into relationships. Genetic counselors need to recognize transference reactions, because they can interfere with building true rapport with clients. Counselors should maintain a neutral professionalism to engage clients appropriately and should also seek advice from mental health colleagues.

- *Countertransference*—Counselors who do not recognize that the client is reacting to his/her (faulty) first impressions may begin to react to the client's actions or words in a way that actually reinforces the client's impressions. For example, in the wake of a client's hostility due to transference (because the counselor reminds the client of his ex-wife) a counselor might become defensive or abrupt. This type of counselor response might be exactly how the client's ex-wife used to react, hence reinforcing the client's first impression. By continuing this faulty dynamic, the counselor decreases the likelihood of forming a true connection with the client.

- *Projection*—A counselor might say something that triggers a memory or emotion within a client that then affects the client's response (often to the puzzlement of the counselor). Thus, a client who feels guilty about not staying in touch with relatives may become defensive when the counselor asks for basic family history information and a client whose relatives continually harp on the importance of screening may snap at the counselor who mentions the screening guidelines. In both cases, it is the clients' past experiences (and their strong emotional reactions to these experiences) that has triggered their responses. Projection can also occur when the client shares a story with which the genetic counselor strongly identifies. For example, a client may talk about the stress of dealing with a child who has been diagnosed with an eating disorder and severe depression. A counselor, who has a child with similar issues, may unwittingly make responses that are personally relevant rather than formulating responses based on the client's experiences or feelings.

10.2.2.11. Help Client with Decisions and Actions

During the cancer counseling sessions, clients may be asked to consider certain actions or decisions. These can include decisions about whether to have genetic testing, how best to tell relatives about their increased cancer risks, or whether to undergo prophylactic surgery. Counselors should remain value neutral and nondirective while presenting options to clients. To help clients with the decision-making process, counselors may wish to utilize the following strategies:

- Allow the client to talk through the issue without jumping to possible solutions
- Ask how the client has dealt with other difficult situations or decisions
- Ask if the client has one or more support person(s) to help make these types of decisions
- Seek to understand the client's motivations and concerns that are likely to be driving the decision-making process
- Remind the client that decisions rarely have to be made urgently; there is usually plenty of time to consider all of the ramifications and alternatives

- Provide the client with additional resources for information and support

10.2.3. THE GENOGRAM ASSESSMENT TOOL

A genogram is a tool that depicts a client's relationships with other close relatives and also illustrates the family's overall supportiveness and communication style. A genogram is constructed by jotting down additional facts next to a relative's pedigree symbol and drawing the appropriate relationship lines between each family member.

Most clients appreciate the opportunity to talk more about themselves and their family relationships. Constructing a genogram gives counselors more information about the client and his or her family and may also uncover issues that would benefit from more discussion or a mental health referral.

Consider the following example:

The client, Susan, is a 25-year-old graduate student in law school. She lives alone but is engaged to be married. Her main reason for seeking genetic counseling is to learn if her future offspring could have increased risks of cancer. Susan reports having a close relationship with her fiancé, but maintains little contact with her parents and has a contentious relationship with her sister, Lisa. Susan reports somewhat bitterly that Lisa has a solid relationship with both parents and that their mother continues to smother Lisa with attention and concern. Susan was 7 years old when her younger sister was diagnosed with cancer and she has vivid memories of the impact this diagnosis had on the household. In contrast, her father's cancer diagnosis last year seems to have had little impact on her. A genogram depicting this family information is shown in Figure 10.1.

Genograms can take as little as 15 minutes to construct if kept to a narrow focus; sample questions for cancer genetic counselors to ask are listed in Table 10.14. The types of information obtained in the construction of a genogram are presented in the succeeding sections.

10.2.3.1. Demographic Data

In addition to obtaining information about each relative's cancer status and current age (or age at death), which is collected as part of the standard genetic pedigree, counselors can ask about each relative's level of education and current or past occupation.

10.2.3.2. Functioning Level

Assessing a person's functioning level involves asking questions about any physical, mental, or emotional limitations or strengths. In addition, the

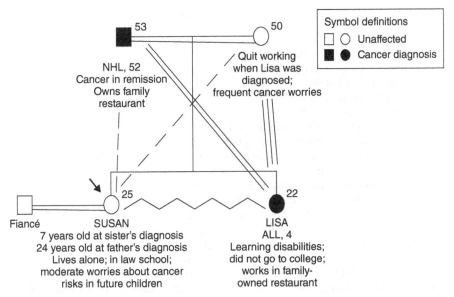

FIGURE 10.1. An example of a genogram. This genogram depicts Susan's nuclear family. See the accompanying text for details of this case example. Refer to Figure 10.2 for a description of the relationship lines used in the genogram. NHL = non-Hodgkin's lymphoma; ALL = acute lymphoblastic leukemia.

counselor can ask how each close relative is dealing with the heightened cancer risks, both emotionally and in terms of screening practices.

10.2.3.3. Critical Family Events

Critical family events are ones that had a major impact on the client and possibly the entire family. Cancer counselors should ask how the cancer diagnoses and deaths in the family might have impacted the client. Counselors may also wish to ascertain how old the client was at the time of the event, because a person's stage of emotional and cognitive development often influences the overall impact of the event. Counselors can also ask about any potential cancer-related anniversary dates that may be influencing the client's current attitudes and decisions. It may also be helpful to document other noncancer critical events such as divorces, moves, or trauma that may have had a long-lasting impact on the client.

10.2.3.4. Family Relationships

Relationships among family members are illustrated by the specific types of lines drawn between two family members (as shown in Fig. 10.2). This

TABLE 10.14. SAMPLE QUESTIONS TO ASK CLIENTS IN THE CONSTRUCTION
OF A GENOGRAM

- Who lives in your household?
- Of the people you have listed, who do you feel:
  - Especially close to?
  - Distant or in conflict with?
  - Overly dependent on?
  - Who helps out when help is needed?
  - To whom do family members confide?

Now I would like to ask a few questions about your relatives who have had cancer
or have died of cancer:

- When was your relative diagnosed with cancer?
- How old was your relative at that time?
- How old were you when your relative was diagnosed with cancer?
- How old were you when your relative died of cancer?
- What did you understand about the diagnosis?
- How involved were you in the care of your relatives?
  How much did this relative's cancer diagnosis impact you?
- How did the family react when a particular family member died? Who took it
  the hardest? Who took it the least hard?
- Have there recently been any major changes in your life?
- Are there any other major events or changes going on in your life right now?
- Are you thinking about making any major changes in your life?
- How stressful would you say your life is right now? What do you think are the
  factors contributing to your level of stress?

Source: McGoldrick et al. (1999).

indicates the level of communication and support that exists between family
members.

10.2.3.5. Current Stressors

The counselors should take note of any major issues or changes that are
contributing to the client's current level of stress. These stressors can include
worries about relatives, parenting difficulties, failed relationships, financial
woes, or the pressures of school or work. This line of questioning may also
pinpoint stressors that are influencing the client's attitudes about cancer
surveillance and prevention strategies.

10.2.4. THE COLORED ECO-GENETIC RELATIONSHIP MAP ASSESSMENT TOOL

It is time to reaffirm the "counseling" aspects of genetic counseling.

(Peters et al., 2006, p. 487)

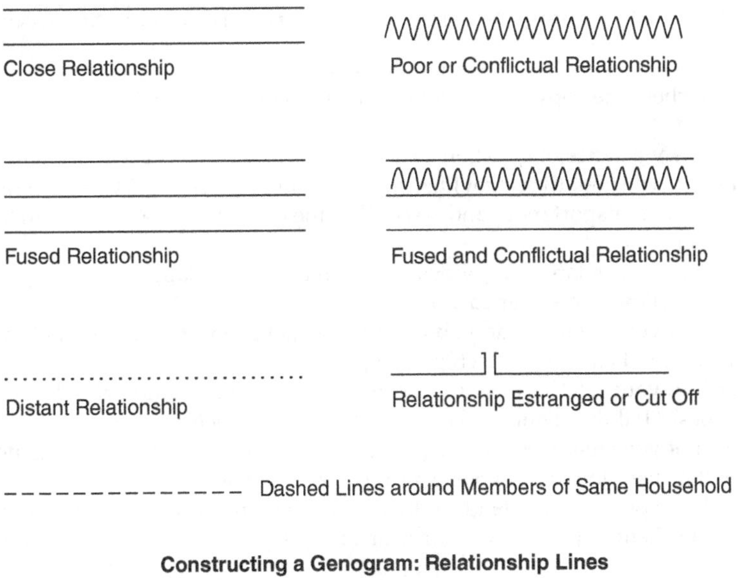

Constructing a Genogram: Relationship Lines

FIGURE 10.2. The types of relationship lines used to construct a genogram. Depending on the client's answers, draw the appropriate relationship line between the two individuals on the genetic pedigree. Source: McGoldrick et al. (1999).

The colored eco-genetic relationship map (CEGRM) is a psychosocial tool designed specifically for use during a genetic counseling session. The CEGRM is a blend of the genetic pedigree, a genogram, and an eco-map.

According to June Peters, a clinically trained genetic counselor and therapist, et al. (2004, p. 258), the purpose of the CEGRM is to:

- increase understanding of the client's social milieu
- bolster client awareness and insight
- foster active client participation and mutuality in the counseling interaction
- encourage the client to share stories about friends and relatives
- address any outstanding emotional issues

Sample questions and instructions for creating a CEGRM are listed in Table 10.15. An example of a CEGRM can be found in Figure 10.3. To create a CEGRM, the counselor hands the pedigree to the client along with packets of small stickers and instructs the client to place specific small stickers near the relevant individuals on the pedigree. For example, the counselor will instruct the client to put a small yellow circle sticker near each relative who provides him or her with emotional support.

TABLE 10.15. SAMPLE QUESTIONS AND INSTRUCTIONS FOR CREATING A CEGRM

Hand the client the copy of the pedigree along with some small stickers or colored pencils.
Ask the client a series of questions, such as:
- Which of your relatives provides you with tangible services? Can be monetary, child care, transportation, and so on (Tell the client to place a green circle near each person.)
- Which of your relatives provides you with emotional support? (Tell the client to place a yellow circle near each person.)
- Which of your relatives do you have a spiritual connection with? (Tell the client to place a red circle near each person.)
- Which of your relatives like to research or gather information about cancer and genetics? (Tell the client to place a silver star near each person.)
- Which of your relatives likes to pass on information about cancer or genetics? (Tell the client to place a green star near each person.)
- Which of your relatives tends to block information about cancer or genetics? (Tell the client to place a red star near each person.)

Source: Peters et al. (2004).

The CEGRM generates an illustrated view of the client's social networks, information exchange patterns, and sources of support that the client and counselor can then view and discuss. This exercise can lead to "aha moments" from clients as they notice unexpected positive or negative patterns, and it can also give counselors a more complete picture of their clients. Creating a CEGRM takes an average of 30 minutes (the range is 13–60 minutes). Clients seem to enjoy creating a CEGRM, viewing it as a welcome break from the informational portions of the sessions.

10.3. PROVIDING ADDITIONAL EMOTIONAL SUPPORT

For some clients, it will be sufficient to explore psychosocial issues within the genetic counseling session. However, certain clients would benefit from in-depth psychological counseling that is beyond the scope of the genetic counselor. Clients should also be made aware of any appropriate patient support organizations, Internet-based resources, and local support groups.

10.3.1. MAKING A MENTAL HEALTH REFERRAL

Clients may benefit from meeting with a mental health professional to discuss their reactions to positive genetic test results or to reduce their fears about being screened. Others may have reached a crisis point in their lives

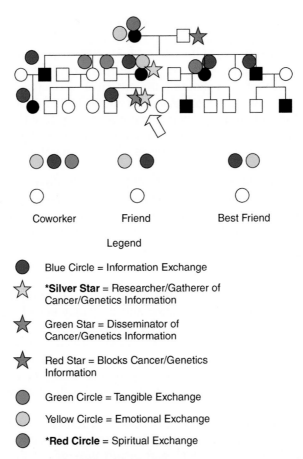

FIGURE 10.3. An example of a colored eco-genetic relationship map (CEGRM). The client is asked to place specific small stickers near the appropriate individuals on the pedigree. (The original reference contains a multicolored version of the genogram, which makes it easier to appreciate the final product.) *Domains added in 2005. Reprinted from *Journal of Medical Genetics*, J.R. Hansford and L.M. Mulligan, vol. 37, p. 818, copyright 2000, with permission from BMJ Publishing Group Ltd.

and could use short-term counseling to help them through a difficult time. Still others may need counseling on a long-term basis to help resolve issues surrounding the death of a family member, an underlying mental health disorder, or their general unhappiness about life.

It is important for genetic counselors to recognize clients who are in need of additional psychological support or intervention. Counselors should have strategies for how to assess a client's level of distress and how to determine the source of the distress (e.g., is it related to the cancer history or due to other life events?). Psychological counseling services can be offered to clients who appear to have high levels of anxiety regarding their cancer risks, have adopted poor coping responses to their risks, or seem to be having significant difficulties in other aspects of their lives. Table 10.16 lists examples of cancer genetic counseling clients who may benefit from a psychological referral. In general, genetic counselors should refer any client who has emotional needs that are beyond what the counselor feels comfortable handling. Common motivations for seeking psychological counseling are listed in Table 10.17. Cancer genetic counselors should have an established system of referral in place, so that they are not scrambling to identify a mental health provider when the need arises.

All cancer genetic counselors should establish alliances with mental health professionals who can review challenging cases, suggest strategies for dealing with fragile clients, and assist in the referral process. Ideally, the mental health professional will have experience dealing with families around chronic or acute illnesses and will possess fundamental knowledge about the inheritance pattern and cancer risks associated with hereditary cancer syndromes.

Clients may be surprised or offended by the suggestion that they consider further psychological counseling and they may even brush aside the suggestion the first time it is brought up. Genetic counselors need to handle these discussions with great sensitivity and tact. The actual referral process can consist of contacting a specific mental health provider and scheduling an appointment on behalf of the client or by providing the client with the provider's telephone number and encouraging the client to call and make an appointment.

Depending on the client's level of distress, counselors may want to set up a series of follow-up phone calls, contact the client's support person on behalf of the client, or page a mental health provider at the hospital for

TABLE 10.16. When Cancer Genetic Counseling Clients May Need a Mental Health Referral

- Clients feel that they will be unable to cope with their genetic test results
- Clients cannot cope with their genetic test results
- Clients express feelings of hopelessness or suicidal ideation
- Clients seem to need more support than they have in their lives (or that the genetic counseling program can provide)
- Clients have significant depression, anxiety, or other mood disorders
- Clients equate positive genetic test results with cancer diagnoses or death
- Genetic testing has triggered intense delayed grief reactions
- Genetic testing has triggered posttraumatic stress reactions
- Clients seem overwhelmed by other major life stressors
- Clients admit to practicing maladaptive coping methods (alcohol, cutting, eating disorder)

TABLE 10.17. Reasons Why People Might Seek Therapy

- Depression or anxiety that does not go away in a reasonable time
- Panic attacks, phobias, or severe fears that interfere with daily living
- Personality disorders and mental illness
- Stress at work, home, or school that feels overwhelming
- Trouble getting to or staying asleep
- Relationship and partner issues
- Eating disorders and weight management
- Trouble with drugs, alcohol, or other addictive behaviors
- Feeling chronically lonely or sad
- Chronic worry, preoccupation, confusion, or disorientation
- Excessive anger, frustration, or problems with physical abuse
- Self-destructive or self-defeating behaviors
- Suicidal thoughts and self-harm
- Trouble making or keeping satisfying relationships
- Job and career issues
- Coping with life-threatening illnesses
- Children's educational and emotional problems
- Domestic violence, traumatic events, or posttraumatic stress disorder
- Issues arising due to sexuality, sexual identity, or sexual orientation
- Dealing with difficult life issues: for example, death, divorce, birth of a child, and so on
- Family issues: for example, parent–child communication, problems with teenagers, and so on
- Life cycle challenges: for example aging parents, changed sexual needs, retirement, and so on
- Personal growth: for example, career changes, dissatisfaction with life

Source: Psychlinks Online (http://forum.psychlinks.ca).

consultation. Clients who are in crisis (especially if suicidal) should be provided with immediate assistance. Clients should be encouraged to go to the local hospital emergency room, which typically has the resources to assess and assist people in emotional crisis. Counselors should also alert the client's oncologist, primary health-care provider, and/or emergency contact person with any serious concerns.

When making a referral, genetic counselors should consider the type of mental health provider that would be most beneficial to the client. There are many types of mental health providers including psychiatrists, psychologists, family therapists, social workers, and grief counselors. Other important factors in making a mental health referral include the provider's expertise and availability, geographic proximity, client preferences, and client's health insurance coverage. Also keep in mind that clients may need to obtain referrals from their primary physicians, especially if they are in health maintenance organizations.

If clients are already in a therapeutic relationship, then it may be helpful for counselors to obtain the client's permission to speak directly with his or her therapist. The genetic counselor can provide information about the hereditary cancer syndrome, including the associated risks of cancer and the implications to the client and his or her family. The therapist can warn the counselor about any additional emotional or family issues which might be relevant and can also suggest ways in which the counselor might be of assistance.

10.3.2. CANCER RISK SUPPORT GROUPS

Clients may also find it beneficial to speak with people who have the hereditary cancer syndrome. There may be great value in having clients' speak to people who have "been there" themselves. Support groups, if available, can be a valuable way for people to connect with others in similar situations. Support group organizations exist for several of the hereditary cancer syndromes (refer to the syndrome entries in Chapter 4). These organizations can provide a variety of support and resources to families. Another excellent resource is the Genetic Alliance (http://www.geneticalliance.org), which provides the contact information for syndrome-specific organizations, including hereditary cancer syndromes.

Increasingly, people are turning to the Internet for information and support. Nowadays, many of the patient and family support organizations have websites that offer the following:

- A detailed description of the genetic condition
- A list of Internet links and other resources
- Personal accounts of individuals and families dealing with the condition
- A forum to seek advice, answers, support, and encouragement

In addition to the specific organization-sponsored Web sites, MD Junction and Yahoo! are two Internet domains that contain discussion groups for people with many different types of health problems or genetic disorders.

Even if clients are not interested in joining a patient support organization or chat forum, they may be interested in speaking to someone on a one-to-one basis. A number of clients are willing to act as resources for individuals who are facing a new diagnosis or positive gene result. Counselors can facilitate these connections by recontacting prior clients and asking whether they would be willing to speak to someone who is facing similar issues. For example a woman who is *BRCA* positive and considering a nipple-sparing mastectomy procedure may wish to speak to someone who actually went through this type of procedure.

Cancer genetic counselors can also consider setting up a support group specifically for people at high risk for cancer. In setting up such a group, there are several issues to consider.

10.3.2.1. Leader(s)

Support groups are usually facilitated by one or two individuals, usually with at least one health-care provider. Groups led by two coleaders often work well, because one person can moderate the discussion while the other person can track the group dynamics. Genetic counselors may benefit from coleading a group with a mental health professional or a cancer survivor. At least one of the coleaders should be trained and/or experienced in facilitating a support group.

10.3.2.2. Group Composition

Support groups are most successful when participants have similar needs and can empathize with one another. Thus, it is important to decide whether the group will be open to everyone interested in a particular topic or limited to a specific subset of people, such as individuals contemplating genetic testing, members of families known to have a hereditary cancer syndrome, or individuals with positive genetic test results. Further considerations include limiting group enrollment to clients of a certain age, gender, and/or cancer status. Group leaders also need to decide whether group membership will be open or closed. In an open group, people come to as many meetings as they like. This allows participants greater flexibility, but can be a logistical nightmare for facilitators. In a closed group, advanced registration is required and the group stays the same for the entire series of meetings. This allows the group to bond but can be problematic if the group fails to gel or too many members drop out prematurely.

10.3.2.3. Timing

Groups can take place on a regular basis (e.g., the first Tuesday of every month) or can be offered as a set series of meetings (e.g., four weekly or biweekly meetings).

10.3.2.4. Format

Group participants are usually seeking both support and information. Facilitators need to allow sufficient time for participants to share stories and vent frustrations. This time can be structured around a specific theme or kept unstructured. To meet the informational needs of group members, the facilitators can devote part of the meeting time to learning about a specific topic.

This can consist of listening to a lecture or panel discussion, watching an educational videotape, or even participating in self-help or role-play exercises.

10.3.2.5. Setting

The group meetings can be held in a hospital conference room or in a more neutral setting, such as a community center. Participants are more likely to attend if the meetings are held in a convenient location with ample parking.

10.4. CASE EXAMPLES

Case 12: "It must be very hard to hear this news."

"Anne Helms," announced the genetic counselor as she entered the crowded waiting room. "Oh that's me!" exclaimed a young woman as she jumped out of the chair and gathered up her cup of coffee, magazine, clinic forms, coat, and scarf.

"Please call me Annie," said the client as she exchanged greetings with the counselor.

On the way to the counseling room, Annie chattered about the weather (bad), the traffic to the hospital (also bad), and how she had been called into work tonight even though it was not her usual shift (really bad). As the counselor invited her to sit down, Annie confided to the counselor that she looked a lot like one of her older sisters—"The good one, not the one I don't talk to." The counselor kept her manner friendly but resisted the impulse to find out more about the family dynamics at the outset of the session.

Instead, the counselor asked Annie what she hoped to get from the counseling session. Annie dumped her stuff on the couch and sat in the chair next to it. "I want to find out what to do about my kids. I'm all set—but I'm worried about them. Plus my mother wanted me to come talk to you."

"When you say you are worried about your children, do you mean because they might have familial adenomatous polyposis (FAP)?" asked the counselor. Annie had been diagnosed with hepatoblastoma at age 15 months, then with colon polyposis in her teens.

"Yeah, I'm worried they might have FAP like me. Lots of my relatives have it." Annie paused and gave the counselor a worried look. "My doctor back home should have sent this information to you. I don't have to repeat it, do I? I'm not sure I can remember it all. My mother keeps track of all that stuff."

The counselor scanned the extensive pedigree of the family's history of colon cancer and assured Annie that she had the information. The counselor did ask if there were any updates or changes to the family history information. Annie shook her head, then brightened and said, "Oh yeah I almost forgot—I'm pregnant again. My mother went through the roof when she found out, but my boyfriend and I are real happy about it. This will be our second child together."

The counselor congratulated the client on the news and added the information to the family tree along with the client's 5-year-old twin sons and two-year-old daughter.

The counselor asked Annie how her children were doing. Annie said that they were all still adjusting to the move to the city but were otherwise alright.

Annie and the counselor talked about testing her children for FAP. They discussed the logistics of the testing process and set up an appointment in a few months' time when Annie's mother was coming for a visit. According to Annie, the mother adored her grandchildren but did not like Annie's boyfriend even though they had been together for the past 3 years.

Annie came to the appointment with the three children and her mother. During the session the counselor asked Annie's mother if she agreed that the children should be tested. "Of course I do. I've been saying it since they were born." Annie's mother went on to say that it would "break her heart" if any of her grandchildren had FAP and that she didn't know how Annie was going to manage with another baby on the way. Annie sent an exasperated look to her mother and said, "Oh and I suppose Sharon is mother of the year?" Annie turned to the counselor to explain. "Sharon is my older sister; she's the perfect one in the family. Maddie and me—we can't do anything right."

"Oh don't be ridiculous," responded the mother.

Before the quarrel escalated further, the counselor changed the topic by asking about Annie's boyfriend who was supposed to meet them at the hospital but had not arrived. Annie said that something must have come up, because he was not answering his cell phone. Her mother shook her head and said that it showed how irresponsible and unreliable he was. The counselor braced herself for an angry retort from Annie, but instead of defending her boyfriend's behavior, she agreed with her mother and they spent the next several minutes complaining about his lack of maturity. Clearly the mother–daughter relationship was a complicated one: adversaries one minute, allies the next.

Annie gave consent for the *APC* tests to be performed and set up a follow-up appointment to receive the results.

About 3 weeks later, Annie returned—alone—to receive the results of the genetic tests. The twin boys were negative for the familial *APC* gene mutation, but the daughter tested positive for it.

Upon hearing the news Annie cried, "Oh no, not my daughter." She then listened silently as the counselor and pediatric gastroenterologist spoke about the implications of the positive test results. Annie shook her head when asked if she had any questions.

After the physician left the room, the counselor tried to get Annie to talk to her—usually an easy task!—but got nothing but silence.

The counselor went over and sat next to Annie on the couch. "Annie, it must be very hard to hear this news. How can I help you right now? Would you like a few minutes to yourself? Would you like to call someone?"

"Could I call my mother?" whispered Annie.

"Sure, that would be fine. I have your mother's phone number right here, would you like me to dial it for you?"

Annie nodded. As soon as the mother answered the phone, the genetic counselor handed the phone to Annie and left the room to give her some privacy.

The counselor walked in the clinic workroom, reviewed the case with the pediatric gastroenterologist, and then paged the program psychologist. She described the case to the psychologist and said that it would be good for the two of them to meet. The psychologist agreed to drop by to introduce himself to Annie and to see if she would be willing to set up an appointment with him.

The counselor returned to the clinic room with a glass of water for Annie. The counselor asked if Annie wanted to talk about her reactions.

"I can't believe it. My daughter is so healthy. I felt sure she was going to be OK," Annie said. "My mother is totally devastated by the news."

The counselor said how sorry she was to have to give her this type of news.

"Now my daughter will have to deal with everything I had to deal with," Annie said in a trembling, quiet voice, almost as though she were talking to herself. She looked around at the exam room with haunted eyes. "It seems like every time I came to a hospital, I got bad news. Every time." It was clear that Annie was reliving her own experiences.

The counselor let her talk. When Annie came to the end of her narrative, the counselor said that the first step of getting this kind of news was getting adjusted to it. "Annie, your daughter may not need to have a lot of doctor's appointments and procedures right now. And she has you to help her through the tough times."

"And my mother. And the rest of my family," said Annie with her first smile of the afternoon. She didn't mention the girl's father, which was a telling point. The counselor made a mental note to discuss his reactions but decided not to broach the subject at this time.

There was a knock on the door and the psychologist entered the room. Annie agreed to talk with the psychologist "for a few minutes" and the counselor left the room. The psychologist later reported that it had been a good meeting and that they planned to meet again next week. The counselor made a note to stop by and say hello to Annie at this appointment.

Case 12 wrap-up: This case describes ways to help clients in dysfunctional families deal with their children's positive test results.

Case 13: "I have one more little favor to ask you..."

Marcia, age 40, had the last appointment of a very long clinic day. Before entering the consult room, the counselor noted the intake history—the client had a new diagnosis of ductal carcinoma *in situ* (DCIS) and a strong family history of premenopausal breast cancer in her mother, maternal aunt, and maternal grandmother.

Marcia acknowledged the counselor's greeting with a cool nod and ignored his attempts at small talk. The family history intake was somewhat of an ordeal. Marcia greeted each set of questions with suspicion and demanded explanations as to why certain questions were being asked. She also refused to provide the names of any of her relatives, but then grew impatient when the counselor did not immediately know to which family member she was referring.

The counselor asked Marcia about her recent DCIS diagnosis. Marcia talked about the doctor who had falsely reassured her that it was nothing to worry about and the surgeon who obtained insufficient cells on the first biopsy and had to repeat the procedure. The counselor did his best to remain friendly and calm even when Marcia made comments like "You won't agree with me since you medical people always stick up for each other, but I received appallingly bad treatment from these doctors."

The counselor made some empathetic responses, focusing on the frustration of the diagnostic process rather than the physician's role in it. As Marcia continued with her narrative, her manner toward the genetic counselor began to thaw.

Marcia related that she had already met with a cancer genetic counselor at another hospital (hence her annoyance at having to retell the family history information). She further related that the other counselor had been rude to her. "That counselor was so rushed for time she didn't make any effort to listen to me or to help me. Clearly you are very good at what you do." The genetic counselor felt flattered by the client's praise and was pleased at the connection he had forged with this somewhat challenging client.

Three weeks later, the counselor attempted to call Marcia with the genetic test results, making sure to follow the client's detailed instructions ("E-mail me first, wait an hour, and then call my home phone number but don't leave a message, then try my cell phone.") Marcia called the counselor on the following day and berated him for not being available when she had finally called back (at 9 P.M.). Although the counselor knew it was unreasonable to expect him to be in the office so late in the evening, he found himself apologizing for not being available when she called.

The counselor disclosed the positive *BRCA1* test results to Marcia and they discussed the result at length. The counselor encouraged Marcia to set up an appointment with one of the program oncologists to discuss the medical management recommendations. Marcia requested an appointment on a nonclinic day and the counselor begged a favor from one of the program oncologists who agreed to meet the client at the special time. Marcia was somewhat appreciative of these efforts to accommodate her, but also asked why all of her physicians had not received notification of the genetic test results. The counselor explained the program's confidentiality practices but said that he would be willing to contact her physicians if she gave him written permission to do so.

After the counselor agreed to send the release form to the client as an e-mail attachment, Marcia said, "Also could I ask you for one more little favor? Could you please call my ex-husband and explain the results to him? I don't wish to speak to him but I think he should have the information since we have a 10-year-old daughter."

The counselor agreed to call the client's ex-husband although he felt a little uneasy about contacting him out of the blue.

Marcia faxed back the form granting permission to share the results with others and instructed the counselor to call her once he had contacted her physicians and ex-husband. One hour later, she left a voice mail message to the counselor wondering why he had not yet done what he had promised he would do.

The counselor sent the results to Marcia's physicians and also called her ex-husband. As the counselor left a message on Marcia's cell phone, he felt relieved to be wrapping up this case.

Everything was fine for a few weeks and then Marcia had a misunderstanding with the gynecologic surgeon and called the counselor to "make it right." At the end of the conversation, she said, "Oh, and I have one more little favor to ask you. Thank you for that family letter you sent me, but would you mind personalizing it? It doesn't make a lot of sense for me to send the same letter to my elderly uncle and my young female cousin. It would take me hours to personalize these letters, but I'm sure it would be easy for you to do, right?" The counselor inwardly groaned at the extra amount of work generated by this one case but was so nervous about telling her "no" that he agreed to write a few different versions of the family letter. Marcia thanked him but then proceeded to call him every day that week wondering why she had not yet received these letters.

It got so the counselor felt a stress headache coming on each time he heard Marcia's voice on the phone. She seemed to make some sort of demand every time she called and it did not matter that the demand was neither reasonable nor in the counselor's purview. The genetic counselor tried hard to meet each of Marcia's demands but he felt drained after each of their interactions. Although he was going above and beyond what he typically did for his clients, he constantly found himself apologizing for not meeting her exacting expectations.

After one particularly difficult interaction with Marcia, he sat down with his genetic counseling colleagues and asked for advice for how to handle this client. They helped him to realize that this client was exhibiting classic borderline behavior. They encouraged him to establish boundaries about what he could and could not do and to let go of his fear of failure since it was unlikely that anyone could meet this client's expectations (hence the number of clinicians whom she had fired over the years).

The counselor began to put limits on what he was willing to do for the client. He learned to say, "I am not able to do that but here is what I can do...." Although Marcia expressed her dissatisfaction with him (and the program), the counselor found that he could tolerate her moods much better now that he was no longer trying to please her.

When Marcia's breast MRI exam got cancelled (due to a snowstorm), she became furious at the medical staff and left the genetic counselor a scathing message that she did not like how the program treated its clientele and that she was switching her care back to the other local hospital.

Although the genetic counselor felt a measure of relief that he would not have to deal with this client again, he did feel badly that it had ended this way. Luckily he worked with supportive genetic counselors who assured him that he had done the best he could do.

Two years later, at a conference held for families with positive *BRCA* results, Marcia greeted the counselor like a long-lost friend. She mentioned that she was thinking of transferring her care back to his program.

Case 13 wrap-up: This case demonstrates the importance of setting clear, professional boundaries when dealing with unreasonable, demanding clients.

Case 14: "You know what I mean?"

When the counselor got back to her office she was surprised to realize that the meeting with her client had lasted almost 2 hours. The female client was at 50% risk for carrying the *VHL* gene mutation, which is known to be in her family, and she had come to the high-risk clinic in order to be tested. However, as the counselor dictated the clinic note, her mind kept returning to the client's poignant story about her mother's steady decline from Alzheimer's disease. The client spoke about the agonizing decision to put her mother in an assisted living center earlier this year. She described the events that led to the family's decision, the disagreements between family members regarding the best course of action, the difficulties of finding an appropriate nursing home, and the continued feelings of guilt and grief regarding the whole situation.

The counselor could certainly identify with the client's story. She began to reminisce about her own mother who had passed away 5 years earlier from Alzheimer's disease. She found herself reliving the many years of worry regarding her mother's declining memory and increasingly erratic behavior, making it impossible for her mother to continue living on her own. Then there was the hassle and stress of finding an appropriate assisted living center and the numerous arguments with her younger sister who couldn't or wouldn't see that there was any problem. In fact, the relationship between the counselor and her sister had never fully recovered.

A few days later, the counselor called the client to let her know that her insurance carrier had agreed to cover the cost of the *VHL* test and that the lab had started the DNA analysis. The client thanked the counselor for this information and also mentioned that she would be out of town all of the following week visiting her brothers and would be visiting her mother for the first time since moving her into the assisted living center. The client spoke about her nervousness regarding the upcoming visit with her mother. As they talked about it, the counselor kept picturing the initial meeting with her mother after moving her to an assisted living center. She remembered how she had held her mother's hands while telling her over and over how much she loved her.

The intensity of that remembered encounter with her mother brought tears to the counselor's eyes and she struggled to maintain her composure as she completed the phone call with the client.

The counselor found herself thinking about this client often over the following week, wondering how emotionally difficult it was going to be for the client to see her mother in the assisted living center for the first time.

When the genetic test result became available the counselor called the client and informed her that she did not carry the familial *VHL* mutation. The client was happy to hear this news and the counselor promised to send a copy of the genetic test result to both the client and the referring physician. The counselor then asked about the client's trip to visit her family and braced herself for an onslaught of grief and emotion.

"Oh, it went great. It was so fabulous seeing all of my nieces and nephews. We had a blast, did all kinds of sightseeing and shopping."

This response was so different from what the counselor expected that she was initially at a loss for what to say next. She wondered if it was too emotionally difficult for the client to speak about seeing her mother again. She asked if the client had visited her mother but said that she would understand if the client was not ready to talk about it.

"I don't mind talking about it at all. Actually, the visit with my mother went better than expected. She even knew who I was—at least at first—so that was nice and I was very impressed with the center and the staff. I only stayed about an hour but that was plenty long enough. Afterwards my brother took me out to dinner at this wonderful restaurant; it is run by an internationally renowned chef."

As the client described the fabulous meal she had eaten at the four-star restaurant, the counselor felt totally disoriented. The counselor realized that the client's visit with her mother had been completely different from what she had been expecting—or what she had personally experienced. She asked about the client's future plans to stay in contact with her mother.

"Oh, I don't know; maybe at some point I will visit again. We were never really that close. I just wanted to make sure I got her into a nice place. Now that I've done that, I feel like my part is done. It's time to focus on the living, you know what I mean?"

The counselor who felt completely differently about the matter searched for an appropriate response and finally said that it was important to make peace with situations like this and that she was glad the client had done so.

Following this conversation, the counselor spent a lot of time thinking about this case and how it had triggered so many emotional reactions and memories in her. She also went back and reviewed the initial counseling session. Now that she was looking at the client's case more objectively, she realized that many aspects of the client's situation were completely different from her own situation. She further realized that it was her questions and comments (not the client's needs) that had caused them to spend so much time discussing the impact of Alzheimer's disease on the family.

The counselor talked over the case with the other program staff members and acknowledged that she had overly identified with this client. The counselor also realized that she was clearly not done grieving the loss of her mother and made an appointment to meet with a grief counselor. She also recognized a need to discuss her family experiences with other people in similar situations (who were not clients!), and she joined an active online support group for relatives of people with Alzheimer's disease.

When the client called the counselor back a few months later to refer two of her cousins for genetic counseling and testing, the client mentioned spending her Christmas holidays with her brothers. However, this time the genetic counselor focused the discussion on what it was like for the client to share her true negative test results with the brother who has von Hippel–Lindau syndrome. Neither the client nor the counselor mentioned Alzheimer's disease at all, which allowed the conversation to remain client-centered and much less emotionally charged.

Case 14 wrap-up: This case describes how important it is to recognize and handle situations in which counselors overidentify with clients' stories.

10.5. Further Reading

Djurdjinovic, L. 2009. Psychosocial counseling. In Uhlmann, WR, Schuette, JL, and Yashar, BM (eds), A Guide to Genetic Counseling. Wiley-Blackwell, Hoboken, NJ, 133–175.

Evans, C. 2006. The psychological processes underlying genetic counseling. In Genetic Counselling: A Psychological Approach. Cambridge University Press, New York, 17–43.

Gettig, B. 2010. Grieving: an inevitable journey. In LeRoy, BS, McCarthy Veach, P, and Bartels, DM (eds), Genetic Counseling Practice. Wiley-Blackwell, Hoboken, NJ, 95–124.

McGoldrick M, Gerson, R, and Shellenberger, S. 1999. Genograms Assessment and Intervention, 2nd edition. W.W. Norton, New York.

Patenaude, A. 2005. Emotional baggage: unresolved grief, emotional distress, risk perception, and health beliefs and behaviors. In Genetic Testing for Cancer: Psychological Approaches for Helping Patients and Families. American Psychological Association, Washington, DC, 109–140.

Peters, JA, Kenen, R, Giusti, R, et al. 2004. Exploratory study of the feasibility and utility of the colored eco-genetic relationship map (CEGRM) in women at high genetic risk of developing breast cancer. Am J Med Genet 130A:258–264.

Peters, JA, Hoskins, L, Prindiville, S, et al. 2006. Evolution of the colored eco-genetic relationship map (CEGRM) for assessing social functioning in women in hereditary breast-ovarian (HBOC) families. J Genet Couns 15:477–490.

Veach, PM, LeRoy, BS, and Bartels, DM. 2003. Listening to clients: primary empathy skills. In Facilitating the Genetic Counseling Process: A Practice Manual. Springer, New York, 51–72.

Weil, J. 2000. Techniques of psychosocial genetic counseling. In Psychosocial Genetic Counseling. Oxford University Press, New York, 53–115.

Veach, PM, LeRoy, BS, and Bartels, DM. 2003. Responding to Client Cues: Advanced Empathy and Confrontation. In Facilitating the Genetic Counseling Process: A Practice Manual. Springer, New York, 150–173.

ETHICAL ISSUES IN CANCER GENETIC COUNSELING

> Often, what counts most in the moral life is not consistent adherence to principles and rules but reliable character, good moral sense, and emotional responsiveness.
>
> *(Beauchamp and Childress, 2001, p. 26)*

This chapter describes the major bioethical principles and tenets that are relevant to cancer genetic counseling. This chapter also provides strategies for approaching and resolving ethical dilemmas and discusses the types of ethical dilemmas that cancer genetic counselors may encounter.

11.1. BIOETHICAL PRINCIPLES AND GUIDELINES

11.1.1. INTRODUCTION TO ETHICS

Ethical norms deal with the universally acknowledged definitions of right and wrong. These ethical norms—for example, do not steal, do not lie, or do not kill another human being—form the basic foundation of moral behavior. Although these norms are, by definition, ones that are recognized across cultures, they are not absolute. There may be times when a person has to make a choice between upholding one principle at the sacrifice of another principle. For example, a person may deliberately tell a lie in order to prevent someone from commiting a murder. Most people would agree that under these circumstances it would be acceptable to tell a lie because it saves a human life. However, is it acceptable for a person to tell a lie in order to prevent someone from stealing something? This becomes a less clear-cut situation and the acceptability of lying will depend on the specific circumstances.

Taken together, the basic ethical principles form the common morality. The common morality is formally defined as the group of ethical norms that are accepted by all morally serious individuals regardless of their ethnic, cultural, or religious affiliations. (Individuals who are amoral deliberately reject all of the ethical principles and individuals who are selectively moral follow some but not all of these principles.) There is a difference between the moral norms that are universally accepted versus those that reflect the views of a specific group or can find exceptions to the accepted norms. Although individuals may believe that their ethical views are representative of the common morality, more often than not, their personal views are specific to a certain community.

Using the tenets of the common morality as the foundation, a governing body then creates the rules, rights, and standards of conduct for its constituents or members. As an example, one broad ethical principle is that a person should not steal from others. A governing body will take this broad principle and create the following:

- a statement of what is meant by the term "stealing," which is specific to the organization, institution, or community
- a description of the various categories of stealing (e.g., shoplifting, copyright infringement, identity theft, or armed robbery)
- a detailed list of the probable consequences if caught stealing (e.g., immediate dismissal, fines, restitution, or jail time)

Therefore, the regulatory information provided by a governing body is much more detailed and germane to the individuals within a specific community compared to the overarching ethical principles. (See Table 11.1

TABLE 11.1. The Definition of Principles, Values, and Other Terms Used in Bioethics

Principles—sources or guides for values, rules, duties, and rights
Values—priorities that are thought to be important and desirable
Rules—specific guidelines of what should (or should not) be done
Ideals—goals to which a moral person aspires
Duties—behaviors that are defined by a person's professional or social role
Virtues—morally and socially desirable characteristics
Rights—justified claims that a person (or group) can make on others or on society

Source: Schmerler (2009, p. 365).

for brief definitions of principles, values, rules, ideals, duties, virtues, and rights.)

Professional ethics (or morality) refers to the standards of conduct that are acknowledged by the members of a specific profession. Cancer genetic counselors are expected to follow the rules and guidelines set forth by the following groups or institutions presented in the succeeding sections.

11.1.1.1. Medicine

As allied health professionals, cancer genetic counselors are bound by the same ethical standards as all health-care providers. Thus, counselors need to follow the strict rules regarding patient confidentiality, informed consent, and conflict of interest.

11.1.1.2. State Licensing Board

In certain states, genetic counselors are licensed health professionals and must follow the state's mandated rules for continuing education and clinical competence.

11.1.1.3. American Board of Genetic Counselors

Cancer genetic counselors who practice in the United States need to follow the rules set forth by the American Board of Genetic Counselors (ABGC) regarding certification eligibility and renewal. Other countries have developed (or are in the process of developing) similar governing boards for genetic counselors and genetic nurses.

11.1.1.4. National Society of Genetic Counselors

Cancer genetic counselors are also expected to follow the ethical guidelines developed by the National Society of Genetic Counselors (NSGC), which is their main professional organization. The NSGC has created a code of ethics that describes appropriate ethical conduct in dealings with clients as well as other colleagues. The entire Code of Ethics can be found on the NSGC website (http://www.nsgc.org). Table 11.2 lists the portion of the NSGC Code of Ethics that pertains to client care.

11.1.1.5. Hospital or Other Place of Employment

Cancer genetic counselors also need to follow the specific rules and regulations of the hospital, laboratory, or agency within which they work. For example, cancer counselors who work in governmental agencies may have very different policies regarding their ability to accept consulting work or honoraria compared to counselors who work in a university medical center or clinical laboratory.

TABLE 11.2. THE NATIONAL SOCIETY OF GENETIC COUNSELORS (NSGC) CODE OF ETHICS: GENETIC COUNSELORS AND THEIR CLIENTS*

The counselor–client relationship is based on values of care and respect for the client's autonomy, individuality, welfare, and freedom. The primary concern of genetic counselors is the interests of their clients. Therefore, genetic counselors strive to:

1. Serve those who seek services regardless of personal or external interests or biases.
2. Clarify and define their professional role(s) and relationships with clients and provide an accurate description of their services.
3. Respect their clients' beliefs, inclinations, circumstances, feelings, family relationships and cultural traditions.
4. Enable their clients to make informed decisions, free of coercion, by providing or illuminating the necessary facts and clarifying alternatives and anticipated consequences.
5. Refer clients to other qualified professionals when they are unable to support the clients.
6. Maintain information received from clients as confidential unless released by the client or disclosure is required by law.
7. Avoid the exploitation of their clients for personal advantage, profit, or interest.

Source: National Society of Genetic Counselors (2006).

*This is an excerpt from the NSGC Code of Ethics.

11.1.2. PRINCIPLE-BASED BIOETHICS

Cancer genetic counseling and testing programs should be guided by the bioethical principles of autonomy, nonmaleficence, beneficence, and justice. These four bioethical principles are described in this section.

11.1.2.1. Autonomy

The principle of autonomy states that a person has the right to choose or decline a specific activity and also has the right to privacy. The principle of autonomy includes four important concepts:

- *Competency*—Individuals must be deemed capable of making autonomous decisions in order to be awarded the rights of decision making and privacy. Individuals are deemed competent if they have the capacity to think rationally and reflectively about an issue and can then make a reasonable decision about it. Nonautonomous individuals include minor children, people with mental disability or illness, and prisoners. A person may also be deemed temporarily incompetent due to illness, substance abuse, or emotional distress.
- *Freedom to decide*—Competent individuals have the right to make their own decisions free from any controlling influences. These

controlling influences can range from subtle manipulation to outright coercion. Coercion is defined as the intentional use of force or threats of harm to control another person. Other types of influence include persuasion, which is an appeal to a person's intellect and good sense; manipulation, which is an appeal to a person's emotions; and bribery, which is the offer of some type of incentive, often financial. For example, a woman with colon polyposis may decide to have *APC* testing because her sister has convinced her that it is the logical thing to do (persuasion) or because her parents have pleaded with her to "look at [your] beautiful children and do it for their sake" (manipulation), or because her brother has offered to pay all of her medical bills if she agrees to be tested (bribery). Even if the woman believes her relatives would be upset with her if she ultimately decides not to be tested, it is not coercion because she has not been threatened or harmed in any way. Relatives and others may try to influence a client's decision about genetic testing, but genetic counselors need to keep testing discussions free from any hint of bias or persuasion. It should also be acknowledged that the importance of autonomy in medical decision making differs from culture to culture. In some cultures, medical decisions may be made by the entire family or by key family decision-makers. Western medicine places great emphasis on individual autonomy. However, in reality, one's insurance coverage and financial means dictates, in large part, the number of health care choices that a person has.

- *Informed consent*—Informed consent is a competent person's autonomous authorization of a medical procedure or participation in a research study. The main purpose of informed consent is to protect individuals from possible exploitation or harm. A consent discussion ensures that the person has received sufficient information about a specific procedure or research study and is able to make an informed decision about it. Informed consent has five main elements:
  - the competence of the client
  - the provider's disclosure of the information to the client
  - the client's understanding of the information
  - voluntariness (absence of controlling influences) as the client makes a decision
  - the authorization by the client regarding the procedure or study
  Underdisclosure or nondisclosure of the risks, limitations, or implications of a procedure or study prevents an individual from making a well-informed decision, thus restricting his/her autonomy.
- *Privacy and confidentiality*—As in other medical specialties, the edicts of privacy and confidentiality are important in cancer genetics. Privacy is defined as a person's right to allow or disallow access to

his or her personal data, which includes personal identifiers, medical record notes, and laboratory test results. A breach of privacy occurs when an unauthorized person has gained access to an individual's personal information, such as when a health-care provider sees a medical chart on the triage desk and leafs through it, even though it does not pertain to one of his or her patients. Individuals who share sensitive or private information about themselves or their relatives with their health-care providers trust that this information will remain confidential. Confidentiality, a subset of privacy, refers to information that one person has disclosed to another with the understanding that the information will not be divulged to anyone else. Cancer genetics programs need to develop policies for how to handle sensitive information such as positive genetic test results, nonpaternity, or other family secrets. A breach of confidentiality occurs if the person to whom information was disclosed in confidence fails to protect the information or deliberately discloses it to a third party without the initial person's consent to do so. There are rare instances in which health-care providers are allowed to breach patient confidentiality, primarily to prevent an immediate, unavoidable harm in the client's first-degree relatives. According to the Institute of Medicine Committee on Assessing Genetics Risks, there are only a few circumstances that might justify disclosure of genetic test results to a third party. (See Table 11.3.) For example, a genetic counselor can consider sharing genetic test results with a client's first-degree relatives if the disclosure of the result would result in averting harm in the relative. This assumes that the knowledge of one's gene status would prevent this harm (a rare circumstance).

11.1.2.2. Nonmaleficence

The phrase in medicine *primum non nocere* (first, do no harm) summarizes the principle of nonmaleficence. A maleficent act is one that thwarts a

TABLE 11.3. CIRCUMSTANCES THAT MAY JUSTIFY PROVIDERS TO DISCLOSE GENETIC TEST RESULTS TO A CLIENT'S CLOSE RELATIVES WITHOUT PRIOR CONSENT

- Attempts to elicit voluntary disclosure have failed.
- There is a high probability of irreversible or fatal harm to the relative if not disclosed.
- The disclosure of the information will prevent harm.
- The disclosure is limited to the information necessary for the diagnosis or treatment of the relative.
- There is no other reasonable way to avert the harm.

Source: Committee on Assessing Genetic Risks, Division of Health Sciences Policy, Institute of Medicine (1994).

person's actions or causes a person to suffer some type of setback. Genetic counselors, along with other health-care providers, have a responsibility to avoid actions that could cause harm to clients. In contrast to beneficence, which is about doing something to prevent harm, nonmaleficence is about *not* doing something in order to avoid harm. For example, cancer testing programs may have a moral obligation not to test individuals who express suicidal ideation. A policy of not testing people who are actively suicidal is an example of nonmaleficence; the programmatic supports and safeguards in place for emotionally fragile individuals who undergo genetic testing are examples of beneficence. Medical malpractice suits focus on a provider's alleged negligence, which is defined as the intentional or unintentional infliction of harm (or risk of harm) to a client.

11.1.2.3. Beneficence

Beneficent acts are ones that aid an individual by either improving the person's situation or by reducing the person's risk of an adverse event. Beneficence includes acts of kindness, charity, and heroism. In keeping with this principle, health-care providers have an obligation to help clients or, at the least, to make sure things do not become worse for them. This means that genetic counselors, along with other health-care providers, are obligated to provide clients with accurate and timely information. Health-care providers who take it upon themselves to make medical decisions on behalf of their clients are termed paternalistic, because it is comparable to a caring father who makes unilateral decisions about his child's welfare but is assumed to have the child's best interests at heart. All paternalistic actions restrict a person's autonomous choices, but in a limited number of circumstances, a paternalistic act of beneficence may be justified. For example, a person who takes away the car keys of a friend who is inebriated has curtailed the friend's autonomy, but few would argue that it was not justified. However, situations that would justify acts of paternalistic beneficence are unlikely to occur in cancer genetic counseling, so counselors should guard against under- or nondisclosing facts or options to clients regardless of the alleged justification. (e.g., a client's terminal illness, a request from the client's spouse).

11.1.2.4. Justice

The principle of justice is the translation of bioethics into public policy. It deals with concepts of equality, liberty, quality care, and quality control. Health-care systems are expected to provide care that is equitable, appropriate, and of high quality regardless of a patient's race, ethnicity, religion, sexual orientation, or ability to pay. An injustice is defined as a wrongful act or omission that denies certain people their deserved benefits. The principle of justice also requires that burdens be distributed fairly; thus, policies should not worsen the plight of those who are already disadvantaged. For this reason, many hospital emergency rooms have policies that they will not turn away any indigent patients who are seriously ill or injured. The principle of justice also contains the following important points:

- *Equals should be treated equally*—Clients who are capable of autonomous decision making should be given similar information and options regarding genetic testing and cancer surveillance. Autonomous clients should also have the freedom of choice regarding providers or services.

- *The authority to make and enforce rules of equitability*—All communities and institutions have rules regarding issues of fairness and accessibility. In the creation of these rules, it is important to answer the following questions:
    - Who has the authority to set up these rules? (e.g., elected officials, special appointed committee)
    - How will these rules be set up? (e.g., open forum, closed committee meetings, group vote)
    - Who will have the authority to enforce these rules? (board of directors, licensing board)
    - How will these rules be enforced? (e.g., honor system, random testing)

- *Distribution of rare resources*—Issues of fairness arise in the allocation of rare resources such as vaccines, platelets, or donated organs. The allocation of these rare resources may require an algorithm that takes into account several factors including a person's immediate need, overall prognosis, and risk of worsening without the resource. The allocation process must be a fair one for everyone, but should also allow those who are most in need to have precedence. For this reason, the most seriously ill patients will jump to the top of an organ transplant list regardless of how long other (more stable) patients have been waiting for an organ donation.

- *Distribution of risks*—When making decisions regarding population-based screening programs or the approval of new drugs, policymakers will consider the potential risks of implementation versus the risks of nonimplementation. Potential costs and benefits are also important to consider.

11.1.3. VIRTUE ETHICS

[We] all recognize that morality would be a cold and uninspiring practice without various emotional responses and heart-felt ideals that reach beyond principles and rules.

(Beauchamp and Childress, 2001, p. 26)

Virtue ethics focuses on a person's moral character that influences one's viewpoints and behaviors. Moral character is a combination of personally held principles, obligations, ideals, beliefs, motives, and emotions. Individuals who behave in ethical ways do so because they have a strong inner moral code. Therefore, virtue ethics is about doing the right thing for the right reason. A person who performs a good deed in hopes of receiving a reward or recognition is not a morally virtuous person (even if the act is a moral one).

Ordinary moral standards can be defined as the common standards that apply to everyone. In a way, these standards are the "moral minimum" that is acceptable to moral individuals. In contrast, extraordinary moral standards exemplify behavior and attitudes that are above and beyond the ordinary moral standard. People who display extraordinary moral behavior can (and should) be admired, but people who do not live up to this ideal of behavior should not be criticized for it.

For example, a toddler slips and falls into a shallow wading pool as an adult is walking by. Rescuing this young child would be the expected action of any moral adult even if the adult cannot swim and does not know the child. Thus, it is an ordinary act of virtue. In contrast, a surfer runs into dangerous ocean currents and is in danger of drowning. The average person on the beach would not be expected to attempt a rescue because of the danger involved in doing so. Anyone who does attempt to rescue the surfer would be praised for the act of heroism because the actions were above and beyond what is reasonably expected. Thus, it would be an extraordinary act of virtue. However, the definition of an extraordinary act depends in part on one's professional expertise. If the person who witnessed the troubled surfer happened to be a certified lifeguard, then that person would be held to a higher standard of obligation in terms of mounting a rescue.

Medical care providers have certain professional obligations regarding the care of clients who have come to them with specific health-related concerns. Clients who feel as though their medical care providers did not take good care of them may lodge complaints with the hospital or may even take the providers to court to sue for damages. Providers who commit a so-called honest mistake (i.e., an error that is somewhat understandable given the set of circumstances) are more likely to be forgiven than providers who commit errors that have resulted in personal gain or that demonstrate a pattern of deception. Mistakes in medicine can be due to:

- *Errors in technique or skill*—such as when a surgeon botches a surgical procedure.
- *Errors in judgment*—such as a misdiagnosis that results in the wrong treatment.
- *Normative errors*—such as when a basic norm of conduct has been violated, thus, raising concerns about the provider's moral character.

TABLE 11.4. Moral Character Traits That Are Important for
Cancer Genetic Counselors

- Compassion
- Conscientiousness
- Discernment
- Fidelity
- Integrity
- Kindness
- Respectfulness
- Trustworthiness
- Veracity
- Wisdom

- *Systems errors*—such as faulty procedures or policies that have culminated in the error.

Medical care providers are expected to be of "good moral character," and this language continues to be used by licensing boards. In fact, as described below, there are several character traits that are relevant for cancer genetic counselors (see Table 11.4).

11.1.3.1. Compassion

Counselors need to treat their clients with compassion, which means treating clients as human beings, not cases. It also means that genetic counselors need to maintain a professional and empathetic manner with all clients, including the clients who are challenging or difficult.

11.1.3.2. Conscientiousness

Genetic counselors should have a strong inner moral compass that allows them to determine whether certain courses of action are right or wrong. Counselors should also have an ability to self-reflect on their prior actions or decisions.

11.1.3.3. Discernment

Discernment has to do with recognizing and understanding the nuances of a specific situation. Discerning medical care providers are ones with excellent clinical skills and finely honed instincts based on one's knowledge and expertise. For example, the discerning cancer counselor knows whether a confused client would benefit from a review of the information or would be better served by exploring the emotional impact of the topic.

11.1.3.4. Fidelity

Fidelity is about acting in good faith and keeping one's promises. Cancer genetic counselors have certain professional obligations to their clients, who in turn trust that the counselors will meet these obligations. For example, genetic counselors who promise to follow up with clients within a certain time frame should make every effort to do so. Failure to do so can be considered a breach of fidelity, which can seriously impair the counselor–client relationship. (Also see the section on trustworthiness.)

11.1.3.5. Integrity

Integrity is about making sound choices that are morally affirming and honorable. It is also about adhering to one's personal moral code. This might involve reminding clients that participation in a clinical research study is voluntary or explaining that a new genetic test is clinically available. A genetic counselor who has concerns that a client is being treated unfairly by another medical provider should strive to advocate on behalf of the client. Counselors who act (or fail to act) in contrast to their inner moral values have compromised their integrity.

11.1.3.6. Kindness

Counselors need to treat their clients in a kind, caring manner. Counselors should demonstrate sensitivity and tact with their word choices and explanations so as not to unduly upset or offend clients.

11.1.3.7. Respectfulness

Counselors should regard their clients (and colleagues) with respect. Counselors may not always agree with their clients' decisions and actions, but they should remain respectful and supportive toward their clients. Counselors should also be respectful toward their genetics colleagues as well as other health-care providers.

11.1.3.8. Trustworthiness

Counselors who are trustworthy have shown that they are worthy of the level of trust that others have placed on them. Clients trust that their genetic counselors will provide them with accurate information and will help facilitate the decision-making process in a way that is supportive and nonjudgmental. Lack of trust is one of the main reasons why clients switch to different medical care providers and why some providers feel compelled to practice defensive medicine.

11.1.3.9. Veracity

Veracity has to do with telling the truth and taking care not to deceive people. It implies a pattern of communicating with honesty, integrity, and credibility. Genetic counselors have an obligation to disclose accurate, comprehensive, and timely information to their clients.

11.1.3.10. Wisdom

Counselors should have a solid foundation of knowledge regarding cancer genetic syndromes, available genetic tests, relevant counseling issues, and available referral sources. In addition to knowing the facts, counselors need to have the skill and sensitivity to know how best to relay this information to clients. Counselors who are wise also know when *not* to say something and also feel comfortable admitting when they do not know the answer to a client's question.

11.1.4. ETHICS OF CARING

The ethics of caring theory states that the moral actions of one person toward another person will differ depending on whether the two people are friends, relatives, strangers, or providers/clients. In other words, it is the *relationship* of the two people that defines the level of care, trust, and obligation between them. Clients who seek cancer genetic counseling expect to receive information about the risk of hereditary cancers and options for genetic testing. Therefore, cancer genetic counselors have an obligation to answer the client's questions and provide information that is up to date and accurate.

The ethics of caring theory grew out of observations from Carol Gilligan, a feminist researcher who suggested that there were gender differences in how children viewed ethical dilemmas. While boys tended to focus on aspects of justice and impartial rights, girls tended to focus on their sense of obligation and desire to care for others. This observation led others to study the importance of attachments and obligations in one's moral actions. Caring theorists also stress the importance of receptivity, responsiveness, and context when facing ethical decisions. (Today, we would be more likely to focus on the spectrum of differences in approaches that may be present among individuals regardless of gender.)

Caring theorists encourage medical care providers to have "attached attentiveness" (e.g., to be attentive, helpful, kind, and caring) to patients who are vulnerable and dependent. Therefore, it is important for counselors to be attentive to clients, but not to become overly involved (enmeshed). Caring theory also places emphasis on *how* actions are performed by medical care providers—for example, willingly, grudgingly, kindly, or carelessly—and considers how a provider's actions may promote or prevent a meaningful provider–client relationship.

11.1.5. Strategies for Being an Ethical Cancer Counselor

This section attempts to take the bioethical principles mentioned earlier in this chapter and create a set of strategies that are appropriate for the ethically minded cancer genetic counselor. (See Table 11.5.) Strategies for being an ethical cancer counselor are presented in the succeeding sections.

11.1.5.1. Have Strategies for Dealing with Ethical Dilemmas

There are a variety of ethical dilemmas that can occur in cancer genetic counseling. Genetic counselors should develop strategies for assessing and resolving ethical dilemmas. More detailed information on resolving clinically based ethical dilemmas can be found in Section 11.2.2.

11.1.5.2. Keep Accurate and Complete Records

Counselors are required to document information in the client's medical record. This includes information regarding client visits, telephone conversations, the genetic pedigree, testing decisions or results, any possible concerns, and plans for follow-up. Clients are best served when the case documentation is accurate and complete.

11.1.5.3. Keep Up to Date with the Latest Advances in Cancer Genetics

The landscape of cancer genetics is constantly changing. In order to provide quality care to clients, it is important for counselors to remain current themselves regarding scientific, medical, psychological, and counseling advances.

11.1.5.4. Know How to Ascertain Client Autonomy

Counselors may encounter clients who are not autonomous and therefore cannot legally consent to medical procedures such as genetic testing.

TABLE 11.5. Strategies for Being an Ethical Cancer Genetic Counselor

---

- Have strategies for dealing with ethical dilemmas
- Keep accurate and complete records
- Keep up to date with the latest advances in cancer genetics
- Know how to ascertain client autonomy
- Practice attached attentiveness
- Respect client confidentiality
- Respect client privacy
- Respect the client's decisions
- Tell the truth but be gentle
- Treat informed consent as a process

Counselors should have strategies in place for ascertaining a client's ability to sign a medical informed consent. Counselors will also need to clarify who is the client's legal guardian and to make sure that the client's legal guardian is included in the informed consent discussions.

11.1.5.5. Practice Attached Attentiveness

Genetic counselors should forge empathetic relationships with their clients. Even in the midst of explaining facts and figures to clients, counselors need to pay attention to the clients' emotional reactions and coping mechanisms.

11.1.5.6. Respect Client Confidentiality

Counselors need to respect client confidentiality by not releasing any client data, especially genetic information, to a third party. Examples of third parties include other medical providers, insurance agents, or the client's relatives. Thus, genetic pedigrees that are sent to another institution for review should not contain any identifiers. Ethical dilemmas can occur when a client shares genetic test results with some but not all relatives. However, unless there are extenuating circumstances, counselors should not share a client's genetic test result with any of the client's relatives without prior permission from the client, preferably in writing.

11.1.5.7. Respect Client Privacy

Counselors should ensure that clients' personal data and genetic information are kept private. This means setting policies about the types of information collected about clients and their relatives, as well as determining which staff members will have access to the client's pedigree and genetic test results. In addition, clients may request that certain personal information be kept "off the record" or request that they undergo genetic testing under a false name. When considering requests of this nature, counselors need to seek solutions that try to accommodate clients (whenever possible) while continuing to comply with hospital regulations and programmatic policies.

11.1.5.8. Respect the Client's Decisions

At times, clients make decisions that differ widely from the standard recommendations (and may be difficult to comprehend). For example, a woman with a *BRCA* mutation may decide to pursue prenatal testing with the plan to terminate the pregnancy of any fetus carrying a *BRCA* mutation (male or female). A postmenopausal woman with a *BRCA* mutation may elect to retain her ovaries despite a strong medical recommendation to have the ovaries surgically removed. Both these types of decisions are outside of what most clients would choose to do, and they may evoke strong reactions in counselors. Even if the decision does not seem to make sense (from a medical standpoint), counselors need to accept that clients have the right to their own decisions and actions. It may also be helpful for counselors to ask clients (in a nonjudgmental way) what led them to make the decisions that they made.

11.1.5.9. Tell the Truth but Be Gentle

It is obviously important for counselors to be honest with their clients, but the dissemination of information should always be accompanied by gentleness, sensitivity, and compassion. Relaying all the syndromic features and screening options in one fell swoop may be overwhelming to some clients. Clients may be quite unprepared to deal with the news that they (and their offspring) could have an inherited cancer syndrome. In these cases, it may be helpful for counselors to help clients to adjust to the news emotionally before continuing to provide more didactic information.

11.1.5.10. Treat Informed Consent as a Process

The purpose of informed consent is to provide sufficient information so that a client can make an informed decision about a specific procedure, test, or study. (Also see Section 11.1.2.1 for the major elements of the consent process.) The consent form—and discussion—should describe the procedure or study as well as its risks, benefits, and alternative options. (Refer to Table 9.2, which lists the major topics to be included in consent discussions for cancer genetic tests.) Having an informed consent dialogue gives clients an opportunity to ask questions and ensures that clients know what it is they are being asked to do.

11.2. STRATEGIES FOR RESOLVING ETHICAL DILEMMAS

Cancer genetic counselors can face an array of ethical problems in their clinical practices. Given the complexities of family relationships, it is not surprising that genetic testing can lead to disagreements and dilemmas among clients and their relatives. In addition, counselors may acquire a certain piece of information and then have to decide whether or not to disclose the information to the client (or the client's relatives).

When it comes to resolving ethical dilemmas there are seldom any right answers. This is one reason why ethical dilemmas can be so daunting. This section suggests ways in which counselors can frame, assess, and resolve ethical dilemmas.

11.2.1. Upholding versus Infringing an Ethical Principle

An ethical dilemma occurs when any course of action will result in the upholding of one ethical principle and the infringement of another ethical principle. As a first step toward approaching ethical dilemmas, genetic counselors should consider when it might be appropriate to choose one ethical principle over another principle.

According to Tom Beauchamp and James Childress (2001, pp. 19–20), the following reasons presented in the succeeding sections can be used to justify upholding one ethical principle at the cost of infringing another ethical principle.

11.2.1.1. There Are Better Reasons to Justify Upholding One Principle over the Opposing Principle

For example, an adult who is severely anemic refuses to undergo a blood transfusion. Although the transfusion is deemed medically necessary, this person's right to autonomous decision making takes precedence over the physician's beneficent recommendation.

11.2.1.2. The Intended Consequence Used to Justify Infringing an Ethical Principle Must Have a Realistic Chance of Being Attained

For example, a clinical trial may be restricted to a certain group of individuals, which infringes the ethical principle of access (justice) for the people who are not eligible for the study (yet could conceivably benefit from participation). However, the study researchers may be able to justify their narrow eligibility criteria as the best way to obtain statistically significant results, which might ultimately benefit the most people.

11.2.1.3. The Infringement of the Ethical Principle Is Considered Necessary, Because There Are No Morally Preferable Alternatives

For example, individuals are prohibited from selling their own kidneys even though they theoretically own all of their body parts. Despite the fact that thousands of people die each year from the lack of donor kidneys, the prohibition ban on selling human organs is deemed necessary because of the high likelihood of abuse if such an action were permitted.

11.2.1.4. The Infringement of the Ethical Principle Is the Least Possible Infringement in Order to Attain the Primary Moral Objective

For example, researchers are allowed to exclude certain groups of people from their study in order to maximize the likelihood of obtaining meaningful results. However, even though it may complicate the implementation of the study, researchers are often required to include people who speak different languages, are of differing ages or genders, and/or have physical impairments that will have no bearing on the study conclusions.

11.2.1.5. Any Potential Negative Effects of the Ethical Principle's Infringement Must Be Minimized

For example, in a randomized clinical trial, the investigators have the ability (and obligation) to halt the study early if the experimental drug leads to unexpectedly strong negative or positive results. Thus, participants in the experimental group can be assured that the study will be prematurely halted if the drug is found to cause life-threatening, serious side effects. In addition, participants in the control group can be assured that they will be allowed access to the experimental drug if it is found to be dramatically effective.

11.2.1.6. Any Decision Made to Uphold One Set of Ethical Principles over Another Set of Ethical Principles Has Been Made Impartially and Fairly

For example, the main purpose of a hospital investigational review board (IRB) is to protect potential study participants by considering the relative risks, benefits, and aims of clinical research studies. Members of the IRB who are involved in a specific study are expected to excuse themselves from the discussions and vote regarding the study protocol, because they are no longer considered to be unbiased and impartial reviewers.

11.2.2. HOW TO EVALUATE ETHICAL DILEMMAS

Facing an ethical dilemma is sometimes referred to as being between a rock and a hard place. In other words, there may not be a perfect solution to the problem (hence the word "dilemma"). However, that is not to say there are no possible resolutions to ethical dilemmas; even nonaction is a response. The aim for cancer counselors is to develop a framework for how to approach and evaluate ethical dilemmas. This section offers a set of strategies that cancer counselors can employ when facing ethical dilemmas. (Also see Table 11.6.)

11.2.2.1. Gather the Facts of the Case

The first step is to gather all of the available data about the ethical case. In a cancer genetics case, this may include gathering information about the client's cancer diagnosis, genetic testing options or results, family dynamics, and the availability of cancer screening. Counselors should ask themselves,

TABLE 11.6. A SET OF STRATEGIES FOR ASSESSING AND RESOLVING ETHICAL DILEMMAS

- Gather the facts of the case
- Get input from all stakeholders
- Ascertain the question(s) being asked
- Determine how and by whom the decision will be made
- Consider and balance the opposing ethical principles
- Brainstorm the possible ways to resolve the dilemma
- Consider the ramifications of each possible course of action
- Use all available resources to help make decisions
- Decide upon a course of action
- Take time to reflect on the case afterwards

Sources: Beauchamp and Childress (2001); Schmerler (2009).

"Are the facts of the case clear? Do I have all the information I need to assess this case?" Having incomplete facts could introduce a source of bias and make it less likely that a fair decision will be reached. And in some instances, counselors might discover that the disagreement is actually based on confusion or misinformation about the facts rather than a clash of ethical values.

11.2.2.2. Get Input from All Stakeholders

In gathering the relevant facts of an ethical case, it is important to obtain information from all of the people who are involved in the case. For example, counselors may find it helpful to speak to the client's spouse, other relctives, physicians, or therapists. Obtaining input from all the people involved in the case ensures that each person's perspective will be represented. It also allows counselors to identify the important people in the case, including the extent of information that they have regarding the issue, and what their stake is in the final outcome of the case. There may be times when it is not feasible to speak directly to everyone who is involved in the case. In these instances, counselors will need to keep in mind that they have gleaned their information from secondary sources.

11.2.2.3. Ascertain the Question(s) Being Asked

Before seeking an answer to an ethical dilemma, it is important to know the exact question that is being asked. It is often useful to write out the question or concern that is at the crux of the ethical dilemma. This is not always as easy as it sounds. If the counselor struggles with phrasing the question or identifying which ethical principles are at stake, then perhaps the facts of the case are incomplete or perhaps the situation does not qualify as a true ethical dilemma. Counselors should also pay attention as to why this particular question is being asked at this particular time. Determining what (or who) is driving the question may be an important element of the case.

11.2.2.4. Determine How and by Whom the Decision Will Be Made

It is useful to know whether the ethical decision-making process will involve informal discussions or formal consultations and whether the counselor needs to initiate any of these discussions. Counselors should also be aware if there are any time constraints or urgency to resolving the case. In addition, it is helpful to recognize who has the final say on a specific ethical dilemma. Is it up to the counselor, the team of providers, or a colleague at a different hospital? Perhaps the final decision rests with the client or one of the client's relatives. Even if counselors do not have the final say in the outcome of the case, they may benefit from conducting these types of ethical case analyses.

11.2.2.5. Consider and Balance the Opposing Ethical Principles

Counselors should develop strategies to evaluate the opposing ethical principles in the case. There are a number of approaches that can be utilized when assessing the opposing principles in an ethical dilemma. One strategy involves assigning values (weights) to each of the ethical principles as a way of comparing and contrasting them. Another strategy involves evaluating the pros and cons of each course of action to identify which is either the most beneficial or the least harmful. Regardless of which strategy is used to assess an ethical case, it may be helpful for counselors to utilize a "reason over emotion" approach while remaining empathetic and compassionate toward the individuals trapped in the dilemma. Counselors can structure their assessment around one or more of the ethical theories by asking themselves the following types of questions:

- What course of action would promote the greatest amount of happiness for the greatest number of people? (consequence-based utilitarianism)
- What are the key ethical principles at stake in this case? How would I prioritize the importance of each ethical principle in this case? (principle-based ethics)
- How would most responsible counselors act in this case? Which course of action is consistent with my inner moral character? (virtue ethics)
- What is the most caring and compassionate course of action I could take? What are my obligations to this client? (caring ethics)

There may not be one perfect solution to the ethical dilemma, but the counselor's course of action does need to be ethically justifiable for both the client and the counselor.

11.2.2.6. Brainstorm the Possible Ways to Resolve the Dilemma

It is helpful to consider all of the different ways to resolve the dilemma. The counselor can start by listing the two main ways to resolve most ethical dilemmas, which can be summarized as "action" versus "no action." Then, the counselor can go on to consider all of the additional possibilities including partial action, action on the part of someone else, compromise, or referral. Even if a certain strategy is not realistic, it may be helpful to write it down during this phase of the analysis.

11.2.2.7. Consider the Ramifications of Each Possible Course of Action

It is important that the resolution of the ethical case be one that the client—and the counselor—can live with. Counselors should consider the potential consequences for each possible course of action or nonaction. Sometimes a certain course of action has unintended (or undesirable) effects. Remember that the resolution of an ethical dilemma often involves choosing the option that is the lesser of two unpleasant options. The counselor can also look for ways to mediate a resolution in the case. For example, if the case involves an ethical dilemma between the client and his or her relative, is it possible for them to come to some type of agreement or compromise?

11.2.2.8. Use All Available Resources to Help Make Decisions

As counselors consider the various options for resolving an ethical dilemma, it is important to determine whether there are any rules or regulations that prohibit or require certain actions. Genetic counselors should also consult their colleagues, published ethical guidelines, and other available resources. (Please see Section 11.2.3 for more specific information on this topic.)

11.2.2.9. Decide upon a Course of Action

The case analysis culminates with coming to a decision about the case and then carrying out the decision. In some cases, counselors may need to inform clients what the program is willing to do and then it is up to the clients to decide whether to stay with the program or go elsewhere. Counselors will also need to consider whether there are any logistical issues or obstacles that need to be addressed before proceeding with the decided-upon action. Lastly, counselors should always document the ethical case carefully in the event that there are any questions about it at a later time.

11.2.2.10. Take Time to Reflect on the Case Afterward

After the case has concluded, it is important for counselors to take the time to reflect on the case. Counselors can consider whether their reasoning of the case and ultimate course of action brought about the desired outcome. Counselors can also reflect on whether anything could or should have been done differently and whether any programmatic changes need to be made in order to avoid similar situations in the future. Counselors are also encouraged to share their insights and lessons learned with other providers so that all may benefit from the experience.

11.2.3. GETTING HELP WITH ETHICAL DILEMMAS

Struggling with ethical dilemmas can be difficult and counselors may feel quite alone as they deal with these types of cases. Yet there are several resources that may be helpful in the evaluation and resolution of ethical dilemmas. These resources include the following presented in the succeeding sections.

11.2.3.1. Ethical Codes and Professional Guidelines

When considering possible ways to resolve ethical dilemmas, counselors should be guided by the NSGC code of ethics (refer to Table 11.2 for an excerpt of this document). Counselors should also seek out the clinical standards of care and ethical guidelines that have been developed by other medical organizations, such as the National Institutes of Health, the American Society of Human Genetics, the American College of Medical Genetics, and the American Society of Clinical Oncology. Table 11.7 provides another useful set of guidelines regarding pre- and posttest counseling developed by David Smith et al. (1998).

11.2.3.2. Colleagues and Others

Counselors may find it extremely beneficial to discuss the case with colleagues. Colleagues may be able to help the counselor reason through the case, provide much needed emotional support, suggest additional resources, and point out alternative ways to resolve the case. Some ethical cases raise questions that are best answered by outside providers or other types of professionals. Counselors may find it helpful to discuss the elements of ethical cases with physicians, nurses, lawyers, clinical bioethicists, psychologists, or members of the clergy.

11.2.3.3. Hospital Ethical Review Boards

Most major medical centers have standing or ad hoc Ethical Review Boards (EABs). Counselors can request formal, and sometimes informal, ethical consultations from these hospital EABs. The counselor would provide the EAB with details of the case (orally or in writing) and then the EAB would

TABLE 11.7. ETHICAL GUIDELINES FOR GENETIC COUNSELORS PROVIDING
PREDICTIVE TESTING

- Professionals should consider ethical issues from the inception of every testing, counseling, and research program, and they should provide consultands with information that is appropriately tailored to the stage of the testing–counseling program the consultand has reached. To the extent possible, ethical dilemmas should be anticipated and the counselor should try to prevent them from arising.
- Genetic testing should be accompanied by both pre- and posttest counseling conducted by persons with competencies in medical genetics, laboratory analysis, counseling, and the psychosocial impact of genetic information.
- Protocols are useful guidelines for the appropriate conduct of presymptomatic testing. Justifications for departure from a protocol must relate to the rationale for that protocol.
- Genetic counselors are ethically obligated to maintain consultands' confidentiality.
- In deciding whether to refuse or postpone testing, genetic counselors should exercise professional judgment based on clinical observation and the consultand's history.
- Consultands should remain free to reject disclosure of test results and other diagnostic information unless their decision not to know their status poses a significant risk to others.
- The fact that testing a consultand will reveal the genetic status of other persons who prefer not to know their status is not, by itself, a sufficient reason to delay testing.
- Genetic testing of symptomatic children to make or confirm a diagnosis may be performed subject to general ethical and legal rules governing medical care for children.
- Presymptomatic genetic testing should only be performed on children when all of the conditions set out in paragraphs A, B, and C are met:
  A A presymptomatic test should be given to a child only if both of the child's parents who are reasonably available have consented to the testing. If only one parent is reasonably available, that parent must consent to the testing.
  B If the child has or can be provided with a reasonable understanding of the proposed genetic test and its implications, the child's assent to genetic testing must be sought.
  C There must be a reasonable possibility that testing will enable the child to receive a real demonstrable benefit.

Source: Smith et al. (1998, pp. 131–163). Printed with permission.

conduct its own case analysis and render recommendations accordingly. Recommendations made by the EAB are seldom binding, but the written reports are generally quite thoughtful and useful. Counselors are encouraged to seek EAB consultations for ongoing cases as well as completed cases that had less than optimal outcomes.

11.2.3.4. Other Types of Ethics Committees

Many professional organizations have ad hoc or standing ethics committees that are available to their membership for consultation. For example, the NSGC has an ethics committee that can provide confidential feedback and recommendations to members regarding specific ethical issues. The advantages to utilizing this type of ethics committee is that its scope of understanding in regards to clinical cancer genetic issues may be greater than the average hospital EAB and it may also be easier to keep confidential any sensitive ethical dilemmas regarding coworkers.

11.3. TYPES OF ETHICAL DILEMMAS IN CANCER GENETIC COUNSELING

> Genetic counseling, with its emphasis on education and empowerment, took root from concepts of autonomous choice.
>
> *(Offit and Thom, 2007, p. 435)*

Cancer genetic counselors are well versed in dealing with ethical dilemmas, which is fortunate since these types of situations are not uncommon in clinical cancer genetics. This section offers examples and discussions/strategies for 17 specific ethical dilemmas that cancer genetic counselors might face. This section ends with a brief overview of the professional/societal issues that might impact on the counselor's ability to provide quality cancer genetic counseling services.

11.3.1. ETHICAL QUESTION #1: INCOMPLETE CONSENT

Question: A counselor is not able to fully describe all elements of genetic testing (due to time constraints, client ailments, or other factors). Is it appropriate for the counselor to continue the consent process in this circumstance?

Discussion: It may be appropriate to continue the consent process in these circumstances if, in the counselor's professional judgment, sufficient information has been provided. Ideally, counselors would have an hour or longer to discuss all of the ramifications of testing with clients who are fully engaged in the discussion. In reality, this is often not feasible. Counselors need to ensure that they cover the main elements of testing—especially the ones that are most relevant to the clients' situations—even if in-depth discussions are not possible. It is helpful for counselors to be aware of any time constraints or other limiting factors (e.g., clients' health) at the outset in order to optimize the session. Determining what clients want and expect from genetic testing can also help guide the encounters. In addition to giving clients copies of the written consent forms, counselors can provide testing factsheets and encourage the clients to recontact them if there are any further questions. Counselors can also arrange to have follow-up interactions with clients to review or expand on the information.

11.3.2. ETHICAL QUESTION #2: INADEQUATELY UNDERSTOOD CONSENT

Question: A counselor is concerned that the client does not adequately understand the testing discussion (due to emotional distress, language barrier, or other factors). Is it appropriate for the counselor to continue the consent process?

Discussion: It is sometimes difficult to ascertain whether clients truly understand the information being presented to them. In these situations, counselors must rely on their best professional judgment as to whether clients have sufficient understanding of the test in order to proceed with the consenting process. Counselors should try to minimize language problems by utilizing interpreters and avoiding technical jargon. Counselors should also be aware of any emotional reactions or defenses that might be interfering with the clients' abilities to process the information. Counselors can ask clients to reiterate certain points in order to ascertain comprehension or to uncover misconceptions. Counselors can also make arrangements to follow up with clients, so that they can answer further questions and review information.

11.3.3. ETHICAL QUESTION #3: PRESSURE / COERCION

Question: A client shares with the counselor that he/she is being pressured (by relatives, medical care providers, or others) to undergo the genetic test. Upon hearing this information, is it appropriate for counselors to continue the consent process?

Discussion: True coercion involves some type of harm or the threat of harm; however, there are many other types of more subtle pressure, including persuasion and manipulation. Some clients will admit that they have been "talked into" genetic testing, often by one of their relatives or physicians. Counselors need to remind these clients that, in fact, they do have a choice as to whether to proceed with testing at this time. Counselors can also describe possible alternatives to testing (e.g., offering genetic testing to other relatives or undergoing cancer screening without having the genetic test). Some clients will be grateful for the chance to defer or decline testing. Other clients may decide that their family obligations or their trust in their physicians' opinions trump their qualms about being tested. Even so, they may have appreciated the chance to consider alternative options. Counselors can also explore with clients the motivations for why certain people are pressuring them to be tested. Are they motivated by self-interest or do they believe that testing is in the clients' best interests? Do the individuals involved have a realistic view about what testing will tell them? Is there any type of misunderstanding between the clients and these other individuals? Counselors who do encounter situations of actual coercion (which is rare) should immediately halt the discussions and request assistance from the appropriate individuals (e.g., program director, referring physician, or hospital security).

11.3.4. ETHICAL QUESTION #4: LACK OF AUTONOMY

Question: A counselor has doubts as to whether the client has the authority or capacity to consent to a specific genetic test. Is it appropriate for the counselor to continue the consent process for testing?

Discussion: If counselors have any doubt regarding their clients' abilities to authorize genetic testing, then these concerns should be raised early in the process (preferably prior to the appointment). Possible strategies include asking clients whether they typically make their own medical decisions (and if they sign their own medical documents), checking with the clients' relatives or primary care physicians, and reviewing the situation with the program directors or colleagues. Counselors are advised not to proceed with genetic testing discussions if they have any major concerns about the clients' authority to provide legal informed consent.

11.3.5. ETHICAL QUESTION #5: CONFLICT OF INTEREST

Question: The counselor has a bias or vested interest in whether the client agrees to have the genetic test. Is it appropriate for the counselor to continue the consent process for testing?

Discussion: Counselors should be aware of their own biases in order to guard against being persuasive or directive in their discussions about genetic testing. It is only natural for counselors to have personal opinions regarding the decisions that clients are making. However, counselors should maintain a neutral and nonjudgmental stance in terms of clients' decisions to be tested. Counselors who have a possible vested interest in whether the clients' are tested should disclose these potential conflicts of interest to clients, preferably at the outset. If there is a definite conflict of interest, then the counselors should excuse themselves from the testing discussions and arrange for other staff members to conduct the consent process.

11.3.6. ETHICAL QUESTION #6: UNAUTHORIZED TESTING

Question: The counselor contacts the client with genetic test results and the client says that he/she never authorized this test. What should be the counselor's next step(s)?

Discussion: Situations of this kind often stem from miscommunications. Counselors should (calmly) remind clients of their previous conversations and agreed-upon plans of action. It is also important for counselors to listen to the clients' version of events, which will often illuminate the source of the confusion. It may also be helpful to apologize to clients for the misunderstanding; this is different from admitting that errors were made. However, if errors were made on the part of the testing program, then these errors should be acknowledged and rectified as soon as possible. Counselors may want to follow up these conversations by sending a letter summarizing the events and most recent conversations along with copies of the previously signed consent forms. Depending on the clients' reactions or level of outrage, it may also be helpful to refer them to other program personnel or the family relations department at the hospital. (This issue also underscores why it is important for counselors to carry adequate malpractice insurance.) To prevent these types of miscommunication problems, counselors should always provide clients with copies of the consent forms, maintain copies of the signed consent forms in the hospital charts, and keep accurate and complete clinical notes. In cases where the genetic tests are complicated or will take a long time to complete, it may be helpful to check in with clients once in a while and review the tests that are in progress.

11.3.7. ETHICAL QUESTION #7: REQUEST FOR ANONYMOUS TESTING

Question: A client asks to undergo a clinical genetic test using a false name. Is it appropriate for the counselor to grant this request?

Discussion: In general, it is not appropriate for counselors to arrange genetic tests using falsified names, addresses, and/or dates of birth. Clinical genetic tests are considered to be highly accurate, at least in part, because of the two or more matching identifiers on the specimen tubes and laboratory requisition forms. Utilizing false information, even with the best intentions, can create doubt and confusion among the health care providers and others regarding the accuracy of the genetic test report. Keeping the genetic test results outside of the clients' medical records may also be problematic (see next example). Counselors should also determine whether the hospital has policies in place that forbid the ordering of anonymous tests; when in doubt, consult with the hospital attorneys. Counselors should warn clients not to lie to their insurance companies regarding genetic test results as this could invalidate their insurance policies. However, counselors can also remind clients that their medical records already contain information about the family history of cancer, so that the genetic test results may not be completely "new" information. Counselors can also explore the clients' motivations and concerns and reassure them regarding the low likelihood of genetic discrimination.

11.3.8. Ethical Question #8: Omitting Test Results from the Medical Record

Question: A client asks that his/her clinical genetic test results be kept out of the hospital medical record. Is it appropriate for the counselor to grant this request?

Discussion: In general, clinical genetic test results should be treated like all other medical tests. This means that the genetic test results belong in the clients' hospital medical records. Placing the genetic test results in the clients' medical records ensures that all of the clients' health care providers will have access to the test results and will be able to make the appropriate medical management recommendations. Keeping the genetic test results out of the clients' medical records forces other health care providers to rely on client recall rather than the official laboratory reports, thus increasing the possibility of error. The counselor should also determine whether the hospital has policies in place mandating the placement of test results in the clients' medical records; when in doubt, the counselor should consult the hospital attorneys. When encountering these types of requests, it may be helpful for counselors to explore the clients' concerns, stress the benefits/policy of placing the test results in medical records, and highlight the privacy protections of all medical information.

11.3.9. Ethical Question #9: Dispensation of Undisclosed Test Results

Question: A counselor is unable to reach a client to disclose his/her positive genetic test results. What is the counselor's obligation regarding these results?

Discussion: It is always disquieting to be the holder of positive genetic test results. First of all, it is important to determine the reason(s) for why it was not possible to disclose these results. In many cases, it is due to logistical reasons: the clients may be unavailable or their contact information is incorrect. Counselors can attempt to reach clients via alternate telephone numbers or email addresses. Sending letters through regular mail may also be helpful, since the post office may have a new address on file and can forward the mail. These correspondences can either ask the client to call in to the program to receive the results (preferred) or can include information regarding the test result. If the clients are simply not returning voice mail or messages, then perhaps they prefer not to learn their genetic test results at this time. This is often a temporary situation and clients will typically call back in a few days or weeks. If counselors do not hear back from the clients, then they can consider placing the test results in clients' medical records so that it can be accessed by their providers. (This strategy also makes it much easier to find the results if and when the clients do recontact the testing program.) Alternatively, counselors can hold on to the genetic test results (in a separate folder or in shadow charts) for a temporary or indefinite amount of time. It is important for programs to have policies in place for how to handle undisclosed genetic test results, and it is advisable to have these policies included in the testing consent forms.

11.3.10. ETHICAL QUESTION #10: UNINTENDED (AND SENSITIVE) GENETIC INFORMATION

Question: Genetic test results inadvertently reveal that the familial relationships are different from what the client initially reported (such as nonpaternity or adoption). Should the counselor disclose this information to the client?

Discussion: At times, DNA results inadvertently reveal information regarding family relationships, including cases of nonpaternity, adoption, consanguinity, or incest. This information may significantly impact clients' risks for carrying familial gene mutations and for developing inherited cancers. However, disclosure of these "family secrets" may have serious repercussions on clients and their families that extend well beyond the scope of cancer counseling. For this reason, the American Society of Human Genetics has made the recommendation that nonpaternity not be revealed unless it is the sole purpose of testing. Therefore, it is suggested that counselors not disclose inadvertent genetic information to clients *unless* there is a compelling reason to do so. For example, if clients are making decisions to have invasive clinical procedures based on erroneous risk information, then it may be important to share this information with them. These types of disclosures, if performed, should be conducted with great tact and gentleness and should include the chance that other conclusions might also be possible. The testing consent form should include a statement regarding the possibility that genetic testing can sometimes reveal these types of inadvertent results.

11.3.11. ETHICAL QUESTION #11: DUTY TO WARN

Question: A client has been identified as carrying a deleterious gene mutation associated with high risks of cancer, but has not shared this information with any of his/her relatives. Does the counselor have an obligation to disclose this information to any or all of the client's relatives?

Discussion: Counselors are bound by the same strict confidentiality rules that govern all physician–patient relationships. Therefore, it is expected that counselors will keep private client information away from all third parties, unless the clients have requested that the information be shared. In the scenario listed above, a client with a deleterious gene mutation has not shared information with other relatives. This is an unfortunate situation since other blood relatives are presumably at high risk for carrying the gene mutation and may not be aware of their cancer risks or the recommendations for cancer screening. However, since the counselors' primary relationships are with their clients, not the clients' relatives, then the counselors' primary obligations are to their clients. Of course, this issue is complicated in genetics since it could be argued that the client *is* the family. Counselors need to make sure that clients understand that their positive genetic test results have ramifications for other blood relatives. This might include the heightened risks of certain cancers, the possibility of targeted genetic testing, and the availability of cancer detection or prevention strategies. Counselors can explore with clients the potential barriers to sharing the information with other relatives and can offer to help them in these efforts by writing family letters or holding family meetings. Sometimes, clients simply need time in which to become accustomed to the news before they are emotionally ready to disseminate the information through the family. The timing and methods by which clients notify their relatives should be theirs to decide. Even if clients ultimately decide not to share their genetic test results with relatives, counselors generally need to honor these decisions. There are very few instances that justify a breach of client confidentiality. For the most part, duty to warn obligations have to do with the notification of risk to first-degree relatives in cases where the hereditary cancer syndrome has close to 100% risks of cancer <u>and</u> there are medical interventions that could ameliorate these risks <u>and</u> the provider has the means of contacting these relatives. Counselors who believe that a particular situation might warrant disclosure of clients' test results to their relatives should seek input from the program directors, other colleagues, the hospital lawyer, and/or an Ethical Advisory Board. Of course, if counselors do not have contact information for the clients' relatives, then this issue may be a moot point.

Counselors should also be aware of the existing legal precedents regarding duty to warn. In *Pate v. Threlkel* (661 So.2d 278 (Fla 1995)), the Florida court considered whether the surgeon who operated on a patient for medullary thyroid carcinoma (MTC) should have done more than inform the patient that her daughter was also at risk. The patient's daughter was not told of her risks and subsequently developed MTC. The court ruled that the surgeon—who was not the patient's regular physician—had sufficiently notified the family by informing the patient of the risks to her offspring.

In *Safer v. Estate of Pack* (677 A. 2d 1188 (N.J. 1996)), the Appellate Court debated whether the physician who treated a man with colorectal polyposis should have informed the patient that his daughter could also be at risk for developing polyposis. Twenty-six years after the patient died, his daughter presented with colorectal cancer and polyposis. The court ruled that the physician should have warned the patient regarding the heritable nature of polyposis. Since the patient's daughter was a minor at the time, notifying the patient (her father) would have been deemed sufficient. The court further stated that physicians have an obligation to take "reasonable steps" to warn at-risk relatives regarding cancers that are potentially preventable.

11.3.12. ETHICAL QUESTION #12: DUTY TO RECONTACT

Question: A counselor has seen a number of clients over the past several years who might be candidates for a newly available genetic test—if the clients knew about it. What are the counselor's obligations regarding recontacting previous clients?

Discussion: In general, it is the clients' main team of physicians (internist, gynecologist, and, possibly, oncologist) who have the responsibility of recognizing when their patients should be seen again by specific specialists, including cancer genetic counselors. Counselors do have obligations to provide updated information to clients with whom they are still working. However, it is unclear how much obligation cancer counselors have regarding recontacting previous clients. For most testing programs, it would be a logistical nightmare to think about having to track down all of the former genetic counseling clients. For this reason, clients should be encouraged to stay in contact with the high-risk program over time, especially if there are changes in the clients' personal or family histories. If a major genetic discovery warrants some type of recontact effort, then genetic counselors can consider sending out a mass mailing to all previous and current clients. This approach is preferred to flagging certain clients for notification, because the sorting process can be quite time-intensive and runs the risk of omitting some clients who are at risk. The mass mailing can include general information about the new genetic discovery and its possible clinical relevance (without focusing on any particular clients) and provide a telephone number for how to obtain more information.

11.13.13. ETHICAL QUESTION #13: CLIENTS WITH EMOTIONAL VULNERABILITY

Question: A client wants to proceed with genetic testing, but the counselor is concerned about the client's ability to cope with a positive genetic test result (due to responses made in the session, previous suicidal ideation, or an untreated mental health disorder). Is it appropriate for the counselor to defer this client's genetic test?

Discussion: Counselors may encounter clients who are emotionally unstable or vulnerable. Counselors may be concerned that the genetic testing process—and the genetic test results—could further exacerbate the clients' emotional issues. However, it is the clients, not the counselors, who ultimately make the decisions about testing. In general, counselors should not deny or defer testing for clients who are appropriate candidates for testing and who wish to be tested. However, counselors do need to raise their concerns with clients. Counselors can explore with clients what it would be like to learn their test results and discuss ways in which the testing program could provide additional emotional support to them. Counselors may find it beneficial to review these types of cases with colleagues who have mental health expertise. Counselors can also encourage clients to set up appointments with mental health providers and can help facilitate these referrals. If clients are frankly suicidal or they are in the midst of major depressive, manic, or psychotic episodes, then counselors should halt the discussions and facilitate getting the clients the help that they need. In general, hospital emergency rooms are best equipped to deal with situations of this nature. Depending on the circumstances, it may also be appropriate for counselors to page the psychiatrist on call at the hospital or to contact the clients' providers or support persons. (See Section 10.3 for more information about providing additional emotional support to clients.)

11.3.14. ETHICAL QUESTION #14: COMPETING RIGHTS OF FAMILY MEMBERS

Question: A client wants to have a genetic test, but his/her at-risk parent or identical twin sibling has declined testing. Does the counselor's primary obligation lie with the person who wants testing or the person who does not want testing?

Discussion: Counselors' primary obligations lie with the individuals who are their clients. Therefore, if clients wish to be tested—even after counselors have discussed the ramifications of these results to other relatives and the possible strain on family relationships—then it is appropriate to test them. In general, relatives who decline cancer genetic tests do not have the right to block other relatives from being tested. Since many of the cancer genetic tests are clinically available, it may not even be necessary (although it is always preferred!) for the initial testing in a family to be performed in relatives who have had cancer. Counselors can discuss these situations with clients and can explore ways in which clients and their relatives might reach some type of agreement or compromise. While it is important to be empathetic to clients who are dealing with these types of difficult family issues, counselors should do their best to stay out of the middle of family quarrels. Counselors can encourage the clients and their relatives to work out these issues themselves, preferably before the testing appointments.

11.3.15. ETHICAL QUESTION #15: OWNERSHIP OF TEST RESULTS FOR DECEASED CLIENTS

Question: A client underwent genetic testing, but died before his/her genetic test results became available. To whom do these genetic test results now belong?

Discussion: Counselors may receive genetic test results for clients who have recently passed away. These genetic test results will need to be disclosed to the clients' designated recipients and placed in the clients' medical records. Counselors should follow the instructions regarding disclosure that were (hopefully) arranged in advance. At the initial testing visits, counselors should routinely ask clients to designate one or more people to whom results should be disclosed in the event that they are no longer available. If this issue was not discussed in advance, then the genetic test results are typically disclosed to the client's surviving spouse. If the client was not married at the time of death, then the next-of-kin designate may be the executor of the client's estate or the client's adult children. It is important to realize that different hospitals and states may have different rules regarding this issue. When disclosing test results to grieving family members, counselors need to be especially sensitive regarding the timing and method of sharing the test results. There may also be complicated family dynamics that could complicate the dissemination of positive genetic results to at-risk relatives. Counselors can also offer to assist the clients' spouse or relatives in these efforts.

11.3.16. ETHICAL DILEMMA #16: COUNSELING COMPLEXITIES WHEN TESTING CHILDREN

Question: The parents have requested a specific genetic test on behalf of their child/adolescent, despite the lack of proven medical benefits to obtaining this information. Should the counselor agree to test this child/adolescent?

Discussion: Parents routinely make medical decisions on behalf of their underage children (age 17 or younger unless they are emancipated). Unless the parent's course of action has potentially life-threatening consequences, medical providers (including genetic counselors) are expected to accede to parental requests. This policy is made with the assumptions that parents want what is best for their child and that they are in the position of knowing their child best. However, these test requests do need to make sense from a clinical standpoint. Therefore it may be useful to consider the cancer syndrome in question when considering requests to test children:

- It is certainly appropriate to test children for hereditary cancer syndromes that are associated with childhood malignancies and for which early detection or prevention strategies are available. Examples of conditions that meet these criteria include Familial Adenomatous Polyposis, Hereditary Retinoblastoma, Juvenile Polyposis, and Multiple Endocrine Neoplasia, type 2.

- It may also be appropriate to arrange testing for hereditary cancer syndromes that are associated with childhood malignancies and for which early detection or prevention strategies *might* be helpful.

Examples of these conditions include Hereditary Leiomyomatosis–Renal Cell Cancer syndrome, Hereditary Paraganglioma–Pheochromocytoma syndrome, and von Hippel Lindau syndrome.

- It is unclear whether it is useful to test children for syndromes that are associated with childhood malignancies, but for which carriers are easy to identify (such as in Blue Rubber Bleb Nevus syndrome or Cutaneous Malignant Melanoma) or the screening may not be of medical benefit (such as in Li-Fraumeni syndrome). Even in Li-Fraumeni syndrome in which many organs are at risk and the screening options are limited, some physicians may argue that it is useful to know a child's *TP53* gene status in order to determine the level of aggressiveness needed to work up vague symptoms or problems.

- It is generally deemed inappropriate to test children for syndromes that are not typically associated with childhood malignancies or childhood screening of any kind. Examples of these syndromes include Hereditary Breast-Ovarian Cancer syndrome and Lynch syndrome. Explaining why certain tests are not typically performed in childhood may lessen the parents' interests in having these tests performed. The parents should also be reminded that proceeding with testing at this juncture takes away the child's future choice to elect not to be tested. Since a fair number of adults decide not to be tested for inherited cancers, this is not an insignificant issue.

Testing programs should develop policies regarding the testing of children for hereditary cancer syndromes, although it is a good idea to have some built-in flexibility to these policies, in the event that there are extenuating circumstances. Counselors should also discuss the possible psychological impact of testing. There may be significant psychological benefits to the child and family to obtain these genetic test results at this time. Of course, there are also very real concerns about the potential risks of testing, including increased anxiety, lowered self-esteem, and changed family relationships. Therefore, counselors should carefully discuss the potential risk and benefits of testing with the parents and explore whether this is an appropriate time in the child's life to be tested. Children's ages help dictate their involvement in the testing process. Older children and adolescents should be included in the testing discussions and can also be asked to provide assent to testing, which is a nonbinding agreement.

11.3.17. ETHICAL DILEMMA #17: EMBRYO TESTING FOR HEREDITARY CANCERS

Question: A couple requests prenatal testing or preimplantation genetic diagnosis (PGD) for a cancer syndrome, which has variable cancer risks and is not associated with childhood malignancies. Is this an appropriate referral for a reproductive genetic testing center?

Discussion: Prenatal genetic testing and PGD are currently available, and these procedures have been performed for a variety of hereditary cancer syndromes. Regardless of the specifics of the hereditary cancer syndrome, clients may have been profoundly impacted by the cancer diagnoses in themselves or their relatives. Counselors should inform clients about the options, limitations, and risks and benefits of prenatal genetic testing and PGD. For individuals or couples who are interested in pursuing these types of tests, counselors should refer them to the appropriate reproductive testing centers in order to obtain more specific information about these options. Prenatal genetic testing is usually covered by group health insurance plans, but for the most part, PGD is available only to individuals or couples who have considerable financial means or excellent insurance coverage.

11.4. ISSUES OF JUSTICE

Justice refers to the principle of fairness and equitability, both at the level of the individual and at the level of society. This section describes the problems regarding the access to genetic testing and also mentions some of the other professional and social issues that potentially impact the public (our genetic counseling clients in the broadest sense).

11.4.1. INEQUALITY OF ACCESS TO GENETIC TESTING

If cancer genetic counseling and testing is considered to be a valuable service (and I contend that it is!), then it is important that individuals of all socioeconomic and ethnic groups have equal access to these services. This is clearly not happening at the current time. Due to the expense of the laboratory analyses, cancer genetic testing has become an option for people who either have excellent health care insurance or have the ability to pay out-of-pocket for these tests. Even the ability to offer free or reduced-cost genetic counseling services has become more limited as hospital administrators worry about balancing hospital budgets.

In an effort to begin addressing this problem, the American Society of Clinical Oncology has issued the following recommendation: "Individuals with substantial high risk of hereditary cancer should have access to genetic counseling, testing, screening, and surgical interventions."

Improving access and increasing interest is a complex issue with multiple factors. As we enter into the age of preventative care and genomic medicine, it behooves us to ensure that the genetic and genomic advances benefit everyone. This applies to all areas of medical care and is not necessarily unique to genetics.

11.4.2. PROFESSIONAL / SOCIETAL ISSUES

In addition to providing ethical genetic counseling to clients and families, genetic counselors may wish to advocate for one or more of the issues that impact our ability to provide quality genetic services to the public. These professional/societal issues include cancer screening disparities in underprivileged populations, direct-to-consumer testing, gene patenting, genetic discrimination, universal health care coverage, reproductive freedom, and state licensure for genetic counselors.

Advocacy efforts can include making presentations to lawmakers and others, writing newspaper editorials, correcting misinformation portrayed in the media, sending letters of concern to biomedical companies, insurance companies, or governmental officials, and volunteering in cancer awareness campaigns or fund-raising efforts. These efforts can be done as an individual genetic counselor as part of a large effort either through the National Society of Genetic Counselors or other professional or consumer organizations.

11.5. FURTHER READING

Beauchamp, TL, and Childress, JF. 2001. Principles of Biomedical Ethics, 5th edition. Oxford University Press, New York.

Bryant, J, Baggott la Valle, L, and Searle, J. 2005. Introduction to Bioethics. Wiley, Chichester, UK.

Committee on Assessing Genetic Risks, Division of Health Sciences Policy, Institute of Medicine. 1994. Social, Legal, and Ethical Implications of Genetic Testing. Andrews, LB, Fullaiton, JE, and Hltzman, NA, eds. National Academy Press, Washington, D.C., 247–289.

Harris, M, Winship, I, and Spriggs, M. 2005. Controversies and ethical issues in cancer-genetics clinics. Lancet Oncol 6:301–310.

National Society of Genetic Counselors (NSGC). 2006. NSGC Code of Ethics. http://www.nsgc.org/advocacy/NSGCCodeofEthics/tabid/155/Default.aspx.

Schmerler, S. 2009. Ethical and legal issues. In Uhlmann, WR, Schuette, JL, and Yashar, BM (eds), A Guide to Genetic Counseling. Wiley, Hoboken, NJ, 363–400.

Schneider, KA, Chittenden, AB, and Branda, KJ. 2006. Ethical issues in cancer genetics 1) Whose information is it? J Genet Couns 15:491–504.

Smith, D, Quaid, K, Dworkin, R, et al. 1998. Early Warning: Cases and Ethical Guidelines for Presymptomatic Testing in Genetic Diseases. Indiana University Press, Bloomington, IN.

Veach, PM, Leroy, BS, and Bartels, DM. 2003. Behaving ethically. In Facilitating the Genetic Counseling Process: A Practice Manual. Springer, New York, 222–241.

APPENDIX A   SPECIFIC TUMOR TYPES AND ASSOCIATED SYNDROMES

Tables A.1–A.10 list various tumor types and the possible associated hereditary cancer syndromes. Keep in mind that these tables list all associated features, even ones that are uncommon. Keep in mind that these tables should not be used as a diagnostic tool.

Please refer to Chapter 4 for the clinical criteria of each hereditary cancer syndrome listed in the following tables. The resources used to compile these tables are those listed in the Chapter 4 bibliography.

The following cancer syndrome abbreviations are used in the Appendix A tables.

Abbreviation	Name of Inherited Cancer Syndrome
A-T	Ataxia Telangiectasia
ALPS	Autoimmune Lymphoproliferative syndrome
BWS	Beckwith–Wiedemann syndrome
BHDS	Birt–Hogg–Dubé syndrome
BS	Bloom syndrome
BRBNS	Blue Rubber Bleb Nevus syndrome
HBOCS	Breast–Ovarian Cancer syndrome hereditary, includes BRCA2-related cancers
CNC	Carney complex
DBA	Diamond–Blackfan anemia
FAP	Familial Adenomatous Polyposis, includes 5q22 deletion syndrome
FA	Fanconi anemia
HDGC	Gastric cancer Hereditary diffuse
GIST	Gastrointestinal stromal tumor, familial
JPS	Juvenile polyposis syndrome, includes Hereditary Mixed Polyposis syndrome (HMPS)

Continued

Counseling About Cancer, Third Edition. Katherine A. Schneider.
© 2012 Wiley-Blackwell. Published 2012 by John Wiley & Sons, Inc.

Abbreviation	Name of Inherited Cancer Syndrome
HLRCC	Leiomyomatosis and renal cell cancer, hereditary, includes Fumarate Hydratase Deficiency (FHD)
LFS	Li–Fraumeni syndrome
LYNCH	Lynch syndrome includes Constitutional Mismatch Repair deficiency syndrome (CMMR-D)
CMM	Melanoma, Cutaneous Malignant
MEN1	Multiple Endocrine Neoplasia, type 1
MEN2	Multiple Endocrine Neoplasia, type 2, includes MEN2B syndrome
MAP	MYH-Associated Polyposis
NB	Neuroblastoma, familial
NF1	Neurofibromatosis, type 1
NF2	Neurofibromatosis, type 2
NBCCS	Nevoid Basal Cell Carcinoma syndrome
PGL-PCC	Paraganglioma–Pheochromocytoma, syndrome, hereditary
PJS	Peutz–Jeghers syndrome
PHS	PTEN Hamartoma syndrome, includes Bannayan–Riley–Ruvalcaba syndrome (BRR)
HPRCC	Renal cell carcinoma, hereditary papillary
RB	Retinoblastoma, hereditary
RTS	Rothmund–Thomson syndrome
TSC	Tuberous sclerosis complex, includes TS/Polycystic Kidney disease (PKD) syndrome
VHL	von Hippel–Lindau syndrome
WAGR	(Wilms' aniridia, genitourinary, and retardation) Denys-Drash syndrome (DDS)
WS	Werner syndrome
WT	Wilms' tumor, familial, includes Frasies syndrome (FS)
XP	Xeroderma pigmentosa, includes XP/Cockayne syndrome (CS), XP/trichothiodystrophy (TTD), and Cerebro-oculo-facial-skeletal syndrome (COFS)

TABLE A.1. CARDIOVASCULAR AND RESPIRATORY SYSTEMS: TUMORS AND OTHER ASSOCIATED FEATURES

Tumor Site	Type	Syndrome
Heart	Cardiac fibroma	NBCCS
	Cardiomegaly	BWS
	Cardiomyopathy	BWS
	Congenital defect, unspecified	FA
	Myxoma (atrium)	BWS, CNC
	Premature atherosclerosis	WS
	Rhabdomyoma	TSC
	Structural defects	BWS
	Ventricular septal defect	DBA

Continued

TABLE A.1. CARDIOVASCULAR AND RESPIRATORY SYSTEMS: TUMORS AND OTHER ASSOCIATED FEATURES—*CONTINUED*

Tumor Site	Type	Syndrome
Larynx	Carcinoma	BS
Lung	Carcinoma	RB, XP, BS, PJS, HPRCC
	Cysts	BHDS, NBCCS
	Lymphangiomyomatosis (LAM)	TSC
	Pneumothorax (spontaneous)	BHDS
	Pulmonary disease, chronic	BRBNS
Pharynx	Hemangioma	BRBNS

TABLE A.2. CENTRAL NERVOUS SYSTEM: TUMORS AND OTHER ASSOCIATED FINDINGS

Tumor Site	Type	Syndrome
Brain	Unspecified type	FA, LFS, LYNCH, XP
	Astrocytoma	CMM, NF1, NF2, LFS
	Astrocytoma, subependymal giant cell	TSC
	Choroid plexus carcinoma	LFS
	Ectopic calcifications of the falx cerebri	NBCCS
	Ependymoma	FAP, NF1, NF2, LFS, MEN1
	Gangliocytoma (dysplastic)	PHS
	Ganglioneuroma	BWS, NB
	Glial nodules, subependymal	TSC
	Glioblastoma	LYNCH, LFS
	Glioma	ALPS, A-T, FAP, NF1, NF2, XP, LYNCH (CMMR-D)
	Hemangioblastoma, cerebellar	VHL
	Hamartoma, glial	TSC
	Medulloblastoma	A-T, FAP, BRBNS, LFS
	Microcephaly	XP (XP/CS; COFS), HLRCC (FHD)
	Meningioma, cranial	MEN1, NF2, NBCCS, WS
	Primitive neuroectodermal tumor (PNET, medulloblastoma)	A-T, FAP, NF1, RB, LFS, NBCCS
	Schwannoma, vestibular (acoustic neuroma)	CNC, NF2
	Triton, malignant	LFS
Nervous system	Malformations, arteriovenous	JP
	Neuroblastoma	BWS, LFS, NB
	Neuropathy	NF2
Spinal cord	Hemangioblastoma, spinal	VHL
	Meningioma, spinal	NF2
	Neurofibroma, subcutaneous	NF1, NF2
	Peripheral sheath, malignant (malignant schwannoma)	MEN1, NF1

Continued

TABLE A.2. CENTRAL NERVOUS SYSTEM—*CONTINUED*

Tumor Site	Type	Syndrome
Other	Autism	PHS, TSC
	Compulsive overeating	BWS
	Developmental delay	PHS (BRR), RB (13q), HLRCC (FHD)
	Hyperactivity	TSC
	Learning disabilities or mental retardation	BS, BWS, FAP (5q22), NF1, TSC, WT (WAGR), XP
	Lhermitte–Duclos disease	PHS
	Neurological problems	XP (XP/CS; COFS), HLRCC (FHD), A-T
	Seizures	A-T, TSC, NF1, HLRCC (FHD)
	Vertigo	NF2

TABLE A.3. CIRCULATORY AND LYMPHATIC SYSTEMS: TUMORS AND OTHER ASSOCIATED FINDINGS

Tumor Site	Type	Syndrome
Anemia	Aplastic	FA, RTS
	Hemolytic	ALPS
	Hypoplastic (congenital)	DBA
	Hypergammablobulinemia	ALPS
	Iron deficiency	BRBNS
	Pancytopenia, progressive	FA
	Thrombocytopenia	ALPS
	Unspecified	JPS, PJS
Leukemia	Acute, unspecified	AT, DBA, BS, FA, LFS, LYNCH (CMMR-D), WS, XP
	Acute lymphoblastic	BS, LFS
	Acute lymphocytic	AT, LFS
	Acute myelogenous	FA, WS
	Juvenile myelomonocytic	NF1
	Chronic lymphocytic	A-T
	Unspecified	A-T, WS
Lymphoma	Hodgkin	ALPS, LFS, LYNCH (CMMR-D)
	Non-Hodgkin, unspecified	ALPS, A-T, LYNCH (CMMR-D), LFS
	Non-Hodgkin, B cell	ALPS, A-T
	Non-Hodgkin, T cell	ALPS, LYNCH (CMMR-D)
	Unspecified	BS
Other	Bone marrow failure	FA
	Chromosomal breakage	BS, FA
	Guillain–Barre disease	ALPS
	Immunodeficiency	ALPS, A-T, BS
	Lymphomesenteric cysts	NBCCS
	Myelodysplasia	BS, RTS
	Vascular problems	NF1

TABLE A.4. CONNECTIVE TISSUE: BENIGN AND MALIGNANT TUMORS

Tumor Site	Type	Syndrome
Bone	Bowen disease	RTS
	Chordoma	TSC
	Disease	NF1
	Ewings sarcoma	RB
	Joint contractures	XP (COFS)
	Keratocyst, jaw	NBCCS
	Osteoma, jaw	FAP, MAP
	Osteochondromyxoma	CNC
	Osteoporosis	WS
	Osteosarcoma	LFS, NF1, RB, RTS, WS
	Osteosclerosis (fingers or toes)	WS
	Skeletal abnormality	FA, NF1, NBCCS, RTS
Soft tissue	Calcification	WS
	Collagenoma	BHDS, MEN1
	Desmoid	FAP, MAP
	Fibroma/Fibroadenoma	BWS, PHS
	Leiomyoma	MEN1
	Leiomyosarcoma	LFS
	Lipoma	FAP, MEN1, PHS, BHDS
	Liposarcoma	LFS
	Muscle weakness	NF2
	Neurofibroma	CNC, NF1, NF2
	Rhabdomyoma, fetal	NBCCS
	Rhabdomyosarcoma	BWS, NF1, LFS
	Sarcoma, unspecified	LFS, NF1, RB, WS, WT
	Spinal muscular atrophy	A-T
Other	Abdominal Wall Defect	BWS
	Acromegaly	CNC
	Advanced bone age	BWS
	Asymmetric overgrowth	BWS
	Gigantism	BWS
	Hand/Feet abnormalities, including digit malformations	DBA, FA, JP, NBCCS
	Macrocephaly	NBCCS, PHS
	Marfanoid body habitus	MEN2 (MEN2B)
	Premature aging	WS, XP (XP/CS)
	Short stature, growth deficiency	BS, DBA, RTS, WS, FA, NF2, XP (COFS; XP/CS)

TABLE A.5. ENDOCRINE SYSTEM: BENIGN AND MALIGNANT TUMORS

Tumor Site	Type	Syndrome
Adrenal gland	Adenoma	FAP, MEN1, TSC, HLRCC
	Adrenocortical carcinoma	BWS, LFS, MEN1
	Adrenocortical cytomegaly	BWS
	Angiomyolipoma	TSC
	Pheochromocytoma	PGL-PCC, MEN2, NF1, VHL
Extra-adrenal gland	Paraganglioma	PGL-PCC, TSC, VHL
Parathyroid	Adenoma	MEN2, TSC
	Hyperplasia	MEN1, MEN2
Pituitary gland	Adenoma	CNC, MEN1
	Pituitary hyperplasia	BWS
Thyroid	Adenoma	ALPS, CNC
	Carcinoma, anaplastic	WS
	Carcinoma, follicular	FAP, PHS, WS
	Carcinoma, medullary	MEN2
	Carcinoma, nonmedullary	ALPS, CNC, LFS, MEN1, WS, FAP, MEN2, PHS, PGL-PCC, PJS
	Carcinoma, papillary	FAP, MEN2, PHS, WS
	Hyperthyroidism	MEN2
Other	Carcinoid	NF1, VHL, MEN1
	Diabetes	WS, BWS, BS, FA, NF1, VHL

TABLE A.6. GASTROINTESTINAL SYSTEM: TUMORS AND OTHER ASSOCIATED FINDINGS

Tumor Site	Type	Syndrome
Ampulla of Vater	Periampullary carcinoma	FAP
Bile duct	Carcinoma	FAP, WS, HBOCS (BRCA2), HPRCC
Colon/rectum	Carcinoma	BS, FAP, JPS, LFS, HPRCC, LYNCH, MAP, PJS
	Carcinoma, signet ring	HDGC, LYNCH
	Hemangioma	BRBNS
	Polyp, adenoma	BWS, BS, FAP, JPS, PJS, LYNCH, MAP
	Polyp, hamartoma	PHS, PJS
	Polyp, hyperplastic	JPS (HMPS)
	Polyp, juvenile	JPS
	Polyposis, adenomatous	FAP, MAP (>100 polyps)
	Polyposis, hamartomatous	PJS
Esophagus	Carcinoma,	BS, LFS, PJS

Continued

Tumor Site	Type	Syndrome
Intestinal tract	Carcinoid	MEN1, NF1
	Desmoid	FAP, MAP
	Ganglioneuroma	MEN2
	Hamartomas	NF1
	Hemangioma	BRBNS
	Obstruction	BRBNS, JP, PJS
	Polyposis, hamartomatous	PJS
	Stromal tumor (GIST)	MEN1, PGL-PCC, NF1, GIST
Gallbladder	Carcinoma	HBOCS (BRCA2)
Liver	Adenoma	FA, VHL
	Carcinoma	ALPS
	Cysts	VHL
	Hemangioma	VHL
	Hepatobiliary	LYNCH
	Hepatoblastoma	BWS, FAP
	Hepatocellular carcinoma	FA, WS
Pancreas	Adenoma	VHL, TSC
	Carcinoma	CNC, HBOCS, FAP, JPS, LFS, LYNCH, PJS, HPRCC, CMM, PJS
	Cysts	VHL
	Hemangioma	VHL
	Insulinoma	MEN1
	Islet cell hyperplasia	BWS, MEN1
	Islet cell tumor (gastrioma)	MEN1, TSC, VHL, HDGC
	Neuroendocrine	VHL, MEN1
Small intestine	Carcinoma	FAP, JPS, LYNCH, MAP, PJS
	Carcinoid (includes Gastrinoma)	MEN1, NF1
	Polyp, adenoma	MAP, FAP
	Polyp, hamartoma	NF1
	Polyp, juvenile	JPS
	Polyposis, hamartomatous	PJS
	Stromal tumor (GIST)	GIST, NF1
Spleen	Adenoma	VHL
	Angioma	VHL
	Cysts	VHL
Stomach	Carcinoma	A-T, BS, FAP, JPS, LFS, HBOCS (BRCA2), LYNCH, PJS, HPRCC, WS, XP
	Carcinoma, diffuse (signet ring)	HDGC
	Carcinoid	MEN1, VHL
	Desmoid	FAP
	Hemangioma	BRBNS
	Polyp, fundic gland	FAP, MAP
	Polyp, hamartoma	PJS
	Polyp, juvenile	JPS
	Stromal tumor (GIST)	GIST
	Ulcer, peptic	MEN1

TABLE A.7. HEAD AND NECK: TUMORS AND OTHER ASSOCIATED FINDINGS

Tumor Site	Type	Syndrome
Ear	Endolymphatic sac (ELST)	VHL
	Vestibular schwannoma	NF2
	Earlobe crease/ear pit	BWS, FA
	Hearing loss, progressive	NF2, VHL, XP, FA
	Tinnitus	NF2, VHL
	Vertigo	VHL
Eye	Acromic patch	TSC
	Aniridia	WT (WAGR)
	Atrophy, eyelid	XP
	Cataract	NF2, RTS, WS, XP
	Coloboma	NBCCS
	Congenital hypertrophy of the retinal pigment epithelium (CHRPE)	FAP, MAP
	Corneal anomalics	MEN2, XP (COFS)
	Epithelioma, eyelid	XP
	Eyelash, loss	XP
	Glaucoma, congenital	DBA
	Hamartoma	TSC
	Hamartoma, iris (lisch nodule)	NF1
	Hemangioma/hemangioblastoma	BRBNS, VHL
	Keratitis	XP
	Leukoria (white spot)	RB
	Melanoma, ocular	HBOCS, CMM, XP
	Optic glioma	NF1
	Papilloma, conjunctival	XP
	Pinealoblastoma	RB
	Photophobia	XP
	Retinal degeneration	XP (XP/CS)
	Retinal hamartoma	NF2
	Retinal phakoma	TSC
	Retinal angioma	VHL
	Retinoma	RB
	Retinoblastoma	RB
	Retinopathy, melanoma associated	CMM
	Sebaceous carcinoma (eyelid)	RB
	Squamous cell carcinoma	
	Telangiectasia	A-T, XP
	Uvea, inflammation	ALPS
Face	Dysmorphic features	FAP (5q22), MEN2 (B), NBCCS, RB (13q), WS
	Infraorbital creases	BWS
	Midfacial hypoplasia	BWS
	Milia	NBCCS
	Palsy	NF2
Jaw	Osteoma	FAP, MAP

Continued

Tumor Site	Type	Syndrome
Mouth	Carcinoma, unspecified	XP
	Carcinoma, squamous cell (tongue)	ALPS, RTS, XP, CMM
	Cleft lip and/or palate	BWS, DBA, HOGC
	Hyperpigmentation (lips, mucosa)	PJS
	Macroglossia	BWS
	Mucosal papillomatosis	PHS
	Mucosal neuroma	MEN2
	Papules, oral	BHDS, PHS
	Trichilimmoma	PHS
Nose/Sinus	Melanoma, nasal mucosa	WS
	Nasal cavity tumor	RB
	Nasopharyngeal angiof.broma, juvenile	FAP
Teeth	Absent or supernumerary	FAP
	Dental cysts	MAP
	Dental problems/abnormalities	NBCCS, RTS, TSC
Other	Abnormal voice	WS, BS
	Characteristic facies	BS, FA, WS

TABLE A.8. REPRODUCTIVE SYSTEM: BENIGN AND MALIGNANT TUMORS

Tumor Site	Type	Syndrome
Breast	Adenoma	ALPS, BWS, CNC
	Carcinoma (female)	ALPS, A-T, BS, HBOCS, HDGC, LFS, CMM, NF1, PJS, PHS, WS, XP
	Carcinoma (male)	HBOCS, PHS, LFS, PJS
	Carcinoma, lobular	HBOCS, HDGC
	Carcinoma, medullary	HBOCS
	Carcinoma, triple negative	HBOCS
	Ductal carcinoma *in situ*	HBOCS
	Fibrocystic disease	PHS
	Myxoma	CNC
	Papilloma	CNC
	Phyllodes, malignant	LFS
Sarcoma		
Cervix	Adenoma malignum (sex cord tumors with annular tubules, SCTAT)	PJS
	Unspecified type	BS, FA
Germ cell	Gonadal	LFS
	Gonadoblastoma	BWS, CNC
	Hypogonadism	FA, WS
	Sertoli–Leydig cell	WT (FS), HLRCC
Fallopian tube	Carcinoma	HBOCS, PJS

Continued

TABLE A.8. REPRODUCTIVE SYSTEM—*CONTINUED*

Tumor Site	Type	Syndrome
Ovary	Carcinoma, mucinous	PJS
	Carcinoma, unspecified	LFS, LYNCH, MEN1
	Carcinoma, serous	HBOCS
	Cyst adenomas	HLRCC
	Dysgerminoma	A-T
	Fibroma	NBCCS
	Sarcoma	NBCCS
	Sex cord tumor, granulosa	PJS
Peritoneum	Papillary serous carcinoma	HBOCS
Prostate	Carcinoma	HBOCS, LFS, PJS, XP
Testes	Epididymis, cystadenomas	VHL
	Sex cord stromal tumors	CNC, HLRCC, PJS
Uterus	Broad ligament, cystadenoma	VHL
	Carcinoma	A-T, LFS, LYNCH. PHS, PJS, XP
	Hemangioma	BRBNS
	Leiomyoma (fibroid)	HLRCC, PHS, CNC
	Leiomyo Sarcoma	HLRCC, LFS
Vulva	Carcinoma	FA
Other	Genitalia, Hyperpigmentation	PJS
	Genitalia, malformation	WT
	Male pseudohermaphroditism	WT (DDS, FS)
	Sterility/Reduced fertility	BS, CNC (males), FA, WS

TABLE A.9. SKIN: TUMORS AND ASSOCIATED FINDINGS

Tumor Site	Type	Syndrome
Skin	Acrochordon	TSC, BHDS
	Adenoma, sebaceous	LYNCH, MAP
	Angiofibroma	BHDS, MEN1, TSC
	Angioma	XP
	Atrophy, cutaneous and subcutaneous	WS
	Café au lait spot	A-T, CNC, FA, LYNCH (CMMR-D), NF1, BS, NF2
	Carcinoma (unspecified)	ALPS, BS
	Carcinoma, basal cell	A-T, NBCCS, RTS, XP
	Carcinoma, sebaceous	LYNCH, RTS
	Carcinoma, squamous cell	FA, XP, CMM
	Carcinoma, spindle cell	RTS
	Collagenoma	MEN1, BHDS
	Cyst, sebaceous	FAP

Continued

Tumor Site	Type	Syndrome
	Cyst, epidermoid	FAP, NBCCS
	Ephelides (freckles)	CNS, XP
	Epithelioma	LYNCH, XP
	Erythema	BS, CNC, RTS
	Fibrofolliculoma	BHDS
	Fibroma	PHS, BHDS
	Fibroma, ungual	TSC
	Hyperkeratosis	WS
	Ichthyosis	XP (XP/TDD)
	Keratocanthoma	LYNCH, XP
	Keratoses, acral	PHS
	Keratoses actinic	RTS, XP
	Leiomyoma, cutaneous	HLRCC
	Lentigine	CNC
	Macule, (black-blue, melanotic)	CNC, PJS
	Melanoma	A-T, LFS, CMM, RB, XP, HBOCS, WS
	Melanoma, acral lentiginous	WS
	Myxomas, cutaneous	CNC
	Neurofibroma, cutaneous	NF1
	Neurofibroma, myxoid	CNC
	Nonmelanoma skin cancer	LFS
	Nevi, blue (hemangioma)	BRBNS, CNC
	Nevi, compound	CNC
	Nevi, dysplastic	CMM
	Palmoplantar pits	NBCCS, PHS
	Papules, papillomatous	PHS
	Pigmentation, abnormalities	FA, PJS, CNC, GIST, WS, BS
	Pilomatricoma	MAP
	Poikiloderma	RTS, XP
	Scleroderma	WS
	Shagreen patch	TSC
	Telangiectasia	A-T, JPS, XP, BS
	Trichilimmoma	PHS
	Trichodiscoma	BHDS
	Ulceration	WS
	Xerosis (dry skin)	XP
	Vitiligo	A-T
	Warty dyskeratosis	RTS
Hair	Premature graying	WS
	Premature thinning of scalp hair	WS
	Sparse hair, eyebrows, lashes	RTS
Other	Hair, brittle	XP, (XP/TDD)
	Premature aged appearance	WS, XP
	Ultraviolet radiation sensitivity	A-T, BS, FA, RTS, XP, WS

TABLE A.10. URINARY TRACT: TUMORS AND ASSOCIATED FINDINGS

Tumor Site	Type	Syndrome
Kidney	Adenoma, unspecified	VHL
	Adenoma, papillary	HPRCC
	Angioma	VHL
	Angiomyolipoma	TSC
	Carcinoma, unspecified	BS, PGL-PCC, LFS, PJS, XP
	Carcinoma, chromophobe	TSC
	Carcinoma, clear cell	BHDS, PHS, TSC, VHL
	Carcinoma, collecting duct	HLRCC
	Carcinoma, papillary	BHDS, TSC
	Carcinoma, papillary type I	HPRCC
	Carcinoma, papillary type II	HLRCC
	Carcinoma, tubulo-papillary	HLRCC
	Chromophobe	BHDS
	Cyst, unspecified	VHL, TSC
	Cyst, sebaceous	NBCCS, TSC
	Cyst, dermoid	NBCCS
	Glomerulo merulo sclerosis	WT (FS)
	Hypoplasia	DBA
	Lipoma	TSC
	Malformation	FA, BWS
	Nephrocalcinosis	BWS
	Nephro genic rests	WT
	Nephromegaly	BWS
	Oncocytic hybrid	BHDS
	Oncocytoma	BHDS, TSC
	Sclerosis, diffuse mesangial	WT (DDS)
	Severe polycystic kidney disease, infantile	TSC (TS/PKD)
	Structural abnormalities	BWS
	Wilms tumor	BWS, BS, LFS, NF1, WT, TSC
Renal pelvis	Carcinoma, transitional cell	LYNCH
Urogenital	Malformation	WT (WAGR, DDS, FS)
Ureter	Carcinoma, transitional cell	LYNCH

APPENDIX B   REVIEW OF BASIC PEDIGREE SYMBOLS

This appendix offers a brief primer on how to construct a genetic pedigree. Figure B.1 depicts the basic symbols used to depict the individuals in the pedigree. These standardized symbols indicate several factors, including whether the individual is:

- A proband or relative
- Male or female
- Affected or unaffected
- Alive or deceased

Figure B.2 depicts the relationship lines used to construct a genetic pedigree. These relationship lines depict whether the client's relative is a sibling, child, parent, or more distant relative.

Counseling About Cancer, Third Edition. Katherine A. Schneider.
© 2012 Wiley-Blackwell. Published 2012 by John Wiley & Sons, Inc.

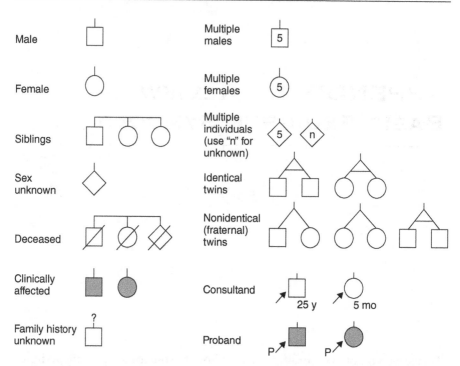

FIGURE B.1. The standardized pedigree symbols. These pedigree symbols are widely used in all clinical genetic specialties, including cancer genetics. (Printed with permission from Bennett, RL, 2010. Getting to the roots: recording the family tree. In The Practical Guide to the Genetic Family History. Wiley-Blackwell, Hoboken, NJ, p. 56).

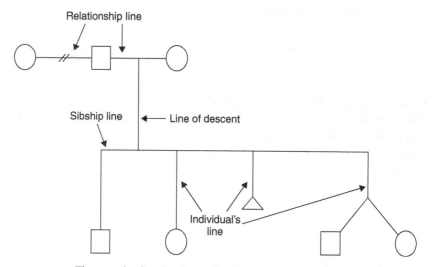

FIGURE B.2. The standardized relationship lines of pedigrees. These relationship lines are used to construct genetic pedigrees. (Printed with permission from Bennett, RL, 2010. Getting to the roots: recording the family tree. In The Practical Guide to the Genetic Family History. Wiley-Blackwell, Hoboken, NJ, p. 49).

INDEX

Note: Page numbers in *italics* refer to figures, those in **bold** to tables.

ABL oncogene, 59
absolute risk, 282
access to genetic testing, 442–443
accuracy, laboratory, 317
acute lymphoblastic leukemia (ALL),
    detection of, 24
adduct, 53
adenocarcinomas
    characteristics of, 197
    FAP-related, 208
    intramucosal, 197
    MAP-related, 216
    in situ, 197
    types of colorectal, 197–198
adenomas
    characteristics of, 195
    and CRC incidence, 194
    development of, 59
    in Lynch syndrome, 213
    precancerous, 196
    screening for premalignant, 181
    sessile, 196
    tubular, 195
    tubulovillous, 196
    types of, 194–195, *195*
    villous, 195
adjuvant therapy, for CRC, 206–207
adoptions, in family history, 244
adrenal cortical carcinoma (ACC), 103, 177
adrenal gland
    syndromes associated with, **454**
    tumors of, **454**
Adult Lhermitte-Duclos disease (LDD), 128

African Americans, cancer in, 4, 4–5, 6–7, **7**
age, 276
    and anxiety during counseling sessions,
      373
    and breast cancer incidence, 153, **154**
    in cancer etiology, 11
    in cancer history, 228–229
    and cancer incidence, 8
    in colorectal cancer, 191
    and inherited forms of cancer, 247–248
alcohol use
    and breast cancer incidence, 154
    in cancer etiology, 15
    in colorectal cancer, 191
allogeneic transplant, 43
ALPS. *See* autoimmune lymphoproliferative
    syndrome
American Board of Genetic Counselors, on
    ethics, 411
American Cancer Society (ACS), 291
    on colon cancer screening, 199, **200**
    guidelines for breast cancer of, 162
    preventive guidelines for CRC of, 200
American Joint Committee on Cancer
    Staging (AJCCS), 34
American Society of Clinical Oncology, 442
American Society of Human Genetics, 436
ampulla of Vater
    syndromes associated with, **454**
    tumors of, **454**
Amsterdam II criteria
    for HNPCC, 106, 107
    for Lynch syndrome, 214

Counseling About Cancer, Third Edition. Katherine A. Schneider.
© 2012 Wiley-Blackwell. Published 2012 by John Wiley & Sons, Inc.

anaplastic tumors, 33
  anatomical features, of malignant cells,
    47–48
anemias, syndromes associated with, **452**. See
    also Diamond-Blackfan anemia; Fanconi
    anemia
aneuploidy, in oncogene activation, 63
anger, client's response as, 358–359
angiogenesis, process of, 51
anonymous testing, request for, 434
anxiety
  baseline, 372
  client's response as, 359
  test results and, 342
APC genetic testing, 91, 401
APC mutation, in FAB, 209
apoptosis, defined, 51
areola, of breast, 152, 152, 153
Arimidex (aromatase inhibitor), 169
Aromasin (aromatase inhibitor), 169
ascending colon, anatomy of, 188, 188
Ashkenazi Jewish ancestry, 173, 232
  and Bloom syndrome, 83
  and breast cancer incidence, 155–156
  FAP in, 93
  and HBOCS, 84, 85
Asian women, cancer in, 6
ataxia telangiectasia (A-T), 75–77
  cancer risks of, 76
  clinical features of, 76
  diagnostic criteria for, 76
  resources for, 77
  syndrome subtypes for, 77
atomic bombings, Hiroshima or Nagasaki,
    158
attentiveness, practice attached, 422
authority, justice and, 416
autoimmune lymphoproliferative syndrome
    (ALPS), 77–78
  cancer risks associated with, 77
  clinical features of, 78
  diagnostic criteria for, 77–78
  resources for, 78
  syndrome subtypes of, 78
autologous transplant, 43
autonomy
  client, 421–422
  lack of, 433
  principle of, 412–414
autopsy report, in cancer history, 241

bacteria, carcinogenicity of, 15–16, 16
Bannayan-Riley-Ruvalcaba (BRR) syndrome.
    See PTEN hamartoma syndrome

barium enema, for CRC, 202
basal cell nevus syndrome. See nevoid basal
    cell carcinoma syndrome
Bean syndrome. See blue rubber bleb nevus
    syndrome
Beckwith-Wiedemann syndrome (BWS), 71,
    78–80
  cancer risks with, 79
  clinical features of, 80
  diagnostic criteria for, 79–80
  resources for, 80
behavioral problems, in cancer history, 230
beneficence, principle of, 415
benign tumors
  hormones excreted by, 32
  location and size of, 31–32
best-case/worst-case scenarios, 334–335
Bethesda criteria, for Lynch syndrome, 106,
    107, 214
BHDS. See Birt-Hoge-Dubé syndrome
biases, in risk communication, 286
bile duct
  syndromes associated with, **454**
  tumors of, **454**
billing policies, of genetic testing
    laboratories, 317
biochemistry, of malignant cells, 48
bioethics
  ethics in, 409–410, **410**, **411**
  principle-based, 412–416, **414**
biological therapy
  for breast cancer, 169–170
  for CRC, 206
biology, cancer
  carcinogenesis, 52–59, 54, 56, **57**, 58
  epigenetic mechanisms, 70–73
  malignant cells, 47–52, **48**, 49
  oncogenes, 59–64, 60, 64
  tumor suppressor genes, 64–70, **66**, 68, 69
biopsy
  of breast mass, 165
  for CRC, 203
  to diagnose cancer, 25
  sentinel node, 170
birth certificate, 244
birth defects, in cancer history, 230
Birt-Hoge-Dubé syndrome (BHDS), 80–82
  cancer risks with, 80–81
  clinical features of, 81
  diagnostic criteria for, 81
  resources for families, 82
bladder
  syndromes associated with, **460**
  tumors of, **460**

bladder carcinoma, *RAS* oncogene in, 62
blastomas, 30
blood tests, for CRC, 203
blood vessels
    of colon, 190
    of rectum, 190
Bloom syndrome (BS), 82–83
    cancer risks with, 82
    clinical features of, 83
    diagnostic criteria for, 82–83
    resources for, 83
Bloom syndrome (BS) Registry, 82
blue rubber bleb nevus syndrome (BRBNS),
    83–84
    cancer risks with, 83–84
    clinical features of, 84
    diagnostic criteria for, 84
    resources for, 84
BMPRIA mutations, 98, 99
body mass index (BMI), and CRC, 194
bone
    syndromes associated with, **453**
    tumors of, **453**
bone marrow toxicity, chemotherapy
    associated with, 41
bone marrow transplantation, 42–43
boundaries
    establishing, 405
    respecting, 386–387
brain
    syndromes associated with, **451**
    tumors of, **451**
brainstorming
    in decision making, 334–335
    to resolve ethical dilemmas, 428
brain tumors
    FAP-related, 208
    LFS-related, 178
BRCA mutations, 175, 304, 346
BRCA1/2 mutations, 85, 86, 173
BRCA1/2 testing, 335, 404
BRCA1-related tumors, 172
BRCA2-related tumors, 172
breast
    atypical hyperplasia in, 154–155,
        155
    basic anatomy of, 151–153, *152*
    syndromes associated with, **457**
    tumors of, **457**
breast cancer
    case examples, *304*, 304–306
    case history, 258–262, *262*
    diagnosing of, 164–166, **167**
    family history for, 232, **234**
        follow-up questions about, **233**
        global incidence of, 10
        in HBOCS, 172
        HDGC-related, 175
        inflammatory breast, 161
        intraductal, 159
        invasive, 159–161
        LFS-related, 177
        PHS-associated, 182–183
        PJS-related, 180
        preventive guidelines for, 163
        recurrent, 171
        risk factors for, 153–158, *154*, **154**, **155**, 184
        screening and prevention guidelines for,
            162, 162–164, **163**
        staging of, 170–171
        syndrome of, 171–175, **172**
        treatment for, 166, 168–171
        warning signs of, 163, **163**
breast conditions, benign, and breast cancer
        incidence, 154–155, **155**
breast lesions, benign, 158–159
breast-ovarian cancer syndrome, hereditary
        (HBOCS), 84–87,
        171–172, **172**, 303
    cancer risks with, 85
    case example, *347*, 347–349
    case history, 258–262, *262*
    clinical features of, 86
    counseling client at low risk for, 290, *290*
    diagnostic criteria for, 85–86
    family history assessment for, 173
    incidence of, 171–172, **172**
    management of, 173–175, **174**
    resources for, 87
    syndrome subtypes of, 86
    tumor types, 172–173
breast tissue, anatomy of, 151
BWS. *See* Beckwith-Wiedemann syndrome

café au lait spots (macules), in NFI,
    118
Canale-Smith syndrome. *See* autoimmune
        lymphoproliferative syndrome
cancer
    anxiety producing types, 373
    autosomal dominant pattern of, 248
    common forms of, 25, **26**
    diagnosis of, 23–27, **24**, **26**
    etiology of, 10–11, **11**, **12**
        modifiable risk factors, **12**, 13–18, *14*, **16**,
            17
        nonmodifiable risk factors, 11–13, **12**
    excess of multifocal or bilateral, 248

cancer (cont'd)
    excess of multiple primary, 248–249
    LFS-related, 178
    primary, 30–31
    prior experiences with, 373
    rare, 248
    recurrence of, 31
    sporadic forms of, 251
    terminology
        cell type, 30
        site of origin, 27
        tissue type, **27**, 27–30
cancer cells
    features of, 47–48, **48**, 49
    functional properties of, 48–52, 50
cancer clusters, 19–20, 251
cancer genetic counselors. See also genetic
        counselors
    ethical, **421**, 421–423
    moral character traits of, 418, **418**
cancer genetics, advances in, 421
cancer risk counselors, 357
cancer story, in genetic counseling session,
        23. See also stories
cancer syndromes. See also hereditary cancer
        syndromes
    counseling about likelihood of,
        290, 290, 292, 292–293, 293, 295, 296
    identification of, 222–223
    in risk communication, 283
candor, in risk communication,
        288
carcinoembryonic antigen (CEA) tumor
        marker, 166
carcinogenesis
    stages of, 53–57, 54, 56, **57**
    two-hit model of, 57
    Vogelstein's multistep process of, 58, 58–59
carcinogens
    broad exposures to, 251
    in cancer history, 232
    in digested food, 191
    environmental, 232
    exposures to, 20–21
    in family business, 251
    identification of, 13–14
    job-related, 232
carcinoid tumors, in MEN1, 113
carcinomas
    defined, 28
    by organ system, **28**
cardiovascular system
    syndromes of, **450**
    tumors of, **450**

caretaker genes, 65, **66**, 66
caring, ethics of, 420
caring theorists, 420
Carney complex (CNC), types I and II, 87–89
    cancer risks with, 87
    clinical features of, 88
    diagnostic criteria for, 87–88
    resources for, 89
Carney-Stratakis syndrome. See
        paraganglioma-pheochromocytoma
        syndrome
carrier test, purpose of, 313
case examples
    breast cancer, 304, 304–306
    client family with FAP, 298–301,
        299
    client with melanoma, 301–303,
        302
    DCIS, 403–405
    genetic counseling
        cancer etiology in, 18–21
        about DCIS, 403–405
        about FAP, 400–403
        VHL gene mutation, 405–407
    of genetic testing, 346–356
    HBOCS, 347, 347–349
    LFS, 352–356, 354
    Lynch syndrome, 349–352, 350
case histories
    breast cancer, 258–262, 262
    Lynch syndrome, 262–266, 264, 265
    paraganglioma-pheochromocytoma
        syndrome, 255–258, 257, 259
CDH1 mutations, 297, 298
CDKN2A mutation, 110
cell cycle
    and cancer predisposition genes, 49
    checkpoints, bypassing, 50
    regulators, 61
cell proliferation, 50, 50
cellular differentiation, 33, 34, 48–50
central nervous system (CNS)
    syndromes associated with, **451**
    tumors of, **451**
cerebellar dysplastic gangliocytoma, PHS-
        related, 183
cerebro-oculo-facial-skeletal syndrome
        (COFS), 144
certainty, in risk communication, 283
cervix
    syndromes associated with, **457**
    tumors of, **457**
character traits, moral, 418, **418**
check-ins, in risk communication, 286

chemotherapy
    action of, 41
    for breast cancer, 169, 170, 171
    for CRC, 205–206
    cytoxic agents, 42
    first clinical use of, 42
    goal of, 41
    hormonal agents, 42
    side effects of, 41
children
    cancer incidence in, 4, **4**
    mortality rates for, **4**
    testing of, 440–441
Chompret's criteria, for *TP53* testing, 103
choroid plexus carcinoma, 103
chromoendoscopy, 176
chromosomal anomalies, in cancer etiology, 13
chromosome 17p13, *TP53* gene on, 67–68, *68*
chromosome rearrangement, and inactivation of tumor suppressor genes, 67
chronic medical conditions, in cancer etiology, 12–13
circulatory system, 55
    syndromes associated with, **452**
    tumors of, **452**
C-KIT mutations, 97
clients
    age of, 311
    assessing interest in testing of, 321–322
    cancer status of, 310
    collecting family history from, 242
    deceased, ownership of test results for, 439–440
    determining eligibility of, 309–311
    a priori risks for, 311
    psychosocial features of
        common emotional responses, 357–362, **358**
        coping strategies, 362–371, **364**
        risk perception of, **274**, 274–278
        test results for, 323
        understanding genetic tests of, 324
        with emotional vulnerability, 438–439
client understanding, in risk communication, 281
clinical certification, requirements for, 317
clinical examination
    of breast, 164
    for CRC, 202
clinical laboratories, 316
clinical record, pedigree in, 225. *See also* pedigree

Cockayne syndrome (CS), 129
code of ethics, of NSGC, **412**, 429
coercion/pressure for genetic testing, 432–433
cognitive functioning, and risk perception, 274
colectomy, 205, 298
    in classic FAP, 209–210
    prophylactic, 211, 215
colleagues, as ethical resource, 429
colon
    anatomy of, 187–191, 188, *188*, *190*
    syndromes associated with, **454**
    tumors of, **454**
colon cancer. *See also* familial adenomatous polyposis
    JPS-related, 211–212
    Lynch syndrome-related, 216
    Vogelstein's model of, *58*, 58–59
colonization, 57
colonography, computed tomography, 202
colonoscopy, 199, 211
    procedure, 201
    side effects of, 201
colorectal cancer (CRC)
    diagnosing, 201–203, **204**
    etiology of, 12–13
    intramucuosal, 197
    invasive, 197–199
    Lynch syndrome associated with, 106–107, 108
    metastases in, 203
    personal history of, 194
    PHS-related, 183
    PJS-related, 180
    recurrent, 207
    risk factors for, 191–194
    risk of, 200–201
    screening and prevention guidelines for, 199–201, **200**, **201**
    syndromes, **206**, 207–217, **208**, **210**, **212**, **215**, **218**
    treatment by stage, 206–207
    treatment of, 204–206
    warning signs of, 199, **201**
colorectal lesions, benign, 194–197, *195*
colorectal walls, anatomy of, 189
colored eco-genetic relationship map (CEGRM), 392–394, *393*, **394**, *395*
colostomy, 205
comfort, for cancer counseling clients, 361
communication, family, 378. *See also* risk communication

comparisons, in risk communication, 280
compassion, of genetic counselors, 418
competency, autonomy and, 412
competing rights of family members, 439
computed tomography (CT) colonography, 202
confidentiality
    autonomy and, 413–414, **414**
    of cancer pedigree, 236
    in genetic testing, 321, 436–438
    respecting client, 422
conflict of interest, 433
congenital hypertrophy of retinal pigment epithelium (CHRPE), 209
connective tissue
    of breast, 152
    syndromes associated with, **453**
    tumors of, **453**
conscientiousness, of genetic counselors, 418
constitutional mismatch repair-deficiency (CMMR-D) syndrome, 108
control, loss of, 361
coping resources, in psychological assessment, 336
coping strategies, 362–371, **364**
    accepting responsibility, 363–364
    anxious preoccupation, 364
    cognitive avoidance, 365
    compulsions, 469
    confrontive, 365
    denial, 365–366
    development of, 363
    displacement, 366
    distancing, 367
    escape-avoidance, 367
    of families, 376
    fatalism, 367
    fighting spirit, 367
    holistic practices, 370–371
    humor, 368
    intellectualism, 368
    magical thinking, 368
    obsessions, 469
    planning, 469
    positive reappraisal, 469
    projection, 369–370
    in psychosocial assessment, 382, **382**
    rationalization, 370
    regression, 370
    relying on social support, 370
    seeking approval from caregivers, 371
    self-controlling, 371
        spiritual, 370–371
        stoic acceptance, 371
coping styles, and risk perception, 275
costs, of genetic testing, 319–321
counseling sessions
    elements of, 267–271, **268**
    impact of clients' fears on, 371–374, **372**
    risk information in, 273
    setting tone for, 226
counseling visits
    results disclosure in, 337–338
    for testing program, 318
    types of, 271–272, 272
counselor, empathy of, 238
counselor-client relationship, basis of, **412**
countertransference, in genetic counseling, 388
Cowden syndrome. See PTEN hamartoma syndrome
cryotherapy, 44
cues
    in psychosocial genetic counseling, 384
    in risk communication, 285
cultural differences, in risk communication, 287
culture. See also ethnicity
    and cancer-related fears, 374
    and genetic testing, 324
    and risk perception, 274–275
customer service, of genetic testing laboratories, 318
cystosarcoma phylloides, 158, 161
cysts, breast, 158

daily activities, impact of cancer fears on, 374–375
data, in risk communication, 281–282
dates, in cancer history, 228–229
death, leading causes of, 5, **5**, 8, **10**, 10
death certificate, in cancer history, 241
deceased clients, ownership of test results for, 439–440
decision making
    assisting client with, 334–335
    autonomy and, 412–413
    and ethical dilemmas, 427
    and ethical principles, 425
    goals of, 333
    impact of cancer-related fear on, 375
    respecting client's, 422
        dedifferentiation, 49

deletion
  and inactivation of tumor suppressor
    genes, 66
  in oncogene activation, 63
deletion 5q22 syndrome, 92
demographic data, on genogram assessment
    tool, 390
denial, versions of, 365–366
Denys-Drash syndrome (DDS), 142. *See also*
    Wilms tumor
depression, test results and, 342
descending colon, anatomy of, 188, *188*
descriptions, qualitative, in risk
    communication, 280
desmoid disease, hereditary. *See* familial
    adenomatous polyposis
desmoid tumors, 91, 92, 209, 211
detection, cancer, 23–24
  common warning signs, 24, **24**
  elusive premalignant cells in, 25
  imperfect screen methods in, 25
  lack of warning signs in, 24
diabetes, in colorectal cancer, 191
diagnosis
  in cancer history, 227–228
  client's misunderstanding of, 245
  in risk communication, 283
diagnostic test, purpose of, 313
Diamond-Blackfan anemia (DBA), 89–90
  cancer risks with, 89
  clinical features of, 90
  diagnostic criteria for, 89–90
  resources for, 90
diet
  in cancer etiology, 15
  in cancer incidence, 11, **11**
  in colorectal cancer, 191
diethylstilbestrol (DES), cancers associated
    with, 18
differentiation, 48–50
digital rectal exam, 202
disability, fear of, 359
discernment, of genetic counselors, 418
disclosure, results. *See also* test results
  client reactions to, 341–343
  and client's needs, 338–339
  follow-up counseling visit for,
    271–272, *272*
  follow-up for, 340–341
  of genetic tests, 319
  mode of, 337–339
  strategies for, 339–341
  topics covered during, 338

disfigurement, fear of, 359
displacement, as coping strategy, 366
DNA, role of adduct in, 53
DNA analysis, in pretest counseling, 325–327
DNA methylation, 71–72
DNA repair genes, *49*, 51, 68–70, *69*
DNA sequencing, 36, 37
DNA testing, 321
donor eggs/sperm, in family history, 244
double contrast barium enema, for CRC, 202
Down syndrome, cancer associated with, 13
ductal carcinoma *in situ* (DCIS), 159, 403–405
ducts, of breast, 152, *152*
duties, in bioethics, **410**
  duty to recontact, 438
  duty to warn, 436–438
dying, fear of, 359–360
dysplastic nevus syndrome. *See* melanoma,
    cutaneous malignant

ear
  syndromes associated with, **456**
  tumors of, **456**
ectoderm, 27, 28
embryo
  testing, for hereditary cancers, 441–442
  tumor origins in, 27, **27**
EMG syndrome. *See* Beckwith-Wiedemann
    syndrome
emotional state, assessing, 226, 336
emotional vulnerability, clients with, 438–439
emotions
  anger, 358–359
  anxiety, 359
  common emotional responses, 357–362,
    358
  fear of disability, 359
  fear of disfigurement, 359
  fear of dying, 359–360
  grief, 360, **360**
  guilt, 360–361
  and interest in testing, 323
  loss of control, 361
  in psychosocial assessment, **379**, 379–380,
    381
  in psychosocial genetic counseling, 386
  resiliency, 361
  in risk communication, 288
  in risk perception, 275
  sadness, 361–362
  shame, 360–361
empathy, in psychosocial genetic counseling,
    383, 383–384

encouragement, for cancer counseling clients, 361
endocrine system
  syndromes associated with, **454**
  tumors of, **454**
endoderm, 27, 28
endolymphatic sac tumors (ELSTs), 137, 138
endometrial cancer
  with Lynch syndrome, 105
  screening for, 216
endoscopy
  indications for, 216, 217
  procedures, 297
ENG gene, 99
environmental pollution, cancer etiology associated with, 18
enzymes, of cancer cells, 51
EPCAM gene, 351
EPCAM (TACD1) gene, 214
epidemiology, cancer, statistics in, 1–10, 3, 4, **4–10**
epigenetic mechanisms
  DNA methylation, 71–72
  genomic imprinting, 70–71
epigenetic silencing, in inactivation of tumor suppressor genes, 67
equality, justice and, 416
Erin Brockovich (film), 19
esophagus
  syndromes associated with, **455**
  tumors of, **455**
ethical codes, **412**, 429
ethical dilemmas
  anonymous testing, request for, 434
  children, testing of, 440–441
  clients with emotional vulnerability, 438–439
  competing rights of family members, 439
  conflict of interest, 433
  duty to recontact, 438
  duty to warn, 436–438
  embryo testing for hereditary cancers, 441–442
  inadequately understood consent for genetic testing, 432
  incomplete consent for genetic testing, 431–432
  lack of autonomy, 433
  pressure/coercion for genetic testing, 432–433
  resolving, 423
    evaluation for, 425–429, **426**
    getting help with, 429–431, **430**
    upholding principles, 424–425
  strategies for dealing with, 421
  test results, for deceased clients, ownership of, 439–440
  test results, omitting from medical record, 435
  test results, undisclosed, dispensation of, 435–436
  unauthorized testing, 433–434
  unintended/sensitive genetic information, 436
ethical principles, opposing, 427
ethics
  of caring, 420
  introduction to, 409–410, **410**, **411**
  virtue, 416–420, **418**
ethnicity
  and breast cancer incidence, 155
  in cancer etiology, 11–12
  in cancer history, 232
  and cancer-related fears, 374
  and cancer survival rates, 6–8, **7**
  and colorectal cancer incidence, 192
  incidence rates and, 4, 4–5
  mortality rates and, 6–8, **7**
  and risk perception, 274–275
events, and genetic testing decisions, 322–323
Ewing's sarcoma, 30
experience
  in risk communication, 287–288
  and risk perception, 276–277
eye
  syndromes associated with, **456**
  tumors of, **456**
  in xeroderma pigmentosum, 144

face
  syndromes associated with, **456**
  tumors of, **456**
facts, in risk communication, 282
fallopian tubes
  syndromes associated with, **457**
  tumors of, **457**
familial adenomatous polyposis (FAP), 90–93, 109, **206**, 208
  attenuated, 90, 92
  cancer risks with, 90–91
  case examples of clients with, 298–301, *299*
  clinical features of, 92
  diagnostic criteria for, 91–92
  family history for, 209

genetic counseling for, 400–403
management of, 209–211, **210**
resources for, 93
syndrome subtypes for, 92–93
tumor types, 208–209
familial atypical mole melanoma (FAMM)
    syndrome, 303. *See
    also* melanoma, cutaneous malignant
familial cluster of cancer, 250–251
familial medullary thyroid carcinoma
    (FMTC). *See also* multiple endocrine
    neoplasia, type 2
    clinical criteria for, 114
    syndrome, 113
families
    communication about cancer of, 378
    coping strategies of, 376
    effect of genetic information on, 375–378,
        376
    and genetic testing, 332–333
    interest in testing of, 322
    obligations of, 377
    relationships within, 377
    roles of, 377
    stories of, 377
    and test results of client, 344–345
family dynamics
    cancer and, 242–243
    pedigree indicating, 225–226
family events, on genogram assessment tool,
    391
family history
    analysis of, 237
    and breast cancer incidence, 156
    classification of, 250–251
    collecting, 222, 232–238, **233–235**
    and colorectal cancer incidence, 192, **192**
    in counseling session, 269
    as counseling tool, 238–239
    different cancer syndromes in, 224
    and existing family relationships, 238
    false information in, 245–246
    in HBOCS, 173
    in HDGC, 176
    incomplete, 242–243
    in JPS, 212
    in LFS, 178
    in Lynch syndrome, 214
    in MAP, 217
    in PHS, 183
    in PJS, 181
    questionnaire for, 239
    unavailable information for, 243–245

family interactions, and risk perception, 275
family members. *See also* relatives
    competing rights of, 439
    in risk assessment, 291, 294, 296–297
family relationships, on genogram
    assessment tool, 391–392, **393**
family stories, 226
FANC-A gene, 94
Fanconi anemia, 93–95
    cancer risks with, 94
    clinical features of, 94
    diagnostic criteria for, 94
    resources for, 95
    syndrome subtypes for, 94–95
fear, in psychosocial assessment, 382
fecal immunochemical test (FIT), 202
fecal occult blood test (FOBT), for CRC, 202
Femara (aromatase inhibitor), 169
fibroadenomas, of breast, 158
fibrocystic breast disease, 155
fibrous tissue, of breast, 152
fidelity, of genetic counselors, 419
figures, in risk communication, 282
five-year survival rates, 6–8, **7**
FLCN genetic analysis, 81
flexibility, in risk communication, 284
fluorescence *in situ* hybridization (FISH), 36
follow-up
    in cancer history, 229
    planning for, 270
food contaminants, cancers associated with,
    18
founder mutation testing, in pretest
    counseling, 327–328
5-FU (fluorouracil), 205
Frasier syndrome (FS), 142. *See also* Wilms
    tumor
fumarate hydratase (FH) gene, 100
functioning level, on genogram assessment
    tool, 390–391

Gail model, for lifetime risk of breast cancer,
    156–157
gallbladder
    syndromes associated with, **455**
    tumors of, **455**
gambler's odds, in risk communication, 279
Gardner's syndrome. *See familial
    adenomatous polyposis
gastrectomy, prophylactic, 176
gastric cancer, 10, 105. *See also* Lynch
    syndrome
gastric cancer, diffuse, 175, 176

gastric cancer, hereditary diffuse (HDGC), 95–96, 171, 175–176
  cancer risks with, 95
  clinical features of, 96
  diagnostic criteria for, 95–96
  family history assessment for, 176
  incidence of, 171, 175
  management recommendations for, 176, **177**
  pedigree of client at risk for, *296*
  resources for, 96
  tumor types, 175–176
gastrointestinal (GI) system
  PJS-related tumors of, 180
  syndromes associated with, **454–455**
  tumors of, **454–455**
gastrointestinal stromal tumor (GIST), 197, 198–199, 237
gastrointestinal stromal tumor (GIST), familial, 97–98
  cancer risks with, 97
  clinical features of, 97
  diagnostic criteria for, 97
  resources for, 98
gatekeeper genes, 65, **66**, 66
gender
  and anxiety during counseling sessions, 373
  and breast cancer incidence, 156
  in cancer etiology, 12
  and colorectal cancer incidence, 192
gender differences, in global cancers, 8, **8**
gene amplification
  in inactivation of tumor suppressor genes, 67
  in oncogene activation, 63
gene silencing
  epigenetic, 70–73
  mechanisms, 72–73
gene therapy, 44
Genetic Alliance, 398
genetic analysis, 35
genetic counseling. *See also* case examples
  effective psychosocial, 383, **383**
    active listening in, 385, **385**
    asking questions in, 385–386
    clients' rationale in, 386
    emotional expression in, 386
    empathy in, 383
    helping client with decisions and actions, 389–390
    monitoring client reactions in, 387
    professionalism in, 388–389

    resistant clients in, 387
    respecting boundaries in, 386–387
    verbal and nonverbal cues in, 384
  ethical dilemmas in, 431–442
  pretest
    about accuracy and limitations, 329–330
    about making decisions, **333**, 333–335
    possible results, 325–329
    psychological assessment for, 335–337
    about risks and benefits, **330**, 330–333, **331**
  use of pedigrees in, 225
genetic counselors, ethical guidelines for, 429, **430**. *See also* cancer genetic counselors
Genetic Insurance Nondiscrimination Act (GINA) (2008), 331, **331**
genetic predisposition
  and breast cancer incidence, 156
  and colorectal cancer, 193
  inheritance of, 225
genetics
  cancer, 421
  of malignant cells, 48, *49*
genetic testing. *See also* disclosure; test results
  access to, 442–443
  anonymous, request for, 434
  arranging for, 269
    choosing laboratory, 315–318
    client's interest and readiness, 321–325
    determining client eligibility, 309–311
    explaining testing process, 318–321, **319**
    selecting right tests, 311–314, **312**
    selection challenges, 314–315
  clinically available, **312**
  consent for, 431–433
  cost of, 319–321
  counseling visit for, 271, *272*
  determining need for, 224
  discussing with client, 321
  ethical dilemmas in, 431–442
  in family history, 241
  follow-up to, 345–346
  justice, issues of, in, 442–443
  limitations of, 314–315
  logistics of, 319
  post-results discussions, 343–346
  in risk assessment, 291, 294, 297
  timing issues for, 323–324
  unauthorized, 433–434
genogram assessment tool, 390–392, *391*, **392**
genomic imprinting, 70–71

genomic instability, 52
genomic rearrangement testing, in pretest counseling, 328–329
germ cell
  syndromes associated with, **457**
  tumors of, **457**
goals, for counseling sessions
  client's, 268–269
  counselor's, 268
Gorlin syndrome. *See* nevoid basal cell carcinoma syndrome
grading of tumors
  based on cell differentiation, 33, *34*
  histological, 32–33, **33**
Gray units (Gy), 40
grief, 360, **360**
group, cancer risk support, 399
group counseling, 20
growth factor receptors, 61
growth factors, 60
guaiac test, for CRC, 202
guilt, 360–361

hair, conditions associated with, **459**
hamartomas
  of breast, 158
  characteristics of, 196
  PHS-related, 183
  PJS-related, 180
  screening for, 181
HBOCS. *See* breast-ovarian cancer syndrome, hereditary
head and neck
  syndromes associated with, **456**
  tumors of, **456**
heart
  syndromes of, **450**
  tumors of, **450**
Helicobacter pylori infection, 96, 175
hemorrhagic telangiectasia (HHT), 99
Herceptin (trastuzumab), 170
hereditary cancer syndromes
  abbreviations for, 449–450
  ataxia telangiectasia, 75–77
  autoimmune lymphoproliferative syndrome, 77–78
  Beckwith-Wiedemann syndrome, 78–80
  Birt-Hoge-Dubé syndrome, 80–82
  Bloom syndrome, 82–83
  blue rubber bleb nevus syndrome, 83–84
  breast-ovarian cancer syndrome, hereditary, 84–87
  Carney complex, types I and II, 87–89

case histories for, 255–266, *257*, *259*, *262*, 264
cutaneous malignant melanoma, 109–111
Diamond-Blackfan anemia, 89–90
embryo testing for, 441–442
and environmental risk factors, 249–250
familial adenomatous polyposis, 90–93
familial neuroblastoma, 116–117
Fanconi anemia, 93–95
gastric cancer, 95–96
gastrointestinal stromal tumor, 97–98
hereditary papillary renal cell carcinoma, 130–131
hereditary retinoblastoma, 131–133
juvenile polyposis syndrome, 98–100
leiomyoatosis renal cell cancer, 100–101
Li-Fraumeni syndrome, 101–104
Lynch syndrome, 105–109
MEN1, 111–113
MEN2, 113–115
multiple mutations in, 314
MYH-associated polyposis, 115–116
neurofibromatosis, type 1, 118–119
neurofibromatosis, type 2, 119–121
nevoid basal cell carcinoma syndrome, 121–123
nonmalignant features of, 249, **249**
oncogenes associated with, **62**
paraganglioma-pheochromocytoma syndrome, 123–125
pedigree of family at low risk for, 254, *254*
Peutz-Jeghers syndrome, 125–127
PTEN hamartoma syndrome, 127–130
Rothmund-Thomson syndrome, 133–134
testing for, in children, 440–441
and 3-2-1 rule, 250
tuberous sclerosis complex, 134–136
tumor suppressor genes associated with, **66**
von Hippel-Lindau syndrome, 137–139
Werner syndrome, 139–141
Wilms tumor, 141–143
xeroderma pigmentosum, 143–145
hereditary mixed polyposis. *See* juvenile polyposis syndrome
hereditary nonpolyposis colorectal cancer (HNPCC), 92
heredity, in cancer etiology, 12
heuristics, and risk perception, 275–276
histology, 32–33

history, cancer
analysis of, 237
classification of, 250–251
client fabrication in, 245–246
collecting, 221–226, 222, 223, 232, **235**, 242–246
historian for, 236–238
interpreting, 246–250
purposes of, 222–226
survey of, 236–238
history, patient, elements of, 227–232, **228.** *See also* family history; personal history
H19 genes, 79
HNPCC. *See* Lynch syndrome
Hodgkin's disease, 30
hope, of cancer counseling clients, 361
hormonal therapy, 42, 169, 170, 171
hormones, and breast cancer incidence, 157
hospitals
ethical review boards of, 429–430
ethics and, 411
hospital summary notes, in cancer history, 241
hydatidiform mole, 70
hysterectomy, indications for, 216

ideals, in bioethics, **410**
identity, sense of, 362
IGF2 genes, 79
I1307K mutation, 93
images, visual, in risk communication, 283–284
imaging studies, to diagnose cancer, 25
immunodeficiency, syndromes associated with, **452**
immunohistochemistry (IHC) test, in Lynch syndrome, 107, 108
immunotherapy, 44–45
imprint organizing center, 72
inadequately understood consent for genetic testing, 432
incidence
cancer
and age, 8
in children, 4, **4**
common forms of, 2, **3**
gender differences in, 2, **3**
geography of, 5
global, 8–10, **8–10**
in U.S., 2–5, **3**, *4*, **4**
use of term, 1–2
incomplete consent for genetic testing, 431–432

industrialized countries, and cancer incidence, 8, 10, **10**
infancy, juvenile polyposis of, 99
infectious agents, in cancer etiology, 15–16, **16**
infiltrating ductal carcinoma, of breast, 160
infiltrating lobular carcinoma, of breast, 160
inflammatory bowel disease (IBD)
and colorectal cancer, 193
pseudopolyps identified with, 196
information
on Internet, 398
and risk perception, 276
informed consent
autonomy and, 413
for genetic testing, 318–319, **319**
as process, 423
inherited cancer syndromes, features of, 246–247, **247**
initiation, of carcinogenesis, 53, *54*
insertions, in oncogene activation, 63
insurance coverage, of genetic testing, 315, 320
integrity, of genetic counselors, 419
International Agency for Research on Cancer (IARC), 14
International Gastric Cancer Linkage Consortium, 96
International Union Against Cancer (IUAC), 34
Internet, information provided by, 398
interview, family history, 226. *See also* family history
intestinal tract. *See also* gastrointestinal system
syndromes associated with, **455**
tumors of, **455**
invasive procedures, to diagnose cancer, 25
inversions, in oncogene activation, 62–63
investigational review board (IRB), hospital, 425
isolation, sense of, 362

justice
issues of, in genetic testing, 442–443
principle of, 415–416
juvenile polyposis, 196
juvenile polyposis syndrome (JPS), 98–100, 207, 211
cancer risks with, 98
clinical features of, 99

diagnostic criteria for, 98–99
family history for, 212
incidence of, 211
management of, **212**, 212–313
resources for, 100
syndrome subtypes for, 99
tumor types, 211–212

Kaposi's sarcoma, 30
kidney
  syndromes associated with, **460**
  tumors of, **460**
kindness, of genetic counselors, 419
Klinefelter syndrome, cancer associated with, 13
Knudson's model of retinoblastoma, 57, *58*

laboratory
  choosing, 315–318
  clinical, 316
  research, 316–317
Lamb syndrome. *See* Carney complex, types I and II
landscaper genes, 66
language, in risk communication, 283
large-cell calcifying Sertoli cell tumor (LCCST), 88
larynx
  syndromes of, **450**
  tumors of, **450**
laser therapy, 44
leader(s), of cancer risk support groups, 399
learning problems, in cancer history, 230
leiomyoatosis renal cell cancer, hereditary (HLRCC), 100–101
  cancer risks with, 100
  clinical features of, 101
  diagnostic criteria for, 100–101
  resources for, 101
  syndrome subtypes for, 101
leiomyomas, 197
leiomyosarcoma, 198
lesions, benign, in cancer history, 230
letters of medical necessity, 320
leukemia, 30
  ALL, 24
  ataxia telangiectasia associated with, 76
  defined, 29
  by organ system, **29**
  syndromes associated with, **452**
licensing boards, state, 411
Liddle's diagnostic test, 88

life stressors, in psychological assessment, 336–337
lifestyle behaviors, impact of cancer fears on, 374–375
lifestyle habits, 231, 251
Li-Fraumeni-like (LFL) syndromes, **102**, 102–103, 104
Li-Fraumeni syndrome (LFS), 101–104, 171, 176–177
  cancer risks with, 102
  case example, 352–356, *354*
  clinical features of, 104
  diagnostic criteria for, **102**, 102–103
  family history assessment for, 178
  incidence of, 177
  management of, **179**, 179–180
  resources for, 104
  syndrome subtypes for, 104
  testing for, 441
  tumor types, 177–178
linitis plastica, 175
listening, active, in effective psychosocial genetic counseling, 385, **385**
liver
  syndromes associated with, **455**
  tumors of, **455**
lobular carcinoma *in situ* (LCIS), 159
lobules, of breast, *152*, 153
low penetrant *RB*, 132
lumpectomy, in DCIS, 170
lung
  syndromes of, **450**
  tumors of, **450**
lung cancer, global incidence of, 8
lung tumors, detection of, 25
lymphatics
  of colon, 190
  of rectum, 190
lymphatic system, 55
  syndromes associated with, **452**
  tumors of, **452**
lymph nodes, biopsy of, 165
lymphomas, 30, 198
  ataxia telangiectasia associated with, 76
  defined, 29
  by organ system, **29**
  syndromes associated with, **452**
lymph vessels, of breast, *152*, 153
Lynch syndrome, 105–109, 193, 213
  cancer risks with, 105–106
  case example, 349–352, *350*
  case history, 262–266, *264*, *265*

Lynch syndrome (*cont'd*)
clinical features of, 108
diagnostic criteria for, 106–108
family history in, 214
incidence of, 213
management of, **215**, 215–216
pedigrees of client at risk for, 292, *292*, *293*
resources for, 109
syndrome subtypes for, 108–109
tumor types, 213–214

macrocephaly, in PHS, 128
malignant cells, features of, 47–48, **48**, *49*
mammography, 164, 179
Manchester Criteria, for NF2, 120
manufacturing, carcinogenic agents in, 17
mastectomy
indications for, 168
nipple-sparing, 398
prophylactic, 180, 184
types of, 168
MDM2 gene, 104
medical care practices, impact of cancer-related fear on, 375
medical care providers, professional obligations of, 417
medical conditions, in cancer history, 230, 231
medical management
following test results, 344
and genetic testing, 332
as option, 270
medical records
importance of, 421
lost, 243
obtaining, 239
omitting test results from, 435
Medicare, genetic testing covered by, 320
medicinal drugs, cancers associated with, 18
medicine
ethics and, 411
mistakes in, 417
medullary carcinoma, of breast, 160
medullary thyroid carcinoma, cancer staging of, 35, **35**
medulloblastomas, 122
melanoma, cutaneous malignant (CMM) syndrome, 109–111
cancer risks with, 109–110
clinical features of, 110–111
diagnostic criteria for, 110
resources for, 111
melanoma-astrocytoma syndrome, 109

melanomas, 198
case examples of client with, 301–303, *302*
defined, 29
ocular, 110
MEN1. *See* multiple endocrine neoplasia, type 1
MEN2. *See* multiple endocrine neoplasia, type 2
mental health history, in psychosocial assessment, **380**, 380–381
mental health professionals, establishing alliances with, 396
mental health referral, making, 394–398, **396**, **397**
mesoderm, 27, 28
metabolism, of cancer cells, 51
metastasis, 30
of cancer cells, 52
in carcinogenesis, *54*, 55, *56*, 57, **57**
defined, 31
metastatic cancer, of unknown origin, 33
methylation, DNA, 70, 71–72
microcalcifications, of breasts, 159
microsatellite instability-high tumor (MSI), and colorectal cancer, 193–194
migration, of cancer cells, 52
mining, cancer etiology associated with, 18
minors
emancipated, 440
testing of, 440–441
mitocycin C chromosome stress test, 94
mitotic nondisjunction, and inactivation of tumor suppressor genes, 67
mitotic recombination, in inactivation of tumor suppressor genes, 67
mixed polyposis syndrome, hereditary (HMPS), 99
MLH1 gene, 194, 214
MOAB 17-1A, 206
molecular studies, examples of, 36, *37*
monitoring client
in psychosocial genetic counseling, 387
in risk assessment, 291–292, 294–295, 297–298
Montgomery's glands, 153
morality, common, 410
mortality rates, 5–8, **5–7**
age and, 5, *5*
for children, **4**, 5, **5**
ethnicity and, 6–8, **7**
gender and, **6**
metastasis, 57
for selected cancers, 6, **7**

mouth
  syndromes associated with, **457**
  tumors associated with, **457**
MRI, breast, 164
MSH2 gene, 214
MSH6 gene, 214
MSI test, in Lynch syndrome, 107, 108
mucinous carcinoma
  adenocarcinoma, 197
  of breast, 160
mucosa, of colorectal walls, 189, *190*
Muir-Torre syndrome, 31, 105, 108
multiple endocrine neoplasia, type 1 (MEN1)
    syndrome, 81, 111–113
  cancer risks with, 111
  clinical features of, 112–113
  diagnostic criteria for, 112
  resources for, 113
multiple endocrine neoplasia, type 2 (MEN2)
    syndrome
  cancer risks with, 113
  clinical features of, 114
  diagnostic criteria for, 114
  resources for, 115
  syndrome subtypes for, 114–115
multiple endocrine neoplasia type 2B
    (MEN2B), 113
Münchausen syndrome, 246
muscularis externa, of colorectal walls, 189,
    190
mutation, 50. *See also specific mutations*
  and inactivation of tumor suppressor
      genes, 66
  initiating, 53
  and signaling networks, 52
  somatic, 53
MYC oncogene, 44
MYH-associated polyposis (MAP), 115–116,
    216
  cancer risks with, 115
  clinical features of, 116
  diagnostic criteria for, 115–116
  family history for, 217
  incidence of, 216
  management of, 217, **218**
  resources for, 116
  tumor types, 216–217

NAME syndrome. *See* Carney complex,
    types I and II
National Cancer Institute (NCI), 291
National Comprehensive Cancer Network,
    291

National Institutes of Health Consensus
    Conference, NF2 criteria of, 120
National Society of Genetic Counselors
    (NSGC), 411, 443
  code of ethics of, 429
  ethics committee of, 431
National Toxicology Agency, U.S.-based, 14
Native Americans, cancer rates among, 4, 5
neoplasms
  defined, 27
  major types of, 28
nervous system
  syndromes associated with, **451**
  tumors of, **451**
neuroblastoma (NB), familial, 116–117
  cancer risks with, 116–117
  clinical features of, 117
  diagnostic criteria for, 117
  resources for, 117
  syndrome subtypes, 117
neuroectodermal tumors, 30
neuroendocrine tumors, 199
neurofibromatosis, type 1 (NF1), 118–119
  cancer risks with, 118
  critical features of, 119
  diagnostic criteria for, 118–119
  resources for, 119
neurofibromatosis, type 2 (NF2), 119–121
  cancer risks with, 120
  clinical features of, 121
  diagnostic criteria for, 120–121
  resources for, 121
nevoid basal cell carcinoma syndrome
    (NBCCS), 121–123
  cancer risks with, 121–122
  clinical features of, 123
  diagnostic criteria for, 122
  resources for, 123
nipple, breast, 152, *152*, 153
nonmaleficence, principle of, 414–415
nonpolyposis, hereditary, 213. *See also* Lynch
    syndrome
nose
  syndromes associated with, **457**
  tumors of, **457**
NSAIDs, and polyp development, 211
nuclear transcription factors, 61
numbers, in risk communication, 278, 283

obesity
  and breast cancer incidence, 157
  in cancer etiology, 15
  and CRC, 194

occupational exposures, in cancer etiology, 17–18, **17**
oncogenes, *49*
  activation of, **62**, 62–64, *64*
  general description of, 59–61, *60*
  hereditary cancer syndromes associated with, **62**
  RET, 64, *64*
oncologist, referral to, 26
osteochondromyxoma of bone, 88
osteosarcoma, 131
outcomes
  in risk communication, 283
  and risk perception, 276
ovarian cancer
  in HBOCS, 172
  monitoring for, 174
ovarian teratoma, 70
ovary
  syndromes associated with, **458**
  tumors of, **458**
overgrowth syndrome, 80

Paget's disease of the breast, 160–161
pancreas
  syndromes associated with, **455**
  tumors of, **455**
papillary carcinoma, of breast, 161
papillomas, of breast, 158
Pap smear, 25
paraganglioma, subtype 1 (PGL1) syndrome, 125
paraganglioma-pheochromocytoma (PGL-PCC) syndrome, 123–125
  cancer risks with, 123–124
  case history, 255–258, *257, 259*
  clinical features of, 124
  diagnostic criteria for, 124
  resources for, 125
  syndrome subtypes for, 124–125
parasites, carcinogenicity of, 15–16, **16**
parathyroid gland
  syndromes associated with, **454**
  tumors of, **454**
parotid gland
  syndromes associated with, **454**
  tumors of, **454**
Pate v. Threlkel, 437
pathology reports, 240
PDGFRA mutations, 97
pedigree
  basic symbols for, 461, *462*
  in cancer history, 232

identifying inheritance patterns with, 224
  relationship lines in, 461, *462*
pedigree, cancer
  and confidentiality practices, 236
  confirming accuracy of, 239–241
  at Dana-Farber Cancer Institute, 222, *223*
  definition of, 222
  example, 222
  for family at high risk, 252
  for family at low risk, 254, *254*
  for family at moderate risk, 253
  general questions for, 232, **235**
  for more than one cancer syndrome, 314
  purposes of, 222–225
  quadrant system, *223*
  standardized nomenclature for, 236
percentages, in risk communication, 278–279
perception, client, in risk communication, 287
peritoneum
  syndromes associated with, **458**
  tumors of, **458**
personal attributes, and risk perception, 276
personal history, and breast cancer incidence, 157
personality
  genetic testing and, 322
  and risk perception, 277
Peutz-Jeghers syndrome (PJS), 125–127, 171, 180
  cancer risks with, 126
  clinical features of, 126–127
  diagnostic criteria for, 126
  family history assessment for, 181
  management of, 181–182, **182**
  resources for, 127
  tumor types, 180
pharynx
  syndromes of, **450**
  tumors of, **450**
PHOX2B gene, 117
physical features, in cancer history, 230
physical inactivity, in cancer etiology, 15
pituitary gland
  syndromes associated with, **454**
  tumors of, **454**
PMS2 gene, 214
PNETs, 122
polychlorinated biphenyls (PCBs), cancers associated with, 18
polyploidy, in oncogene activation, 63

polyposis. *See also* familial adenomatous
    polyposis
  adenomatous, 195
  in FAP, 91
  gastrointestinal, 180
polyps
  adenomatous, 195, 217
  CRC arising from, 194–195
  FAP-related, 209
  hamartomatous intestinal, 128
  histologically confirmed hamartomatous,
    126
  hyperplastic, 196
  inflammatory, 196
  JPS-related, 211–212
  juvenile, 98, 99, 196
  in Lynch syndrome, 213
  MAP-related, 216–217
positron emission tomography (PET) scan, of
    breast, 165
posttraumatic stress disorder (PTSD), 362
poverty, and cancer risk, 7–8
predictive test, purpose of, 313. *See also*
    genetic testing; test results
preferences, client, in risk communication,
    284
preimplantation genetic diagnosis (PGD),
    441–442
prenatal genetic testing, 441–442
preparation, for risk communication, 284–285
pressure/coercion for genetic testing,
    432–433
presymptomatic test, purpose of, 313. *See also*
    genetic testing; test results
prevalence, use of term, 2
Preventive Services Task Force, U.S., 162
principles, in bioethics, **410**
privacy
  autonomy and, 413–414, **414**
  respecting client, 422
PRKAR1A gene test, 88
probability of developing cancer, in risk
    assessment, 291, 293–294, 296
professional guidelines, 429, **430**
professionalism, in psychosocial genetic
    counseling, 388
professional organizations, ethics committees
    of, 431
professional/societal issues in genetic
    counseling, 443
progeria of adult, 139. *See* Werner syndrome
prognosis, in cancer history, 229
progression, of carcinogenesis, *54*, 55

projection
  in case example, 407
  of client, 369–370
  in genetic counseling, 389
proliferation, cell, *50*, *50*
promotion, of carcinogenesis, 53, *54*
proportions, in risk communication, 279
prostate gland
  syndromes associated with, **458**
  tumors of, **458**
proto-oncogenes
  functions of, 59
  major types of, 60
provider-client relationship, 420
providers, for testing program, 318
pseudopolyp, 196
psychosocial assessment, features of, 379–
    382, **379–382**
psychosocial factors, in cancer history, 232
psychosocial issues, exploring, 270
PTCH gene, 122
PTEN hamartoma syndrome (PHS), 127–130,
    158, 171, 182
  cancer risks with, 127–128
  clinical features of, 129
  diagnostic criteria for, 128–129
  family history assessment for, 183
  management of, 184, **184**
  resources for, 130
  syndrome subtypes for, 129
  tumor types, 182–183
PTEN mutations, 183

questionnaire, family history, 239
questions
  about client's reactions, **382**
  in construction of genogram, **392**
  about coping strategies, **382**
  for creating CEGRM, **394**
  in effective psychosocial genetic
    counseling, 385–386
  about emotional responses to cancer risk,
    381
  about emotional well-being, **379**
  for ethical dilemmas, 426–428
  for family history, 232, **233–235**
  about mental health history, **380**
  in risk communication, 288

race, in cancer etiology, 12–13
radiation, in cancer etiology
  ionizing, 16
  ultraviolet, 16

radiation doses, 40
radiation exposure
    and breast cancer incidence, 157–158
    and CRC, 194
radiation therapy
    aim of, 39
    for breast cancer, 168–169, 170, 171
    for CRC, 205
    effectiveness of, 40
    neoadjuvant, 206
    side effects of, 40
rads, measurement of, 40
raloxifene, 169
ranges, in risk communication, 279
ras oncogene, 59
rate, use of term, 2
rationale, clients', in psychosocial genetic
    counseling, 386
ratios, in risk communication, 280
RB gene, 57
RB1 gene, 132
reassurance, in risk communication, 286
rectum. *See also* colorectal cancer
    anatomy of, 187–191, *188, 189, 190*
    syndromes associated with, **454**
    tumors of, **454**
referrals
    making, 270
    mental health, 394–398, **396, 397**
    to oncologist, 26
relationship lines, in pedigree, 461, *462*
relationships, on genogram, **393**
relative risk, use of term, 2
relatives. *See also* family members
    in cancer history, 231
    cancer in, 228
    communication with, 378
    estranged, 243–244
    false information provided by, 246
    lost, 243
    with related cancers, 246–247
    testing, 310
    and test results, 342–343
relief, for cancer counseling clients, 361
religion, and genetic testing, 324
renal cell carcinoma
    diagnosis of, 25
    PHS-related, 183
renal cell carcinoma, hereditary papillary
    (HPRCC), 130–131
    cancer risks with, 130
    clinical features of, 130
    diagnostic criteria for, 130
    resources for, 131

renal pelvis
    syndromes associated with, **460**
    tumors of, **460**
reproductive system
    PJS-related cancers of, 181
    syndromes associated with, **457–458**
    tumors of, **457–458**
research, pedigrees in, 225
research laboratories, 316
research treatment trials, 33
resiliency, feelings of, 361
resistant clients, in psychosocial genetic
    counseling, 387
resources
    justice and, 416
    providing client with, 289
respectfulness, of genetic counselors, 419
respiratory system
    syndromes of, **450**
    tumors of, **450**
results, of genetic tests, 319. *See also*
    disclosure; test results
retinoblastoma (RB), hereditary, 131–133, 252,
    252
    cancer risks with, 131
    clinical features of, 132
    diagnostic criteria for, 131–132
    resources for, 133
    syndrome subtypes for, 132
retinoblastoma (RB), Knudson's model of,
    57, *58*
retinoid agents, 45
RET oncogene, 64, *64*, 114
rights
    in bioethics, **410**
    of family members, competing, 439
risk
    absolute, 282
    categories for, 251–255
    defined, 273
    justice and, 416
    personalized, 280–281
    uncertain, 255
risk assessment
    of clients
        at high risk, 295–298, *296*
        at low risk, 289–292, *290*
        at moderate risk, 292, 292–295, *293*
    in counseling session, 269
    counseling visit for, 271, *272*
risk communication, 267
    in counseling session, 269
    defined, 284
    effective strategies for, 284–289, **285**

goal of, 273
  presenting information in, 278–281, **279**
  strategies for effective, **281**, 281–289, **285**
risk factors, 10–11, **11**, **12**, 231
  modifiable risk factors, **12**, 13–18, *14*, **16**, **17**
  nonmodifiable risk factors, 11–13, **12**
risk information, strategies for presenting,
    281, 281–289, **285**
risk perception, **274**, 274–278
  and cancer-related fears, 374
  genetic counseling and, 267–271
Rothmund-Thomson syndrome (RTS),
    133–134
  cancer risks with, 133
  clinical features of, 134
  diagnostic criteria for, 133–134
  resources for, 134
RPS19 gene test, 89
rules, in bioethics, **410**

sadness, client's, 361–362
Safer v. Estate of Pack, 437–438
sarcomas
  of breast, 161
  defined, 29
  LFS-related, 178
  by organ system, **29**
schwannomas, 120
scoliosis, and Hodgkin's disease, 157–158
screening
  ACS breast cancer guidelines for, 162, **162**
  in cancer history, 230
  for colon cancer, 200, **200**
  purpose of, 313–314
scrotal cancer, in chimney sweeps, 10
SDHB mutation, 123, 125
SDHC gene mutation, 125
SDHD gene, 71
sedentary lifestyle
  and breast cancer incidence, 157
  in cancer etiology, 15
segmental resection, for CRC, 204
self-breast examination (SBE), 163
sensitive genetic information, 436
serosa, of colorectal walls, 189, *190*
Sertoli cell tumors, 181
sex cord tumors with annular tubules
    (SCTAT), 126, 181
shame, 360–361
sigmoid colon, anatomy of, 188, *188*
sigmoidoscopy, 199, 201
signaling systems, of cancer cells, 52
signal transducers, 61
signet ring adenocarcinoma of stomach, 175

signet ring cell carcinoma, 198
single-site analysis, in pretest counseling, 327
sinus
  syndromes associated with, **457**
  tumors of, **457**
Sipple syndrome. *See* multiple endocrine
    neoplasia, type 2
sister chromatid exchanges (SCE), in Bloom
    syndrome, 82–83
site of origin, 27
skin
  of breast, 153
  in Lynch syndrome, 214
  melanoma of, 11–12
  syndromes associated with, **458**
  tumors of, **458–459**
  in xeroderma pigmentosum, 144
skin lesions, PHS-related, 183
SMAD4 mutations, 98, 99
small intestine
  syndromes associated with, **455**
  tumors of, **455**
societal/professional issues in genetic
    counseling, 443
soft tissue
  syndromes associated with, **453**
  tumors of, **453**
southern blotting, 36
spinal cord
  syndromes associated with, **451**
  tumors of, **451**
spirituality, and risk perception, 277–278
spleen
  syndromes associated with, **455**
  tumors of, **455**
squamous cell (epidermoid) carcinoma, 198
staging
  for breast cancer, 166, **167**
  clinical, 33–35, **35**
  for CRC, 203, **204**, 206–207
state licensing boards, 411
statistics, cancer
  cancer-related mortality, 5–8, **5–7**
  global incidence, 8–10, **8–10**
  incidence in U.S., 2–5, **3**, **4**, **4**
  terminology used in, 1–2
stem cells
  sources of, 43
  transplantation, 42–43
stomach. *See also* gastrointestinal
    system
  syndromes associated with, **455**
  tumors of, **455**
stomach cancer, HDGC-related, 175

stool DNA (sDNA) test, 202
stool guaiac test, for CRC, 202
stories
    family, 226
    response to client's, 233–234, 236
stress
    client response to, 362
    test results and, 342
stressors, on genogram assessment tool, 392
submucosa, of colorectal walls, 189,
        190
suicidal ideation, and ethical decision
        making, 415, 438
sun exposure, and melanoma, 110
support, pedigree indicating level of,
        225–226
support groups, cancer risk, 398–400
support network, in psychological
        assessment, 336
surgery
    for breast cancer, 168, 170, 171
    for catheter placement, 39
    conservative, 39
    for CRC, 204–205
    exploratory, 38
    palliative, 39
    radical, 38
surveillance practices, in cancer history, 230
survival rates, 6–8, 7

TACSTD1 gene, 351–352
tamoxifen, 169
team of providers, for testing program, 318
teeth
    syndromes associated with, 457
    tumors of, 457
telangiectases, 76
teratomas, 30
testes
    syndromes associated with, 458
    tumors of, 458
testing. See genetic testing
test results
    adjustment to, 345
    anticipated impact of, 336
    client's family and, 344–345
    for clients with children, 343
    for deceased clients, ownership of, 439–440
    and follow-up interactions, 345
    implications of, 343–344
    indeterminate negative, 341
    intermediate negative, 325–326, 328, 329
    negative, 329–330, 332

omitting from medical record, 435
positive, 325, 328, 329, 341
referrals to specialists following,
        346
and review of genetics, 345
true negative, 328, 329, 341–342
uncertain, 329
undisclosed, dispensation of,
        435–436
unexpected, 343
variant of uncertain significance,
        326–327
variant result, 348–349
VUS, 342
13q deletion syndrome, 132
thyroid cancers
    PHS-related, 183
    screening for, 185
thyroid gland
    syndromes associated with, 454
    tumors of, 454
timing
    in psychosocial assessment, 381
    in risk communication, 288–289
tissue type, embryonic origins of, 27, 27
TNM staging system, 34–35, 35
    for breast cancer, 167
    for CRC, 204
tobacco exposure, in cancer incidence, 11, 11
tobacco use
    in cancer etiology, 14–15
    and CRC, 194
TP53 mutations, 102, 104, 177, 178, 441
TP53 testing, 103, 353, 354, 355, 441
TP53 tumor suppressor gene, 44
trans-acting factors, loss of, 73
transference, in genetic counseling, 388
transitional cell carcinomas, 30
translocations, in oncogene activation, 62–63
transplant, autologous vs. allogenic, 43
transverse colon, anatomy of, 188, 188
trauma, 362
treatment, cancer, 37–38
    in cancer history, 229
    chemotherapy, 41–42
    cryotherapy, 44
    laser therapy, 44
    radiation therapy, 39–40
    stem cell transplantation, 42–43
    surgery, 38–39
trustworthiness, of genetic counselors, 419
truth telling, 423
TS gene, 136

tuberous sclerosis complex (TSC), 81,
134–136
cancer risks with, 134–135
clinical features of, 136
diagnostic criteria for, 135–136
resources for, 136
syndrome subtypes for, 136
tuberous sclerosis (TS)/polycystic kidney
disease (PKD) contiguous gene
syndrome, 136
tubular carcinoma, of breast, 160
tumor grading
for breast cancer, 166
for CRC, 203
tumor markers, commonly ordered,
26, **26**
tumors
benign, 31–32
classification of
benign or malignant, 31–32
clinical staging for, 33–35, **35**
grading for, 32–33
genetic analysis of, 35
chromosome studies, 36
molecular studies, 36, 37
metastatic, *54*, 55, *56*, 57, **57**
neuroectodermal, 30
neuroendocrine, 199
precancerous, 32
tumor suppressor genes, *49*, 64
categories of, 65–66, 66
general description of, 65
hereditary cancer syndromes associated
with, **66**
inactivation of, 66–67
mismatch repair genes, 68–70, *69*
TP53 gene, 67–68, *68*
Turcot syndrome, 208. *See also* familial
adenomatous polyposis
Turner syndrome, cancer associated with,
13
two-hit theory, of cancer development, 57
tyrosine kinases, nonreceptor, 61

ulcerative colitis, 199
ultrasonography, of breast, 165
unauthorized testing, 433–434
uncertainty, and genetic testing,
332
undisclosed test results, dispensation of,
435–436
unintended/sensitive genetic information,
436

uniparental disomy (UPD), 71
urinary tract
syndromes associated with, **460**
tumors of, **460**
urogenital system, syndromes associated
with, **460**
uterus
in Lynch syndrome, 213
PHS-related tumors of, 183
syndromes associated with, **458**
tumors of, **458**

values, in bioethics, **410**
variant of uncertain significance (VUS),
326–327
veracity, of genetic counselors, 420
verbal confirmation, of cancer history, 240
viral insertion, in oncogene activation, 63
virtues, in bioethics, **410**
viruses
in cancer history, 231
carcinogenicity of, 15–16, **16**
Vogelstein's model, of colon cancer, *58*, 58–59
Von Hippel-Lindau (VHL) syndrome,
137–139
cancer risks with, 137
case example, 405–407
case history, 255–258, *257*, *259*
clinical features of, 138
diagnostic criteria for, 137–138
pedigree of family at risk for, *253*, 253
resources for, 139
syndrome subtypes for, 138–139
Von Recklinghausen disease. *See*
neurofibromatosis, type 1
vulva
syndromes associated with, **458**
tumors of, **458**

WAGR syndrome, 142. *See also* Wilms tumor
warning signs, of breast cancer, 163, **163**
wedge resection, for CRC, 204
well-being, and interest in testing, 323
Wermer syndrome. *See* multiple endocrine
neoplasia, type 1
Werner syndrome, 139–141
cancer risks with, 139
clinical features of, 140–141
diagnostic criteria for, 139–140
resources for, 141
Wilms tumor, 30, 79, 141–143
cancer risks with, 141
clinical features of, 142

Wilms tumor (*cont'd*)
  diagnostic criteria for, 141–142
  resources for, 143
  syndrome subtypes, 142
wisdom, of genetic counselors, 420
word choices, in risk communication,
  285–286
workup, for cancer, 25
WT2 gene, 142

xeroderma pigmentosum (XP), 143–145
  cancer risks with, 143
  clinical features of, 144

diagnostic criteria for, 143–144
  resources for, 145
  syndrome subtypes for, 144–145
XP/CS complex, 144–145
XP genes, 144
XP/trichothiodystrophy (TDD) syndrome,
  145
XP variant, 145
X-ray studies
  in CRC, 203
  double contrast barium enema, 202

Zollinger-Ellison syndrome, 113